Jones'
Clinical Paediatric Surgery
Diagnosis and Management

Jones'
Clinical
Paediatric Surgery

Diagnosis and Management

By the Staff of the Royal Children's Hospital, Melbourne

EDITED BY

John M Hutson AO, BS, MD (Monash), MD, DSc (Melb), FRACS, FAAP (Hon)
Chair of Paediatric Surgery, Department of Paediatrics, University of Melbourne
General Surgeon and Urologist, Royal Children's Hospital, Melbourne

Michael O'Brien MB, BCh, BAO, PhD, FRCSI (Paed), FRACS (Paed)
Paediatric Urologist, Royal Children's Hospital, Melbourne

Alan A Woodward MBBS, FRCS, FRACS
General Surgeon and Urologist, Royal Children's Hospital

Spencer W Beasley MBChB (Otago), MS (Melb). FRACS
Professor of Paediatric Surgery, Christchurch Hospital, New Zealand

SIXTH EDITION

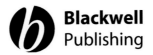

Blackwell
Publishing

© 2008 by Blackwell Publishing
Blackwell Publishing, Inc., 350 Main Street, Malden, Massachusetts 02148-5020, USA
Blackwell Publishing Ltd, 9600 Garsington Road, Oxford OX4 2DQ, UK
Blackwell Publishing Asia Pty Ltd, 550 Swanston Street, Carlton, Victoria 3053, Australia

The right of the Author to be identified as the Author of this Work has been asserted in accordance with the
Copyright, Designs and Patents Act 1988.

Sixth edition 2008
1 2008

Library of Congress Cataloging-in-Publication Data

Jones' clinical paediatric surgery : diagnosis and management / by the staff of the Royal Children's Hospital,
Melbourne ; edited by John M. Hutson ... [et al.]. -- 6th ed.
    p. ; cm.
  Includes bibliographical references and index.
  ISBN 978-1-4051-6267-8
  1. Children--Surgery. I. Jones, Peter G. II. Hutson, John M. III. Royal Children's Hospital.
  IV. Title: Clinical paediatric surgery.
  [DNLM: 1. Surgical Procedures, Operative. 2. Child. 3. Infant, Newborn. 4. Infant.
  5. Pediatrics--methods. WO 925 J76 2008]
  RD137.C55 2008
  617.9'8--dc22
                                                                    2007047283
  ISBN: 978-1-4051-6267-8

A catalogue record for this title is available from the British Library

Set in 9.25/11.5 Minion by Newgen Imaging Systems Pvt Ltd, Chennai, India
Printed and bound in Singapore by Fabulous Printers Pte Ltd

Commissioning Editor: Martin Sugden
Development Editor: Elisabeth Dodds and Laura Murphy
Production Controller: Debbie Wyer

For further information on Blackwell Publishing, visit our website:
http://www.blackwellpublishing.com

Contents

Contributors

Spencer W Beasley, MS, FRACS
Professor of Paediatric Surgery
Christchurch Hospital
Christchurch, New Zealand

Robert Berkowitz MD, FRACS
Department of Otolaryngology
Royal Children's Hospital
Parkville, Victoria, Australia

CA Bevan, MRCPCH
Department of General Surgery
(Trauma unit)
Royal Children's Hospital
Parkville, Victoria, Australia

Thomas Clarnette, MD, FRACS
Department of General Surgery
Royal Children's Hospital
Parkville, Victoria, Australia

Joe Crameri, FRACS
Department of General Surgery
Royal Children's Hospital
Parkville, Victoria, Australia

James E Elder, FRACO, FRACS
Department of Ophthalmology
Royal Children's Hospital
Parkville, Victoria, Australia

Kerr Graham, MD, FRCS(Ed), FRACS
Professor of Orthopaedics
Royal Children's Hospital
Parkville, Victoria,
Australia

Anthony Holmes, FRACS
Diplomate, American Board of Plastic
Surgery; Plastic and
Maxillofacial Surgery Department
Royal Children's Hospital
Parkville, Victoria,
Australia

John M Hutson, AO, MD, DSc, FRACS, FAAP
Professor of Paediatric Surgery
Royal Children's Hospital
Parkville, Victoria, Australia

Bruce R Johnstone, FRACS
Department of Plastic and Maxillofacial
Surgery Royal Children's Hospital
Parkville, Victoria, Australia

Vivek A Josan, FRACS
Department of Neurosurgery Royal
Children's Hospital Melbourne,
Australia

Wirginia J Maixner, FRACS
Neuroscience Centre
Royal Children's Hospital
Melbourne, Australia

Michael O'Brien, PhD, FRCSI (Paed), FRACS (Paed)
Department of Paediatric Urology
Royal Children's Hospital
Parkville, Victoria, Australia

Anthony J Penington, FRACS
Department of Plastic Surgery
Royal Children's Hospital
Parkville, Victoria, Australia

Keith B Stokes, FRACS
Department of General Surgery
Royal Children's Hospital
Parkville, Victoria, Australia

Russell G Taylor, FRACS
Department of General Surgery
Royal Children's Hospital
Parkville, Victoria, Australia

Alan A Woodward, FRCS, FRACS
Department of Paediatric Urology
Royal Children's Hospital
Parkville, Victoria, Australia

Foreword to the First Edition

The progressive increase in the body of information relative to the surgical specialities has come to present a vexing problem in the instruction of medical students. There is not enough time in the medical curriculum to present everything about everything to them, and in textbook material, one is reduced either to synoptic sections in textbooks of surgery or to the speciality too detailed for the student or the non-specialist in complete and authoritative textbooks.

There has long been a need for a book of modest size dealing with paediatric surgery in a way suited to the requirements of the medical student, general practitioner and paediatrician. Peter G. Jones and his associates from the distinguished and productive group at the Royal Children's Hospital in Melbourne have succeeded in meeting this need. The book could have been entitled *Surgical Conditions in Infancy and Childhood,* for it deals with the child and his afflictions, their symptoms, diagnosis and treatment rather than surgery as such. The reader is told when and how urgently an operation is required, and enough about the nature of the procedure to understand its risks and appreciate its results. This is what students need to know and what paediatricians and general practitioners need to be refreshed on.

Many of the chapters are novel, in that they deal not with categorical diseases but with the conditions that give rise to a specific symptom – Vomiting in the First Month of Life, The Jaundiced Newborn Baby, Surgical Causes of Failure to Thrive. The chapter on genetic counselling is a model of information and good sense.

The book is systematic and thorough. A clean style, logical sequential discussions and avoidance of esoterica allow the presentation of substantial information over the entire field of paediatric surgery in this comfortable-sized volume with well-chosen illustrations and carefully selected bibliography. Many charts and tables, original in conception, enhance the clear presentation.

No other book so satisfactorily meets the need of the student for broad and authoritative coverage in a modest compass. The paediatric house officer (in whose hospital more than 50% of the patients are, after all, surgical) will be serviced equally well. Paediatric surgeons will find between these covers an account of the attitudes, practices and results of one of the world's greatest paediatric surgical centres. The book comes as a fitting tribute to the 100th anniversary of the Royal Children's Hospital.

Mark M. Ravitch
Professor of Paediatric Surgery
University of Pennsylvania

Tribute to Mr Peter Jones

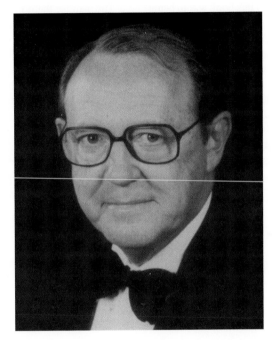

Mr Peter Jones (1922–1995) MB, MS, FRCS, FRACS, FACS, FAAP. The first Australian surgeon to obtain the FRACS in paediatric surgery, and member of RACS Council (1987–1995), Vice-President of the Medical Defence Association of Victoria (1974–1988) and President of the Australian Association of Surgeons (1983–1986). He was legendary as a medical historian and in heraldry, as a great raconteur, but primarily as a great student teacher.

Preface to the Sixth Edition

The objective of the first edition of this book was to bring together information on surgical conditions in infancy and childhood for use by medical students and resident medical officers. It remains a great satisfaction to our contributors that the book has fulfilled this aim successfully, and that a sixth edition is now required. Family doctors, paediatricians and many others concerned with the welfare of children have also found the book useful.

A knowledgeable medical publisher once commented to Peter Jones that this book is not about surgery but about paediatrics, and this is what it should be, as we have continued to omit almost all details of operative surgery.

The plan for the fifth edition has been largely retained, with the inclusion of a list of key points for each chapter. Nearly half of the contributors to this edition are new members of the hospital staff, and bring a fresh outlook and state-of-the-art ideas. We have maintained the previously successful style, while including some new images.

It is now more than 10 years since Mr Peter Jones died, and this book remains as a dedication to him. Peter was a great teacher and it is a daunting task for those who follow in his footsteps. We hope this new edition will continue to honour the memory of a great paediatric surgeon who understood what students need to know.

Acknowledgements

Many members of the Royal Children's Hospital community have made valuable contributions to this sixth edition. The secretarial staff of the Department of Surgery, and particularly Mrs Shirley D'Cruz, are thanked sincerely for their untiring support. Finally, we express our gratitude to Elisabeth Dodds of Blackwell Publishing for bringing this edition to fruition.

Introduction

1 Antenatal Diagnosis – Surgical Aspects

Case 1

At 18-weeks' gestation, right fetal hydronephrosis is diagnosed on ultrasound.
Q 1.1 Discuss the further management during pregnancy.
Q 1.2 Does the antenatal diagnosis improve the postnatal outlook for this condition?

Case 2

An exomphalos is diagnosed at the 18-week ultrasound.
Q 2.1 What further evaluation is required at that stage?
Q 2.2 Does this anomaly influence the timing and mode of delivery?

Antenatal diagnosis is one of the most rapidly developing fields in medical practice. Whilst the genetic and biochemical evaluation of the developing fetus provides the key to many medical diagnoses, the development of accurate ultrasound has provided the impetus for the diagnosis of surgical fetal anomalies. At first, it was expected that the antenatal diagnosis of fetal problems would lead to better treatment and an improved outcome. In some cases, this is true. Antenatally diagnosed fetuses with gastroschisis will be delivered in a tertiary-level obstetric hospital with neonatal intensive care in order to prevent hypothermia, and the results of treatment have improved. In other cases, such as in diaphragmatic hernia, these expectations have not been fulfilled because antenatal diagnosis has opened a Pandora's box of complex and lethal anomalies, which in the past never survived the pregnancy, and were recorded in the statistics as fetal death *in utero* and stillbirth.

Indications and timing for antenatal ultrasound

All pregnancies are now assessed with a mid-trimester ultrasound, which is usually performed at 17–18-weeks'

gestation [Fig. 1.1]. The main purpose of this examination is to assess the obstetric parameters of the pregnancy, but the increasingly important secondary role of this study is to screen the fetus for anomalies. Most anomalies are picked up at 18 weeks, but some only become apparent later in the pregnancy. Renal anomalies are best seen on a 30-week ultrasound as urine flow is low before 24 weeks. Earlier ultrasound examinations may be performed with transvaginal scanning in special circumstances, such as a previous pregnancy with neural tube defect and increasingly to detect early signs of aneuploidy. Magnetic resonance imaging of the developing fetus may be another means of fetal assessment in future.

Natural history of fetal anomalies

Before the advent of ultrasound, paediatric surgeons saw only a selected group of infants with congenital anomalies. These babies had survived the pregnancy and lived long enough after birth to reach surgical attention. Thus the babies coming to surgical treatment were already a selected group, mostly with a good prognosis.

Antenatal diagnosis has brought surgeons into contact with a new group of conditions with a poor prognosis, and at last the full spectrum of pathology is coming to surgical attention. For example, posterior urethral valves causing obstruction of the urinary tract were thought to

Jones' Clinical Paediatric Surgery, 6th edition. By Hutson, O'Brien, Woodward and Beasley. Published 2008 by Blackwell Publishing, ISBN: 978-1-4051-6267-8.

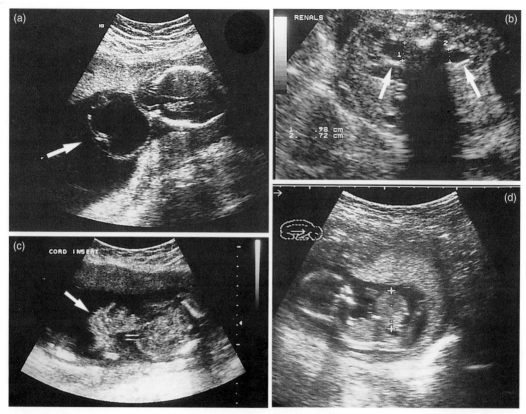

Figure 1.1 (a) Encephalocele shown in a cross section of the fetal head. The sac protruding through the posterior skull defect is arrowed. (b) Bilateral hydronephrosis shown in an upper abdominal section. The dilated renal pelvis containing clear fluid is marked. (c) The irregular outline of the free-floating bowel in the amniotic cavity of a term baby with gastroschisis. (d) A longitudinal section through a 14-week fetus showing a large exomphalos. The head is seen to the left of the picture. The large sac (marked) is seen between blurred (moving) images of the arms and legs.

be rare, with an incidence of 1:5000 male births; most cases did well with postnatal valve resection. It is now known that the true incidence of urethral valves is 1:2500 male births, and these additional cases did not come to surgical attention as they developed intrauterine renal failure with either fetal death *in utero* or early neonatal death from respiratory problems such as Potter's syndrome. It was thought that antenatal diagnosis would improve the outcome of such congenital anomalies, but the overall results have appeared to become worse with these severe 'new' cases being included.

There are similar problems with the antenatal diagnosis of diaphragmatic hernia [Fig. 1.2]. Congenital diaphragmatic hernia was not associated with multiple congenital anomalies when cases presented after birth. Now antenatal diagnosis of diaphragmatic hernia has uncovered a more severe subgroup with associated chromosomal anomalies and multiple developmental defects. It would seem that the earlier the diaphragmatic hernia is diagnosed, the worse is the outcome.

Despite these problems, there are many advantages in antenatal diagnosis. The outcome of many conditions is improved by the prior knowledge of 'congenital' anomalies.

Management following antenatal diagnosis

Fetal management
Cases diagnosed antenatally may be classified into three groups.

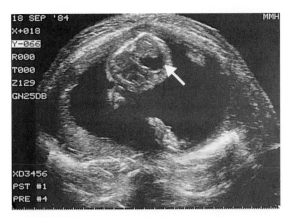

Figure 1.2. Cross section of a uterus with marked polyhydramnios. The fetal chest is seen in cross section within the uterus. The fluid-filled cavity within the left side of the chest is the stomach protruding through a diaphragmatic hernia (arrow).

Good prognosis

In some cases, such as a unilateral hydronephrosis, there is no place for active management, and the main task is to track the progress of the problem through pregnancy with serial ultrasound. A detailed diagnosis is made with the more sophisticated range of tests available after birth, and UTIs are prevented with prophylactic antibiotics commenced at birth. Thus, a child with severe vesico-ureteric reflux may go through the first year of life without any UTIs. If the parents receive counselling by a surgeon experienced in the care of the particular problem, they have time to understand the condition. In the case of cleft lip seen on fetal ultrasound, the parents will have time to understand the nature of the problem by seeing photographs of the condition before and after surgery, and will have the chance to meet other families with this condition. With such preparation, the family can cope better with the birth of a baby with congenital anomalies.

The paediatric surgeon also has an important role to play in advising the obstetrician on the prognosis of a particular condition. Some cases of exomphalos are easy to repair, whereas in others, the defect may be so large that primary repair will be difficult. Moreover, in some fetuses there may be major chromosomal and cardiac anomalies associated with the exomphalos which may alter the outcome. In exomphalos, therefore, the prognosis varies from good to poor. In other conditions, the outlook for a congenital defect may change as treatment improves. Gastroschisis was a lethal condition before 1970, but now management of the disease has changed

and there is a 95% survival rate. In those cases with a good prognosis, fetal intervention is not indicated and the pregnancy should be allowed to run its course. The mode of delivery will usually be determined on obstetric grounds. Babies with exomphalos may be delivered by vaginal delivery if the birth process is easy. In other obstetric circumstances, caesarian section may be indicated to prevent rupture of the exomphalos. There is evidence that spina bifida cases may undergo further nerve damage at vaginal delivery, and caesarian section may be preferred in this circumstance. If urgent neonatal surgery is required, for example, for gastroschisis, the baby should be delivered at a tertiary obstetric unit with a neonatal intensive care unit and neonatal surgical service. In other cases, for example, cleft lip and palate, where urgent surgery is not required but good family and nursing support is important, delivery close to the family's home may be more appropriate. Antenatal planning and family counselling give us the opportunity to make the appropriate arrangements for the birth. A baby born with gastroschisis in the middle of winter in a bush nursing hospital in the mountains, many hours away from surgical care, will have a very different outlook from a baby with the same condition born at a major neonatal centre.

Poor prognosis

Anencephaly, diaphragmatic hernia with major chromosomal anomalies or urethral valves with early intrauterine renal failure are examples of conditions with a poor prognosis. These are lethal conditions, and the outcome is predetermined before the diagnosis is made.

Late deterioration

Initial assessment of the fetal anomaly indicates a good prognosis with no reason for interference, but, later in gestation, the fetus deteriorates and some action must be undertaken to prevent a lethal outcome. An example would be the lower urinary tract obstruction seen in posterior urethral valves. Early in the pregnancy, renal function may be acceptable with good amniotic fluid volumes. However, on follow-up ultrasound assessment, there may be loss of liquor with oligohydramnios as a sign of intrauterine renal failure. There are several ways to treat this problem. If the gestation is at a viable stage, for example, 36 weeks, labour could be induced and the urethral valves treated at birth. If the risks of premature delivery are higher, for example, for 28-weeks' gestation, temporary relief may be obtained by using percutaneous transuterine techniques to place a shunt catheter from the fetal bladder into the amniotic cavity. These catheters tend to become dislodged by fetal activity. A more definitive approach to drain the urinary tract is intrauterine surgery to perform a vesicostomy and allow the pregnancy to continue. This procedure has been performed with success in a few cases of posterior urethral valves. These patients are highly selected and only a few special centres perform intrauterine surgery. At present this surgery is regarded as experimental, and reserved for rare situations, but this may not always be the case.

Antenatal ultrasound has become the most important means of diagnosing fetal anomalies and has given us a valuable means of understanding the natural history of developmental abnormalities.

Surgical counselling

When a child is born with unanticipated birth defects, there is inevitably shock and confusion until the diagnosis is clarified and the family begin to assimilate and accept the information given to them, and make plans for the future. Important treatment decisions have to be made urgently while the new parents are still too stunned to play any sensible part in ongoing care of their baby. Antenatal diagnosis has changed this situation. New parents may now have many weeks to understand and come to terms with their baby's problem. With suitable preparation, they can play an active role in the postnatal diagnosis and treatment choices for their newborn baby.

The paediatric surgical specialist who treats the particular problem uncovered by antenatal diagnosis is in the best position to advise the parents on the prognosis and further treatment of the baby. Detailed information on the management after birth, with photographs before and after corrective surgery, allows the parents to understand and come to terms with the surgical procedures. The opportunity to meet other families with a child treated for the same condition gives time for the pregnant woman and her partner to understand the problem before the birth. Handling and nurturing the baby immediately after birth is an important part of bonding. Parents and nursing staff suddenly confronted with a newborn baby with the unexpected finding of a gross anomaly, such as sacro-coccygeal teratoma, may be afraid to handle the baby who is then taken away to another hospital for complex surgery. Parents in this situation may take many months to relate to the new baby and understand the nature of the problem. Prepared by antenatal diagnosis, the nursing staff and parents realise they can handle and nurture the baby. They understand the nature of the surgery and maintain their bond with the baby, Thus instead of being stunned by the birth of a malformed baby, the new parents can play an active part in the postnatal surgical management and provide better informed consent for surgery.

Key Points

- Antenatal diagnosis with ultrasound has revealed the natural history of some anomalies and made prognosis seem worse (e.g. diaphragmatic hernia, posterior urethra valve).
- Diagnosis before birth has allowed surgical planning (and occasional fetal intervention) as well as time for parents to be informed.

Further reading

Flake AW (2006) Molecular clinical genetics and gene therapy. In: Grosfeld JL, O'Neill JA, Fonkalsrud EW, Coran AG (eds) *Pediatric Surgery*, 6th Edn. Mosby, Elsevier, Philadelphia, pp. 11–20.

Harrison MR (2006) The fetus as a patient. In: Grosfeld JL, O'Neill JA, Fonkalsrud EW, Coran AG (eds) *Pediatric Surgery*, 6th Edn. Mosby, Elsevier, Philadelphia, pp. 77–88.

2 The Care and Transport of the Newborn

Case 1

A 30-week gestation infant is born with gastroschisis.
Q 1.1 What advice would you give the referring institution about the management of this infant prior to transport to a tertiary institution?

Case 2

A 40-week gestation infant develops respiratory distress shortly after birth. A left diaphragmatic hernia is diagnosed.
Q 2.1 List two iatrogenic problems which may occur with positive pressure ventilation.
Q 2.2 How do you avoid these iatrogenic problems?

The care and transport of a sick newborn baby is of critical importance to the surgical outcome.

A detailed preoperative assessment is necessary to detect associated or coexistent developmental anomalies. Vital disturbances should be corrected before operation, and predictable complications of the abnormalities should be anticipated and recognised early.

Respiratory care

The aims of respiratory care are (1) to maintain a clear airway; (2) to prevent abdominal distension; (3) avoid aspiration of gastric contents and (4) to provide supplementary oxygen if necessary. Apnoea, hyaline membrane disease, meconium aspiration and pneumothorax are common medical causes of respiratory distress in the newborn. Surgical causes of respiratory distress include oesophageal atresia and diaphragmatic hernia.

1 Placing the baby in the prone position improves the airways and reduces gastro-oesophageal reflux and the likelihood of aspiration of gastric contents.

2 Suction of the pharyngeal secretions maintains a clear airway, especially in the premature infant with poorly

developed laryngeal reflexes, and in the infant with oesophageal atresia.

3 A nasogastric tube, size 8 French, will prevent life-threatening aspiration of vomitus, provided the tube is kept patent and allowed to drain freely with additional aspiration at frequent intervals. It will also reduce abdominal distension and improve pulmonary ventilation in patients with intestinal obstruction or congenital diaphragmatic hernia.

4 Oxygen therapy, endotracheal intubation and ventilation will be required in the preoperative resuscitation of some neonates with conditions such as congenital diaphragmatic hernia. However, ventilation and oxygen therapy in diaphragmatic hernia is a specialised field best left to experts as barotrauma to the poorly developed lungs will cause bronchopulmonary damage and pneumothorax.

Blood and fluid loss

The blood volume of a full term infant is 80 mL/kg. Blood loss of only 30 mL in a neonate is equivalent to losing 500 mL in an adult. Newborn babies do not tolerate blood or fluid loss well.

Fresh whole blood is cross-matched for major operations in the neonatal period. Blood loss during surgery is kept to a minimum and measured by weighing all swabs and packs used. The haemoglobin concentration in the

Jones' Clinical Paediatric Surgery, 6th edition. By Hutson, O'Brien, Woodward and Beasley. Published 2008 by Blackwell Publishing, ISBN: 978-1-4051-6267-8.

first few days of life is about 19 g/dL and the haematocrit 50–70%. Blood viscosity is relatively high, and blood loss in this circumstance may be replaced in part with blood and in part with a crystalloid solution, which lowers the viscosity of the blood.

Diminished blood volume in a sick neonate with a bowel obstruction will lead to poor peripheral circulation. The baby will be lethargic and pale, with cool limbs, venoconstriction and cyanosis. Acidosis becomes a complicating factor. In this situation a 'bolus infusion' of a crystalloid solution such as Hartmann's solution over 15 min at 10 mL/kg is used for resuscitation. When this is effective, the peripheral circulation will improve dramatically. If this initial infusion is not adequate, further bolus infusions of crystalloid at 10 mL/kg may be given and the clinical response monitored.

Control of body temperature

The sick neonate with a surgical condition is prone to hypothermia, defined as a core body temperature of less than 36ºC. In hypothermia, heat production is stimulated above normal metabolic requirements and may be boosted by thermogenesis from increased metabolism of brown fat deposits. However, if heat loss exceeds heat production, the body temperature will continue to fall, leading to acidosis and depression of respiratory, cardiac and nervous function.

All metabolic functions are altered by hypothermia. Newborn infants, especially the premature, are at risk of excessive heat loss because of the relatively large surface area-to-volume ratio and the lack of subcutaneous insulating fat.

Heat loss occurs from the body surface to the environment by radiation, conduction, convection and the evaporation of water. Excessive heat loss during transport, assessment and operation must be avoided, particularly in conditions such as gastroschisis where the eviscerated bowel provides a very large surface area for evaporation. Heat loss is controlled once the bowel is wrapped in domestic clear plastic wrap to prevent evaporation. Wet packs should never be applied to a neonate as they will accelerate evaporative and conductive heat losses.

Radiant overhead heaters are of particular value during procedures such as intravenous cannulation or the induction of anaesthesia, because they allow unimpeded access to the infant.

Fluids, electrolytes and nutrition

Many infants with a surgical condition cannot be fed in the perioperative period. Intravenous fluids provide daily maintenance requirements and prevent dehydration. The total volume of fluid given must supply maintenance requirements, restore fluid and electrolyte deficits and replace ongoing losses.

Maintenance water requirements are
60–80 mL/kg on day 1 of life
80–100 mL/kg on day 2
100–150 mL/kg on day 3 and thereafter.
Maintenance electrolyte requirements are
Sodium: 3 mmol/kg/day
Chloride: 3 mmol/kg/day
Potassium: 2 mmol/kg/day.
Maintenance joule requirements are
100–140 kJ/kg/day.

These maintenance requirements can be provided in the first week by a solution made up of 5% dextrose in 0.45% sodium chloride (sodium: 35 mmol/L) with the addition of potassium chloride at 20 mmol/L. However, this solution is inadequate for long-term maintenance of body functions as it has many deficiencies, especially in kJ.

Replacement of fluid and electrolyte deficiencies may be necessary in surgical patients, such as those with neonatal bowel obstruction. Before birth, the placenta maintains fluid and electrolyte balance. At birth, electrolyte levels are normal despite long-standing bowel obstruction, and extracellular water levels are relatively high. Persistent vomiting after birth soon causes dehydration and electrolyte imbalance. The degree of dehydration can be measured by the clinical parameters of tissue turgor, the state of peripheral circulation, depression of the fontanelle, dryness of the mouth and urine output. Bodyweight loss also gives an approximation of water loss.

The rule of thumb for estimating water loss is that dehydration of 5% or less of body mass has few clinical manifestations: 5–8% shows moderate clinical signs of dehydration; 10% shows severe signs and poor peripheral circulation. Thus a 3000 g infant who has been vomiting and has a diminished urine output, but shows no overt signs of dehydration, may have lost approximately 5% of body mass and will require 3000 × 5% mL = 150 mL fluid replacement to correct the deficit. Maintenance fluid requirements must be administered also.

Electrolyte estimations are most useful for identifying a deficiency of electrolytes that are distributed mainly in the extracellular fluid, for example sodium, but will not be as reliable for electrolytes that are found mainly in the intracellular space, for example potassium. Fluid and electrolyte deficiency due to vomiting will need to be replaced with a crystalloid solution which contains adequate levels of sodium, for example 0.9% sodium chloride (sodium: 150 mmol/L).

Continuing losses of fluid and electrolytes need to be measured and replaced. Losses may arise from nasogastric tube aspirates in bowel obstruction, diarrhoea from an ileostomy, and the excessive urinary losses which may occur after the relief of urinary obstruction, for example after resection of posterior urethral valves. When the losses are high they are best measured and replaced with an intravenous infusion of electrolytes equivalent to those of the fluid being lost.

Intravenous nutrition will be required when the period of starvation extends beyond 4–5 days. Common indications for intravenous nutrition in the neonatal period include necrotising enterocolitis, extensive gut resection and gastroschisis. The aim of intravenous nutrition is to provide all substances necessary for normal growth and development. Intravenous nutrition may be maintained for weeks or months as required. Complications of prolonged nutrition include sepsis and jaundice.

Oral nutrition is preferred where possible and breast feeding is best. Surgery to the alimentary tract may make oral feeding impossible for a variable period: gut enzyme function may be poor and various substrates in the feeds may not be absorbed. Lactose intolerance is seen commonly and leads to diarrhoea with the passage of acidic fluid stools. Other malabsorptive problems relate to sugars, protein, fat and the osmolarity of the feeds. These can be handled by altering the conformation of the feeds or, in severe cases, by a period of intravenous nutrition to allow the gut enzymes time to recover.

Biochemical abnormalities

Important problems include metabolic acidosis, hypoglycaemia and hypocalcaemia. These are corrected before operation because they may adversely influence the infant's response to anaesthetic agents.

Metabolic acidosis
Metabolic acidosis, which may result from hypovolaemia, dehydration, cold stress, renal failure or hypoxia, increases pulmonary vascular resistance and impairs cardiac output.

Acidosis is corrected by fixing the underlying cause of the acidosis. In some circumstances such as renal failure sodium bicarbonate is also used.

Hypoglycaemia
Hypoglycaemia occurs in the sick newborn, especially if premature. Liver stores of glycogen are small, as are fat stores. Starvation and stress will use up liver glycogen rapidly, and there will be a switch to fatty acid metabolism to maintain blood glucose levels, with consequent ketoacidosis. Gluconeogenesis from amino acids or pyruvate is slow to develop in the newborn, due to the relative inactivity of liver enzymes. A point is soon reached when blood glucose levels cannot be maintained and severe hypoglycaemia will result, causing apnoea, convulsions and cerebral damage. These complications of hypoglycaemia may be prevented by intravenous dextrose infusions. Young babies should not be starved for longer than 4 h before surgery.

Hypocalcaemia
Hypocalcaemia may occur in infants with respiratory distress. The ionised calcium level in the blood maintains cell membrane activity. Hypocalcaemia may cause twitching and convulsions, and can be corrected by slow infusion of calcium gluconate.

Prevention of infection

The poorly developed immune defences of the newborn infant predispose to infection with Gram positive and Gram negative organisms. Infection may spread rapidly, and result in septicaemia. Signs of systemic infection in the neonate include hypothermia, pallor and lethargy.

Early recognition and treatment of infection is aided by bacteriological cultures from the infant's nose, throat, umbilicus and rectum, both on admission to hospital and subsequently on a regular basis. This is important in picking up 'marker organisms' such as multiple antibiotic-resistant *Staphylococcus aureus*. When infection is suspected, a 'septic workup' is performed, taking specimens of CSF, urine and blood for culture and starting appropriate intravenous antibiotics immediately.

Infants undergoing surgery are at special risk of infection, and care must be taken not to introduce pathogenic organisms: this applies particularly to cross-infection in the neonatal ward. Handwashing with antiseptic must be performed before handling any patient. Prophylactic antibiotics may be used to cover major surgery.

Parents

An important part of the care for neonates undergoing surgery is the reassurance and support of the infant's anxious parents. The mother may be confined in a maternity hospital while her baby is separated from her and undergoing major surgery in another institution. Close communication is important in this situation, and the mother and baby should be brought together as soon as possible. The parents should handle and fondle the baby to facilitate bonding and for the infant's general welfare. With goodwill, gentle contact between infant and mother can be achieved, even in difficult circumstances.

General principles of neonatal transport

Transport of a critically ill neonate is a precarious undertaking, and the following principles should be followed:
1 The infant's condition should be stabilised before embarkation.
2 The most experienced/qualified personnel available should accompany the patient.
3 Specialised neonatal 'retrieval' services should be used.
4 Transport should be as rapid as possible, but without causing further deterioration or incurring unnecessary risks to patient or transporting personnel.
5 Transport should be undertaken early rather than late.

Table 2.1 Neonatal surgical conditions requiring transportation

Obvious malformations	Exomphalos/gastroschisis
	Myelomeningocele/encephalocele
	Imperforate anus
Respiratory distress	
Upper airways obstruction	Choanal atresia
	Pierre–Robin syndrome
Lung compression	Emphysematous lobe
	Pulmonary cyst(s)
	Pneumothorax (should have chest drain inserted)
	Congenital diaphragmatic hernia
Congenital heart disease	
Acute alimentary or abdominal emergencies	Oesophageal atresia
	Intestinal obstruction
	Necrotising enterocolitis
	Haematemesis and/or melaena
Ambiguous genitalia	

6 All equipment should be checked before setting out.
7 The receiving institution should be notified early so that additional staff and equipment can be prepared for arrival.

Transport of neonatal emergencies

A list of the more common emergencies is given in Table 2.1. Most infants with these conditions should have transport arranged as soon as the diagnosis is apparent or suspected.

Some developmental anomalies do not require transportation, and specialist consultation at the hospital of birth may suffice (e.g. cleft lip and palate, orthopaedic deformities). Where doubt exists concerning the appropriateness or timing of transportation, specialist advice should be sought.

Choice of vehicle

The choice between road ambulance, helicopter or fixed-wing aircraft will depend on distance, availability of vehicle, time of day, traffic conditions, airport facilities and weather conditions. In general, fixed-wing aircraft offer no time advantages for transfers of under 160 km (100 miles).

Patients with entrapped gas (e.g. pneumothorax or significant abdominal distension) are better not to travel by air. If air travel is necessary, the aircraft should fly at low levels if it is unpressurised; otherwise expansion of the trapped gases with decrease in ambient atmospheric pressure may make ventilation difficult.

Communication

Good communication between the referring and receiving institutions can be crucial to survival and expedites treatment prior to transportation. Any change in the patient's condition should be reported to the receiving unit in advance of arrival. Detailed documentation of the history and written permission for treatment, including surgery, should be sent with the infant. In addition, neonates require 10 mL of maternal blood to accompany them, as well as cord blood and the placenta, if available.

Details of stabilisation procedures can be discussed with the headquarters of the transport team if difficulties arise while awaiting their arrival.

Written permission for transport is required. A full explanation of what has been arranged and why, and an accurate prognosis should be given to the parents. They should be allowed as much access to the infant or child prior to transport as is possible. The parents can be given a digital photograph of the infant, taken before departure or at admission to hospital, if they are to be separated from their infant.

Stabilisation of neonates prior to transfer

Table 2.2 presents neonatal medical conditions that require stabilisation before transport.

Temperature control
An incubator or radiant warmer is used to keep the infant warm. Recommended incubator temperatures are shown in Table 2.3. The infant should be covered except for parts required for observation or access. Axillary or rectal temperatures should be taken half-hourly, or quarter-hourly if under a radiant warmer.

Respiratory distress
Oxygen requirements
Enough oxygen should be given to abolish cyanosis and ensure adequate saturation. Pulse oximeter oxygen saturation levels >97% indicate adequate oxygenation. If measurements of blood gases are available, an arterial PO_2 of 50–80 mm Hg is desirable. Although an excessively high PO_2 is liable to initiate retinopathy of prematurity, a short period of hyperoxia is less likely to be detrimental than a similarly short period of hypoxia.

Respiratory failure
Infants in severe respiratory failure (on clinical grounds or $PCO_2 > 70$ mmHg), or those with apnoea, may require endotracheal intubation and intermittent positive pressure ventilation. Positive pressure ventilation may cause problems in cases of diaphragmatic hernia.

Metabolic derangements
Hypoglycaemia should be corrected by intravenous infusion of glucose. Monitoring of babies at risk should be done with Dextrostix. Intravenous infusion may be by the umbilical, or a peripheral, route.

An infusion of blood or plasma expander at 10–20 mL/kg, i.v. over 0.5–1 h may be required to correct shock.

Acid–base balance should be estimated if facilities are available. Otherwise, a small volume of sodium bicarbonate (3 mmol/kg, slowly i.v.) may be given to an infant who has been asphyxiated severely, has had recurrent hypoxia, or shows signs of poor peripheral circulation. The best way, however, to correct acidosis is to correct the underlying abnormality.

Convulsions should be controlled with phenobarbitone (10–15 mg/kg i.v. or orally) or diphenylhydantoin (15 mg, i.v. or orally).

Specialist advice regarding management of specific conditions should be sought from the transporting agency. For example, in gastroschisis and exomphalos, the exposed viscera should be wrapped in clean plastic wrap to prevent heat loss; moist packs or gauze should never be used. A nasogastric tube with continuous drainage is required for patients with diaphragmatic hernia (Chapter 5), bowel obstruction (Chapter 7) or exomphalos (Chapter 9). In oesophageal atresia, frequent aspiration of the blind upper oesophageal pouch, at 10–15 min intervals, is essential to avoid aspiration (Chapter 6).

Table 2.2 Neonatal medical conditions requiring stabilisation before transport

1 Prematurity
2 Temperature control problems
3 Respiratory distress causing hypoxia and/or respiratory failure
4 Metabolic derangements
   - Hypoglycaemia
   - Metabolic acidosis
   - Hypocalcaemia
5 Shock
6 Convulsions

Table 2.3 Incubator temperature

Baby's weight (Gm)	Incubator temperature (°C)
<1000	35–37
1000–1500	34–36
1500–2000	33–35
2000–2500	32–34
<2500	31–33

Key Points
- Sick neonates need stabilisation before transport.
- Early transport is best done by a specialised team.
- Communication with parents, and with receiving surgical centre is crucial.

Further reading

James AG (1993) Resuscitation, stabilisation and transport in perinatology. *Curr Opin Pediatr* **5**: 150–155.

Pierro A, Eaton S, Ong E (2006) Neonatal physiology and metabolic considerations. In: Grosfeld JL, O'Neill JA Jr., Fonkalsrud EW, Coran AG (eds) *Pediatric Surgery*, 6th Edn. Mosby Elsevier, Philadelphia, pp. 89–113.

Rocchini AP (2006) Neonatal cardiovascular physiology and care. In: Grosfeld JL, O'Neill JA Jr., Fonkalsrud EW, Coran AG (eds) *Pediatric Surgery*, 6th Edn. Mosby Jr., Elsevier, Philadelphia, pp. 146–155.

Teitelbaum DH, Coran AG (2006) Nutritional support. In: Grosfeld JL, O'Neill JA Jr., Fonkalsrud EW, Coran AG (eds) *Pediatric Surgery*, 6th Edn. Mosby Jr., Elsevier, Philadelphia, pp. 194–220.

3 The Child in Hospital

Case 1

Erin, aged 2 years, is seen in the surgical clinic because of an inguinal hernia. During the explanation before filling out the consent form, the surgeon describes the use of 'invisible stitches', a waterproof dressing and local anaesthetic.

Q 1.1 Will the operation be done under local anaesthetic?

Q 1.2 Why are 'invisible stitches' important?

Q 1.3 Why should the dressing be waterproof?

Case 2

Jacob, aged 6 years, attends the surgical clinic very reluctantly because he is apprehensive about an upcoming orchidopexy.

Q 2.1 What are his major fears likely to be?

Great effort should be made to minimise psychological disturbances in children undergoing surgery. The important factors to consider are the age and temperament of the child; the site, nature and extent of the surgical procedure; the degree and duration of discomfort after operation and the time spent in hospital.

Children between 1 and 3 years of age are the most vulnerable, and many procedures should be done in the first year of life, or postponed until 4 or 6 years of age when the child can comprehend and co-operate better.

The temperament and ability of children to cope with stress are infinitely variable; the trust which children are prepared to grant those who care for them is a measure of the confidence they have in their own family circle. Major disturbances within the family may affect the patient's equanimity and the ability of the parents to give support. Elective surgery may need to be deferred for stressful family events such as

- the arrival of a new baby;
- a death in the family;
- shifting to a new house.

Jones' Clinical Paediatric Surgery, 6th edition. By Hutson, O'Brien, Woodward and Beasley. Published 2008 by Blackwell Publishing, ISBN: 978-1-4051-6267-8.

Preparation for admission

Preparation for elective admission is important for children over 4 or 5 years of age and, whether assisted by a booklet (see Further Reading) or advice, is largely in the hands of the parents whose acceptance of the situation is its endorsement in the child's eyes.

The child needs a brief and simple description of the operation, and if something is to be removed, it should be made clear that it is dispensable. Children should also be told that they will be asleep while the operation is performed, that it will be over when they wake and that they will be 'stiff' and a little 'sore' for a day or so, and they should also be told the time when they will be able to go home. It is pointless to say that it will not hurt at all, for honesty is essential to preserve trust.

How the child's questions are handled is just as important as the factual content of the answers; possible sources of fear should be dealt with, and the pleasant aspects suitably emphasised. The amount of information must be adjusted to the child's age and particular needs; more detail will be expected by older children.

Effect of site of surgery

Operations on the genitalia or the body's orifices, including circumcision after the age of 2 years, are more likely to cause emotional upset than other operations of the same magnitude. One or both parents should stay with the child and suitable occupational or play therapy is of considerable value.

Anal and oesophageal surgery should be completed shortly after birth, and subsequent dilatations performed under anaesthesia wherever possible. Many boys who have experienced both operations would prefer, in retrospect, bilateral orchidopexy to tonsillectomy by even the gentlest hands.

Day surgery

Time spent in hospital should be as short as possible. 'Day surgery' with admission, operation and discharge a few hours later is cost-effective, convenient and suitable for at least 80% of elective paediatric surgery.

The greatest advantage is minimizing the psychological impact on the child, which is magnified by sleeping away from home for even one night. There are many other obvious advantages, including minimal disturbances of breast feeding and reduced travelling by parents (i.e. fewer visits to the hospital).

Although surgical technique is important (haemostasis, secure dressings), day surgery has been made safe and acceptable by special anaesthetic techniques: timing and choice of premedication and general anaesthetic agents, minimal trauma during intubation (particularly the use of the laryngeal mask rather than endotracheal intubation), reversal of anaesthesia and long-acting local anaesthetic blocks or caudal analgesia in lieu of the usual postoperative injections of narcotics.

In the most vulnerable 1–3 years age group, day surgery has reduced the likelihood of behavioural disturbances. Suitable operations for day surgery depend on parental attitudes, logistics and careful selection of individual patients.

Ward atmosphere and procedures

Unlimited visiting by parents, living-in quarters for parents and a more understanding and empathetic approach by all who care for children have led to a less formal and more friendly atmosphere in hospital.

The procedures necessary for investigation, or in preparation for operation, should be scrutinised carefully to see whether they are necessary. Blood tests or x-rays are rarely required for elective day surgery.

The induction of anaesthesia is an important source of fear and distress. The presence of a parent is very helpful during most anaesthetic inductions. Effective premedication, skilful intravenous induction and the prompt administration of hypnotics and analgesics after operation keep discomfort to the absolute minimum. Again, the early presence of a parent in the postoperative recovery room will reduce the child's stress as it wakes up from anaesthesia.

Even after major abdominal surgery, some toddlers will be walking within 48 h. They might just as well be playing on the floor or sitting at a table, and today that is where they are, with no subsequent ill effects. The playroom is not required for most postoperative patients, since once they can walk to the toilet and playroom, they can be discharged home. The child usually sets the pace of convalescence, and as a general rule will show no desire to move when they should rest, for example, during a period of paralytic ileus.

Play materials, a day room, television and bright surroundings act as constant stimuli to those who are well enough to be 'up and doing'. Play specialists are involved in the management of children who have a longer hospital stay or require frequent dressing changes (e.g. burns patients), and they significantly reduce the amount of analgesia required.

A single, absorbable subcuticular stitch can be used to close almost all incisions, and avoids the anxiety and time spent in removing sutures. A waterproof dressing allows normal washing, and can be left on until the wound is fully healed.

Parental support

The parents always require consideration, especially when a first-born baby is transferred to a children's hospital on the first day of life. The baby may stay there for several weeks, at precisely the time when the mother's emotions are in turmoil and she would normally be establishing a new and unique relationship. Feelings of guilt at producing an infant with a congenital abnormality, or inadequacy following removal of the infant from her care and the lack of close physical contact, may lead her to have difficulty bonding to her baby and produce an exaggeration of the usual puerperal emotional instability. To help overcome this when separation is unavoidable, the mother should be given a photograph of her baby, and should see the baby again as soon as possible, to be involved in the day-to-day care of the child as much as the illness permits (Chapter 2).

Response of the child

The average child's natural optimism, freedom from unfounded anxiety, remarkable powers of recuperation and apparently short memory for unpleasant experiences can make even major surgery a relatively short and simple matter. Most children are out of bed in 2–3 days and active for much of the day or are already at home by 5 days after many major operations.

Even when minor surgery has been uneventfully concluded, the child may have disturbed behaviour for several months after leaving hospital, and the parents should be made aware of this possibility. Signs of insecurity, increased dependency and disturbed sleep are not uncommon but fortunately are of short duration when met with warm affection, reassurance and understanding by the parents.

The undesirable psychological effects of surgery must be put in proper perspective by mentioning the beneficial effects which so often follow operation: the well-being after repair of an uncomfortable hernia, the freely expressed satisfaction at the excision of an unsightly lump or blemish.

Finally, in many older children there is a detectable increase in confidence and poise which comes from facing, and coping adequately with, an operation. This may be the first occasion on which the child has been away from home, and metaphorically at least, standing on his or her own two feet.

The timing of surgical procedures

Surgical conditions in infancy and childhood can be classified according to the degree of urgency with which treatment should be carried out. Three categories can be distinguished:

1 The immediate group – that is, conditions where immediate investigation and/or definitive operation is required; for example, intussusception; appendicitis.
2 The intermediate group – where treatment is not urgent, but should be undertaken without undue delay; for example, infant inguinal hernia.

3 The elective group – where operation is performed at an optimum age determined by one or more factors which affect the patient's best interests, for example, undescended testis, hypospadias.

The immediate group

Trauma, acute infections, abdominal emergencies and acute scrotal conditions fall into this category. A particularly important subgroup is neonatal emergencies. Most of these are the result of developmental abnormalities causing disorders of function, some of which may threaten life. The best prognosis depends upon early diagnosis and timely transport to a hospital where the appropriate skills and equipment are available (sometimes this is best done where the infant is born, as in a congenital diaphragmatic hernia) (see Chapters 4–11).

The intermediate group

Inguinal hernias are prone to strangulation, especially in the first year of life. For this reason, herniotomy should be performed within a few days of diagnosis in those less than 1 year of age. Investigation of swellings or masses suspected to be malignant should be undertaken within a day or two of their discovery, in close consultation with the regional paediatric oncology service.

The elective group

Factors favouring deferment of operation

Factors which favour deferment of operation, and hence may determine an optimum age for surgery, include
1 The possibility of spontaneous correction or cure. In infants, scrotal hydroceles, encysted hydroceles of the cord, true umbilical hernias and sternomastoid tumours all show a strong tendency to spontaneous resolution. Surgery is only required for those few that persist well beyond the age of natural resolution.
2 Strawberry naevi (intracutaneous capillary haemangiomas) progress and enlarge in the first year of life, but usually involute and fade spontaneously in the ensuing 2–4 years (Chapter 50). In general, they should be left alone to do so, and surgical measures are required rarely.
3 The difficulties posed by minute and delicate structures can be avoided by postponing operation until they are more robust, although this is seldom the sole reason for deferring operation: for example, an undescended testis can be repaired more easily in a 6–12-month-old boy than shortly after birth.
4 The development of co-operation and comprehension with age. Voluntary exercises are important after some

operations, and it may be desirable to defer them until the necessary degree of co-operation is forthcoming.

5 The effects of growth are important in some instances. Chest wall deformities are corrected at adolescence, when chest wall growth is almost complete.

6 Coexistent anomalies and intercurrent diseases, for example, infections, will affect the timing of operations. The situation in each patient should be assessed to establish the order of priorities when there are multiple abnormalities, and to determine whether the treatment of non-urgent conditions should be deferred temporarily.

Factors favouring early operation

Factors which favour early operation rather than deferred treatment include capacity for healing and adaptation in the very young. For example, a fracture of a long bone at birth causes such an exuberant growth of callus that clinical union occurs in 7–10 days, and the subsequent moulding will remove any residual bony deformities.

1 Stimulation of development by early treatment occurs in infants with a congenital dislocation of the hip. When splinting is commenced in the first week of life, this will prevent the secondary dysplasia of the acetabulum and femur, which in the past was thought to be the primary cause of the dislocation.

2 Malleability of infantile tissues is an advantage, for example, in talipes, in which the best results are obtained when treatment is commenced in the first few days after birth.

3 Avoidance of undesirable psychological effects. Often these can be prevented by completing treatment, including repetitive painful procedures, before the memory of past things is established (at about 18 months) or before the child goes to school, where obvious deformities or disabilities are likely to attract attention.

4 Effect on the parents. The family as a whole should be considered, and when it is not disadvantageous to the child, early operation may resolve parental anxiety and prevent rejection of the child.

Key Points

- All hospital and operative procedures are modified to reduce psychological stress in children.
- As much as possible, all painful procedures are done while the child is anaesthetised.
- Invisible stitches, waterproof dressing and local anaesthetic given before waking mean the wound can be left alone postoperatively.
- Day surgery avoids separation anxiety in older children.

Further reading

Frawley G (1999) *I'm Going to Have an Anaesthetic*. Paediatric Anaesthetic Department, Royal Children's Hospital, Melbourne.

McGrath PJ, Finlay GA, Ritchie J, Dowden SJ (2003) *Pain, Pain, Go Away: Helping Children with Pain*, 2nd Edn. Royal Children's Hospital, Melbourne.

Neonatal Emergencies

4 Respiratory Distress in the Newborn

Case 1

Antenatal ultrasonography has revealed a large solid lesion occupying most of the right chest. At birth respiratory distress develops rapidly: a chest x-ray shows a partly cystic and solid lesion in the right lower zone.

Q 1.1 What is the differential diagnosis?

Q 1.2 What treatment is needed?

Case 2

After a breech delivery, acute cyanosis and respiratory distress develops in a term infant. Breath sounds are diminished over the left chest.

Q 2.1 What is the likely problem?

Q 2.2 What emergency treatment may be needed?

When breathing is more rapid than normal in a newborn baby, respiratory distress is confirmed. The degree of distress may be slight initially, but progressive deterioration may culminate in irreversible respiratory failure.

Neonatal respiratory distress is not normally the province of the paediatric surgeon, but it may occur in a specific group of neonatal patients in whom the causes are amenable to surgical correction. Respiratory failure may have developed already when the baby presents, and prompt action can save the infant's life and regain the opportunity for corrective surgery. Those concerned with the care of the newborn must be able to recognise respiratory distress, and the paediatric surgeon must be familiar with its causes and the principles of management.

In only a few cases can a firm diagnosis be made on clinical grounds alone, and x-rays of the thorax and abdomen should be obtained as soon as possible.

Recognition of respiratory distress

The key clinical feature is a raised respiratory rate. Tachycardia is almost invariably present as well, and if the

Jones' Clinical Paediatric Surgery, 6th edition. By Hutson, O'Brien, Woodward and Beasley. Published 2008 by Blackwell Publishing, ISBN: 978-1-4051-6267-8.

pulse rate is more than 200/min the situation is serious. Bradycardia is also a dangerous sign and often portends imminent respiratory failure.

Other cardiovascular signs, such as the presence of apparent 'dextrocardia', and the nature of the peripheral pulses, will provide further clues as to the underlying cause. The abdomen may be scaphoid in babies with a diaphragmatic hernia, but can be distended when there is a pulmonary cause for the respiratory distress. Intestinal obstruction and neonatal peritonitis can cause abdominal distension and lead to respiratory embarrassment. Respiration may be 'laboured' or associated with deformity of the chest wall, or there may be inspiratory (sternal) retraction, indicative of obstruction of the airways.

A surgical cause is present in a minority of babies with respiratory distress, and the surgeon must be familiar with other conditions which enter into the differential diagnosis, for example, hyaline membrane disease and cerebral birth injuries [Table 4.1]. Evidence from antenatal ultrasonography, obstetrical details and any abnormal physical signs will help determine the cause of tachypnoea. A baby who is pale and cyanosed but improves following the administration of oxygen may have a diaphragmatic hernia (Chapter 5). A scaphoid abdomen and barrelled chest with the heart sounds best heard on the right are supportive physical signs, and a chest x-ray

Table 4.1 Causes of neonatal respiratory distress

Types of obstruction	Examples
Upper respiratory tract obstruction	
Nasal	Choanal atresia
Pharyngeal	Pierre–Robin syndrome
	Hamartoma of tongue
Laryngeal	'Infantile larynx'
	Vocal cord palsy
	Subglottic haemangioma
Tracheal	Laryngeal web-cyst
	Tracheomalacia
	Massive cystic hygroma
	Vascular ring
Lower respiratory tract obstruction	Meconium aspiration
	Aspiration of gastric contents
	Lobar emphysema (congenital)
Alveolar disease	Hyaline membrane disease
	Pneumonia
	Congenital heart disease
	Pulmonary oedema
	Diaphragmatic hernia
Pulmonary compression	Pneumothorax
	Diaphragmatic hernia
	Repaired exomphalos or gastroschisis
	Congenital lobar emphysema
	Congenital lung cysts
	Bronchogenic cysts
	Duplication cysts
	Abdominal distension
Neurological disease	Birth asphyxia
	Apnoea of prematurity
	Intracranial haemorrhage
	Convulsions

will confirm the diagnosis. By contrast, an infant with cyanosis and respiratory distress which is relieved by crying may have choanal atresia (Chapter 14).

The principles of management

When respiratory failure is present already, urgent treatment is required, regardless of the underlying cause. Accurate diagnosis of the cause is made on the clinical signs and imaging. The degree of respiratory or metabolic acidosis must be determined as a guide to the resuscitation

required. Where applicable, surgery is undertaken to correct the cause, usually after correction of the physiological disturbances.

Specific conditions

One of the important aspects of neonatal respiratory distress is that many of the causes have a wide clinical spectrum: for example, a diaphragmatic hernia may produce a direct threat to life within minutes of birth, yet on other occasions may cause no distress in the neonatal period and give rise to symptoms only after several weeks (Chapter 5). Congenital cystic adenomatoid malformations and pulmonary sequestration are often diagnosed on antenatal ultrasonography. Choanal atresia is discussed in Chapter 14 and oesophageal atresia in Chapter 6.

Malformations that involve part or whole of one lung and cause respiratory distress in the newborn include congenital lobar emphysema and congenital cysts of the lung, either solitary or multiple. The physical signs are never diagnostic and imaging is required to make the diagnosis. There are considerable variations in the clinical picture, and when there is obvious respiratory distress, surgery is indicated. Resection of the affected segment of lung not only removes functionless pulmonary tissue in which there is little or no gaseous exchange but also allows expansion of the normal areas which have been compressed by the over-distended segment, lobe or lobes.

Congenital lobar emphysema

The underlying abnormality is bronchomalacia from congenital deficiency of the cartilage. It results in expiratory obstruction and trapping of air in the affected lobe, leading to massive distension of a pulmonary lobe.

The cardinal symptom is tachypnoea which is most noticeable when the baby is being fed. Not infrequently there is a dry cough and stridor. Cyanosis is usually an indication for urgent treatment. The mediastinum is displaced and the chest wall over the affected area is prominent and has relatively reduced respiratory excursion; breath sounds are diminished and the percussion note typically is hyper-resonant.

X-rays show an area of increased radiolucency in which there are some bronchovascular markings. There is also downward displacement of the diaphragm on the affected side, and the over-distended lung may herniate across the midline [Fig. 4.1].

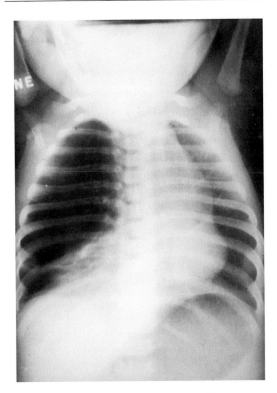

Figure 4.1 Congenital lobar emphysema of the right upper lobe which is over-distended and herniating across the midline.

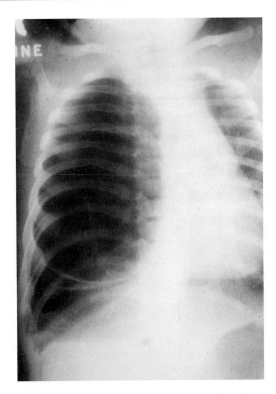

Figure 4.2 Congenital cystic lung. A giant cyst replaces the right lower lobe, compressing the remaining right lung and herniating across the midline to displace the heart and compress the left lung.

The lobes most commonly affected are the left upper lobe or the right middle lobe. The treatment is lobectomy.

Congenital cystic lung

The clinical features are similar to those of lobar emphysema in that respiratory distress often occurs early, but usually it is more urgent and severe. X-rays show a large cyst with a sharply defined border [Fig. 4.2] or an extensive multicystic area. There is compression and collapse of unaffected areas of the lungs and displacement of the mediastinum.

The aim of surgery is to remove the portion of the lung that is functionless and is interfering with the function of the surrounding normal lung. Depending on the distribution of disease, resection of the affected lobe or even pneumonectomy may be required.

Pulmonary sequestration

Pulmonary sequestration is an uncommon malformation in which there is non-functioning lung tissue which

has no connection with the normal bronchial tree, and a blood supply which arises from an anomalous systemic artery, often directly from the aorta [Fig. 4.3; Chapter 49]. It usually occurs on the left side and may be either intralobar or extralobar, depending on whether it shares visceral pleura with the normal lung. It may present as a pulmonary infection, because of its space-occupying effect, or be found incidentally on chest x-ray. The sequestration is resected by a thoracoscopic approach or by open thoracotomy.

Congenital cystic adenomatoid malformation

Congenital cystic adenomatoid malformations (CCAMs) include a range of localised abnormalities in which the bronchiolar tissue is abnormal, with communicating cysts and a relative paucity of cartilage. They may be diagnosed on antenatal ultrasonography as a cystic or solid mass in one part of the lung. Maternal polyhydramnios

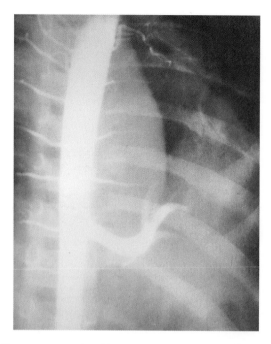

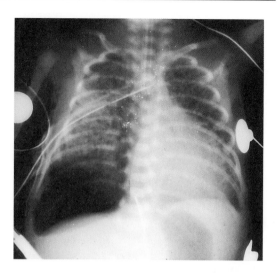

Figure 4.4 Severe pulmonary interstitial emphysema.

Figure 4.3 Anomalous blood supply from the aorta to a left pulmonary sequestration.

and mediastinal shift are common. CCAM presents post-natally in three ways:

1 respiratory distress (60%);

2 infectious complications, for example, recurrent pneumonia (20%);

3 as an incidental finding on chest x-ray (20%).

Many CCAMs observed on antenatal ultrasonography regress and are resolved by term. CCAMs identified post-natally are usually resected.

Mediastinal conditions

Very rarely, large cystic teratomas and duplication cysts cause respiratory distress and should be removed. In the neonate, oesophageal duplication cysts may present with increasing respiratory distress because of their space-occupying effect compressing the normal airways.

Pulmonary interstitial emphysema

This is an acquired condition of extreme prematurity seen in infants where assisted ventilation is required for severe hyaline membrane disease. High ventilatory pressures force air into the lung interstitium, which tracks along peribronchial spaces, producing interstitial cysts which have a characteristic appearance on x-ray

[Fig. 4.4]. Treatment is directed at reducing the ventila-tory pressures. In severe and progressive cases, thoracot-omy may be required to deflate the cysts. Refinements in neonatology have resulted in a significant decrease in the incidence of this condition, such that it is now seen rarely.

Neonatal pneumothorax

Pneumothorax may occur as a complication of diffuse pulmonary disease or of a localised abnormality such as a subpleural emphysematous bleb. The pneumothorax may be suspected on clinical grounds by sudden deterioration in condition, displacement of the trachea or apex beat and a hyper-resonant percussion note, but x-rays are required to confirm the diagnosis.

In neonates, the severity of the symptoms frequently is out of proportion to the size of the pneumothorax. Even a small pneumothorax may be associated with severe respiratory distress when there is pre-existing parenchymal lung disease and little respiratory reserve. Intercostal drainage is urgent.

Haemothorax

Haemothorax is an infrequent complication of haemor-rhagic disease of the newborn and may produce an alarm-ing clinical picture; this is due to mechanical factors which interfere with respiration, and to the reduction of the circulating blood volume. Pleural paracentesis and blood transfusion are required.

Acute respiratory failure in the neonate

Acute respiratory failure occurs when oxygenation and/ or ventilation are impaired sufficiently to be an immediate threat to life. It is usually the result of asphyxia due to

1 birth asphyxia;

2 injuries sustained during birth;

3 developmental anomalies, including congenital heart disease;

4 hyaline membrane disease in the premature infant;

5 increased susceptibility to infection.

The factors in infants which predispose to respiratory failure are summarised in Table 4.2. With limited respiratory reserve, respiratory failure can occur rapidly.

Signs of respiratory failure

In the neonate, especially in the premature neonate, acute hypoxia causes pallor, apnoea, bradycardia, hypotension and lethargy. The clinical signs of hypercapnia – sweating, tachycardia and hypertension are seen rarely, but pulmonary haemorrhage, cerebral haemorrhage, severe hyperkalaemia and hypoglycaemia may all occur as the result of hypoxia.

General management

An infant with incipient respiratory failure requires close observation at all times. Neonates should be nursed in an isolette or under a radiant heater so that the temperature is controlled and observation unimpeded. Handling should be kept to a minimum, as it can increase oxygen consumption dramatically.

The position most favourable in nursing neonates is prone, with hips and knees flexed, and the head turned regularly from one side to the other. This reduces apnoeic episodes, shortens gastric emptying time and reduces the risk of regurgitation and aspiration. The supine position is preferred if bag and mask ventilation or resuscitation is needed.

Oxygen

The method of delivery of oxygen depends upon the age of the infant, oxygen concentration required and the underlying condition. All patients having prolonged oxygen therapy should have continuous oximetry and serial arterial blood gas estimations with adjustment of inspired oxygen concentration to ensure adequate arterial saturation. Premature infants receiving supplementary oxygen therapy are at risk of retinopathy of prematurity, for which frequent blood gas measurements are required to maintain the arterial PO_2 in the range of 6.6–10.6 kPa (50–80 mmHg). In the newborn, gentle suction is performed at intervals to remove pooled secretions and to stimulate coughing. However, pharyngeal and endotracheal suction may cause a sudden fall in P_aO_2, which necessitates an increase in the concentration of oxygen in the inspired gases.

Fluids and feeding

Oral feeding should be suspended in children with severe dyspnoea, but enteral nutrition can be continued via a nasogastric tube. If abdominal distension occurs, feeding must be discontinued to avoid regurgitation and aspiration, and to prevent splinting of the diaphragm, as these may cause additional respiratory embarrassment. Intravenous fluids can supply fluids and parenteral nutrition, but total fluid intake may need to be restricted in some patients with pulmonary disease.

Sodium bicarbonate may be required to correct metabolic acidosis (Chapter 2). Fluid management

Table 4.2 Factors predisposing infants to respiratory failure

Factor	Comment
Metabolic rate	Metabolism per kg is twice that of adults
Respiratory rate	Lung surface area per kg is about the same as for an adult; so the infant has much less respiratory reserve
Compliance	The chest wall of the infant is less able to adjust to a reduction in lung compliance or an increase in airways resistance
Airway calibre	Relatively larger total airways resistance than in older children or adults
Airway obstruction	The narrow airways are more prone to obstruction by oedema and secretions
Temperature control	Temperature regulation is relatively poor in the newborn, especially in the premature. In a cold environment, oxygen consumption may increase two- or three-fold

requires regular biochemical monitoring and an accurate record of fluid balance.

Temperature control

Seriously ill neonates are particularly vulnerable to cold stress, and maintenance of body temperature is of vital importance before, during and after any surgery (Chapter 2). The neonate has a narrow 'thermoneutral' range in which oxygen consumption is minimised and optimal: abdominal wall skin temperature is optimal between 36°C and 36.5°C. Exposure to an environmental temperature of 20–25°C increases oxygen consumption three-fold and may precipitate cardiorespiratory failure. Critically ill neonates should be nursed in open cots with servocontrolled radiant heat so that access to them is not compromised. Insensible water loss may be increased, particularly in infants of very low birthweight, but this can be taken into account when planning fluid replacements.

Monitoring

Respiratory and cardiovascular signs should be monitored, along with the oxygen concentration in the inspired air. Blood for gas analysis is obtained by percutaneous puncture or, more accurately, in samples from an indwelling catheter in a peripheral artery, which can also be used for a continuous record of the arterial pressure. Continuous transcutaneous monitoring of oxygen and carbon dioxide levels is used widely.

Ventilatory support

In neonates, nasotracheal intubation is the preferred type of artificial airway [Table 4.3]. Tubes of appropriate size and composition can be left *in situ* for long periods with minimal adverse effects or complications.

Humidification of dry inspired gases is necessary to reduce the risk of viscid and retained sputum, atelectasis and blockage of the endotracheal tube with inspissated secretions, and to preserve mucociliary function.

Inspired gases should be delivered to the trachea at 37°C, fully saturated with water vapour, using a safe, servocontrolled humidifier. This is an important contribution to maintenance of body temperature, and it reduces insensible fluid losses from the airways.

Regular suctioning of the trachea is necessary to stimulate coughing and to remove accumulated secretions. Suctioning can cause hypoxia and atelectasis and may introduce infection, and various techniques are used to avoid these risks. Gentle 'bagging' with an oxygen-rich mixture is used before and after suction to reduce hypoxia and re-expand the lung. In infants at risk of retinopathy of prematurity, the oxygen concentration in the 'bag' should not be more than 10% higher than the mixture used for ventilation. In older children, 100% oxygen can be used.

Continuous positive airways pressure

This is a technique that employs a distending pressure (5–10 cm H_2O) applied to the airways of a patient who is breathing spontaneously. It is used in pulmonary conditions causing hypoxaemia due to atelectasis, alveolar instability and intrapulmonary shunting. Continuous positive airways pressure (CPAP) increases functional residual capacity and compliance, re-expands areas of atelectasis, decreases intrapulmonary shunting and increases arterial PO_2. In premature infants, CPAP will often improve the regularity of respiratory movements and decrease apnoeic episodes. The technique requires careful control to avoid reduced cardiac output, retention of fluids, rupture of alveoli and pneumothorax.

Table 4.3   Use of nasotracheal tube in neonates

Advantages	Disadvantages
Provides patent airway	Narrows the upper airways
Overcomes airway obstruction	Bypasses natural humidification, heating and filtering of inspired gases
Allows tracheo-bronchial toilet and suction	Prevents coughing and expectoration of secretions
Facilitates continuous positive airway pressure	May cause subglottic irritation and stenosis: a risk which can be minimised by using a tube of the correct size allowing a small air leak during positive pressure ventilation
	Enables mechanical ventilation

Intermittent positive pressure ventilation

Intermittent positive pressure ventilation (IPPV) is used to correct hypoventilation, and sometimes (e.g. raised intracranial pressure, pulmonary hypertension) to produce hyperventilation and to lower $PaCO_2$. Mechanical ventilators have been designed specifically for neonatal use. IPPV is often combined with positive end-expiratory pressure (PEEP). PEEP is used for the same reasons as CPAP, that is, as a means of improving oxygenation. The hazards of IPPV are greater than those of CPAP and related directly to the level of pressure applied. Barotrauma to immature lungs may result in a chronic lung disease in neonates known as bronchopulmonary dysplasia.

Intermittent mandatory ventilation (IMV) is a technique of mechanical ventilation in which a predetermined minute volume is guaranteed even when the patient breathes independently from the ventilator. With infant ventilators, a constant flow is provided during the expiratory phase from which the infant can breathe. It is a technique useful for weaning from mechanical ventilation and is used as a means of minimising barotrauma.

Controlled ventilation involves the use of relaxants and sedatives which paralyse respiratory movements, to completely abolish the work of breathing and improve gas exchange. The technique is useful in critically ill neonates and those with difficult ventilatory problems, but it should only be employed where expert surveillance and sophisticated monitoring are available. Inappropriate pressure settings can cause a pneumothorax with sudden deterioration, and inadvertent disconnection rapidly results in potentially fatal hypoxia.

Key Points

- Neonatal respiratory distress should be diagnosed by tachypnoea, before cyanosis appears.
- A surgical cause is present in the minority, but can be identified by physical examination and chest x-ray.

Further reading

Advanced Life Support Group (1997) Resuscitation of the newborn. In: *Advanced Paediatric Life Support: the Practical Approach*, 2nd Edn. BMJ Publishing Group, pp. 55–61.

Wilson JM, DiFiore JW (2006) Respiratory physiology and care. In: Grosfeld JL, O'Neill JA Jr., Fonkalsrud EW, Coran AG (eds) *Pediatric Surgery*, 6th Edn. Mosby Jr., Elsevier, Philadelphia, pp. 114–133.

5 Diaphragmatic Hernia

Case 1

Within minutes of birth, a full-term infant boy develops increasing respiratory distress and becomes cyanosed. He fails to improve with upper airway suctioning. The pregnancy was uneventful. He looks barrel-chested and his abdomen is scaphoid.

Q 1.1 What is the diagnosis?

Q 1.2 What investigation will confirm the diagnosis?

Q 1.3 What factors determine the outcome in these situations?

Case 2

A newborn infant with a recently diagnosed left-sided congenital diaphragmatic hernia is about to be transferred to a paediatric surgical institution by air. He is currently being ventilated through an endotracheal tube and just maintaining adequate blood gas levels.

Q 2.1 Should his ventilation be increased during transport?

Q 2.2 Should any other manoeuvre be performed to reduce the likelihood of problems during transport?

Q 2.3 If he suddenly deteriorates, what complication may have happened?

Definitions

The diaphragm develops largely from three structures:
1 the pleuroperitoneal membrane;
2 the septum transversum;
3 the marginal ingrowths from the muscles of the body wall.

Congenital diaphragmatic hernia results from failure of formation or fusion of the components of the diaphragm, such that abdominal contents can move through a defect into the chest. Sometimes, failure of muscularisation may produce a thin, weak diaphragm, referred to as an eventration of the diaphragm.

The Bochdalek type is the most common variety of congenital diaphragmatic hernia (1 in 5000 live births) and results from a defect in the posterolateral part of the diaphragm. During intra-uterine development, the small bowel, stomach, spleen and left lobe of the liver pass through the defect in the diaphragm into the chest, limiting the space available for the developing lung. This causes lung hypoplasia, which in many infants is severe enough to produce severe respiratory distress within minutes of birth, and may not be compatible with life.

The Morgagni (retrosternal) type of diaphragmatic hernia is rare, and results from a defect in the anterior midline, just behind the sternum [Fig. 5.1]. It usually contains part of the colon or small bowel, and less commonly, part of the liver.

Occasionally, a hernia may occur through the apex of the cupola or at the periphery adjacent to the costal margin. Oesophageal hiatal hernias also occur and usually produce symptoms of gastro-oesophageal reflux.

Clinical features

Antenatal diagnosis

Most congenital diaphragmatic hernias are diagnosed well before birth, on antenatal ultrasonography. Factors that may indicate a worse prognosis on antenatal scanning (summarised in Table 5.1) may influence counselling of the parents-to-be. Antenatal ultrasonographic diagnosis of diaphragmatic hernias also allows the mother-to-be to be transferred to a tertiary paediatric surgical centre before birth. Successful *in utero* correction of diaphragmatic hernia and fetoscopic tracheal occlusion has been achieved in

Jones' Clinical Paediatric Surgery, 6th edition. By Hutson, O'Brien, Woodward and Beasley. Published 2008 by Blackwell Publishing, ISBN: 978-1-4051-6267-8.

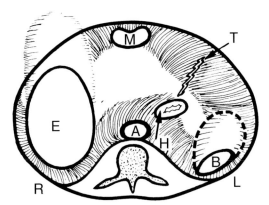

Figure 5.1 Diaphragmatic hernias. Diaphragm as seen from below, showing: [B] Bochdalek left posterolateral defect; [M] anterior or Morgagni type; [H] hiatus for oesophageal and hiatus hernia; [E] large eventration in the tendinous portion of the right cupola; [T] a tear which causes a post-traumatic hernia; [A] aorta.

Table 5.1 Possible antenatal markers of severity

- Early gestational age at diagnosis on ultrasonography
- Lung-to-head ratio (LHR) at 24–26-weeks' gestation <1.0
- Small fetal lung volume on 3D ultrasonography and MRI
- >50% liver in chest on right side
- Liver in chest on left side
- Stomach and spleen in chest on left side
- No hernial 'sac' (difficult to confirm on scanning)

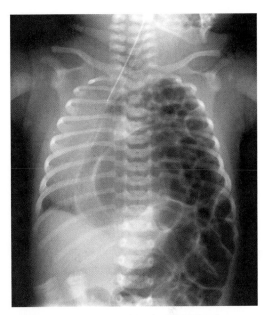

Figure 5.2 X-ray of congenital diaphragmatic hernia (Bochdalek type). Multiple bowel loops fill the left pleural cavity, and the heart is displaced to the right.

a research setting, but the techniques are complex and the indications are still being refined. To date, they have not resulted in improved survival or reduced morbidity compared with modern postnatal techniques.

Postnatal diagnosis

The majority of infants born with a Bochdalek (posterolateral) diaphragmatic hernia become symptomatic at or shortly after birth. Where pulmonary hypoplasia is severe, the infant becomes cyanosed with severe respiratory distress within minutes of birth. In other patients there is tachypnoea, increased respiratory effort, hyperinflated chest and scaphoid abdomen, and heart sounds are on the right side. This is because 85% of posterolateral hernias involve the left hemidiaphragm. The remainder are right-sided (12%) or bilateral (3%). Associated anomalies occur in up to 40%, but most are minor and do not affect survival, for example, undescended testes. The most common serious abnormalities are heart defects.

Unlike posterolateral hernias, most anterior (retrosternal) hernias are symptomless unless strangulation occurs. Very rarely the hernia may protrude into the pericardial cavity rather than into the inferior mediastinum and cause cardiac tamponade, presenting as cardiorespiratory distress in the neonatal period.

Investigation

Diagnosis of a posterolateral hernia is confirmed by a chest x-ray [Fig. 5.2]. In left-sided defects, loops of bowel can be seen in the left chest. The heart is deviated to the right. Little room is left for the lungs, particularly the left lung which is markedly compressed. Sometimes, the appearance may be difficult to distinguish from basal lung cysts, in which case a repeat chest x-ray is performed after a nasogastric tube has been inserted, the tip of which can be seen in the chest. Alternatively, a barium study will show bowel within the thoracic cavity when there is a diaphragmatic hernia.

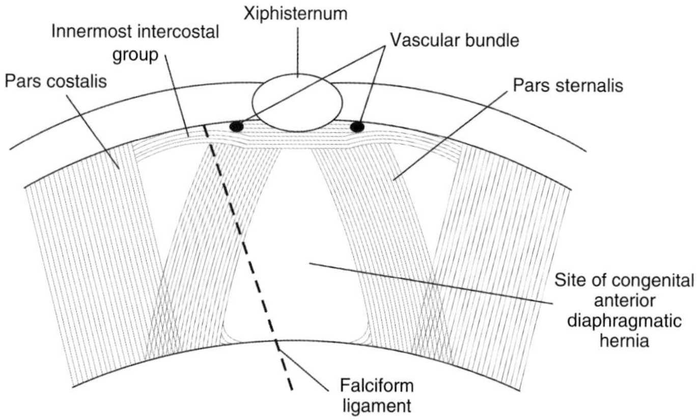

Figure 5.3 Diagram of the diaphragm and its attachment to the sternum, showing the site of an anterior diaphragmatic hernia.

Treatment

Posterolateral (Bochdalek) hernia

Where an antenatal ultrasound examination has identified a diaphragmatic hernia, the best outcomes are achieved if the infant is transferred to a tertiary paediatric surgical centre prior to birth. This is because these infants may develop severe pulmonary distress very quickly after birth, making subsequent transfer difficult and potentially dangerous.

Initial treatment involves intensive cardiorespiratory support and insertion of a nasogastric tube to prevent bowel dilatation within the chest. Care must be taken to avoid hyperinflation and barotrauma of the small hypoplastic lungs. High-frequency oscillatory ventilation in combination with nitric oxide has improved survival rates. Ventilation with a face mask ('bagging') should be avoided as this may force air into the stomach, increasing its volume at the expense of the already compromised lungs. Vigorous endotracheal ventilation should also be avoided because of the risk of causing barotrauma and a tension pneumothorax, which can lead to the rapid demise of the infant. Exogenous surfactant provides no specific benefit in newborns with diaphragmatic hernia. The key to success is careful gentle ventilation that minimises injury to the hypoplastic lungs.

Sudden deterioration of the infant's condition during initial resuscitation or during transport suggests the development of a tension pneumothorax, and this may necessitate prompt drainage by needle aspiration or insertion of an intercostal drain. Fortunately, strict avoidance of hyperventilation and limited inflation pressures have made this complication rare.

Surgery to return the bowel to the abdominal cavity and to repair the defect in the diaphragm is performed when the infant's condition is stable. This may be anywhere between 12 h and 7 or more days after birth. In left-sided defects, a left transverse or subcostal abdominal incision is used. The management of the infant with severe hypoplastic lungs is difficult and may involve high-frequency oscillation or extracorporeal membrane oxygenation. The major cause of death remains pulmonary hypoplasia and pulmonary hypertension. Pulmonary hypertension is due to the small pulmonary vascular bed and to the changing resistance of the pulmonary arterioles: it resolves in most patients with time, provided ventilation does not produce additional lung injury. Survival rates of about 80% are now being reported.

Anterior diaphragmatic hernia

Anterior diaphragmatic (Morgagni) hernias are often diagnosed on an incidental x-ray of the chest in a symptomless patient, but repair is still advisable because of the risk of strangulation of the bowel that protrudes through the defect. This is usually performed as a laparoscopic procedure [Fig. 5.3]. The results are excellent.

> **Key Points**
> - Diaphragmatic hernia is diagnosed antenatally or by chest x-ray in a baby with a barrel chest, scaphoid abdomen and respiratory distress.
> - Ventilatory support, especially during transport, should be the minimum required to prevent deterioration, as hyperinflation with 2° barotrauma is a significant complication.
> - Sudden deterioration is usually caused by tension pneumothorax.

Further reading

Bagolan P, Lasallia G, Crescenzi F, Nahom A, Trucchi A, Giorlandino C (2004) Impact of a current treatment protocol on outcome of high-risk congenital diaphragmatic hernia. *J Pediatr Surg* **39**: 313–318.

Granholm T, Albanese CT, Harrison MR (2003) Congenital diaphragmatic hernia. In: Puri P (ed) *Newborn Surgery*, 2 Edn. Arnold, London, pp. 309–316.

Kays DW (2006) Congenital diaphragmatic hernia: real improvements in survival. *Neo Rev* **7**: c428–439.

6

Oesophageal Atresia and Tracheo-Oesophageal Fistula

Case 1

Mrs W has been admitted to a district hospital where she has delivered a baby boy at 38-weeks' gestation, who despite initial suctioning, appears to be salivating excessively and is very 'mucousy'. He has mild tachypnoea, but is pink.

Q 1.1 What manoeuvre must be undertaken to establish the cause of his excessive drooling?

Q 1.2 Are there any other abnormalities likely to be present?

Q 1.3 What needs to be done before and during transfer to a paediatric surgical institution?

Case 2

Annabel R aged 38 had difficulty conceiving, but now has an infant girl. The baby looks dysmorphic and is noted to have a deformed forearm and thumb abnormalities, and an anorectal abnormality. An orogastric tube could not be passed into the stomach.

Q 2.1 What other abnormalities are likely, and how would they be detected?

Q 2.2 What would you do before proceeding to surgery?

Oesophageal atresia is a congenital anomaly in which there is complete interruption of the oesophagus. This produces a blind upper oesophageal pouch, and a lower oesophageal segment that usually communicates with the trachea through a distal tracheo-oesophageal fistula. Less common variations of the abnormality also occur [Fig. 6.1; Table 6.1].

Pathophysiology

The effect of oesophageal atresia on the infant is that saliva (or milk if the infant has been fed) accumulates in the blind upper oesophageal segment and spills over into the trachea, causing choking and cyanosis, and soiling of the lungs. Gastric contents may be aspirated through the distal tracheo-oesophageal fistula into the bronchial tree.

Pulmonary complications may follow, initially atelectasis, and then pneumonia. Abdominal distension from air passing down the fistula into the stomach may elevate and splint the diaphragm, adversely affecting the infant's ability to ventilate adequately.

Antenatal diagnosis

Sometimes oesophageal atresia is diagnosed on antenatal ultrasonography by the observation of polyhydramnios, a small stomach or abnormal oesophageal contraction with swallowing. Congenital abnormalities known to be associated with oesophageal atresia may also be evident.

Early diagnosis

Oesophageal atresia should be recognised as soon as possible after birth, for delay may lead to aspiration and progressive pulmonary complications. The diagnosis is

Jones' Clinical Paediatric Surgery, 6th edition. By Hutson, O'Brien, Woodward and Beasley. Published 2008 by Blackwell Publishing, ISBN: 978-1-4051-6267-8.

Figure 6.1 The anatomical variants of oesophageal atresia and/or tracheo-oesophageal fistula. The percentage frequency of each variant is shown.

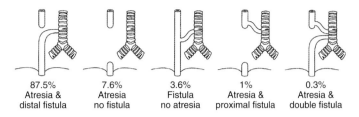

| 87.5% | 7.6% | 3.6% | 1% | 0.3% |
| Atresia & distal fistula | Atresia no fistula | Fistula no atresia | Atresia & proximal fistula | Atresia & double fistula |

Table 6.1 Frequency of associated abnormalities in oesophageal atresia

Abnormality	Percentage
Cardiac	25
Gastrointestinal (including anorectal)	22
Vertebral/skeletal	20
Renal	15
Chromosomal (usually Trisomy 18 and 21)	7

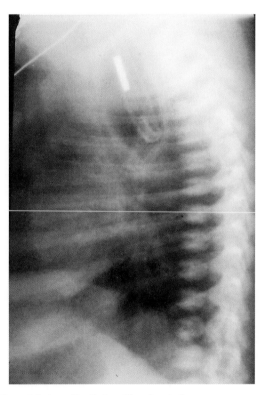

Figure 6.2 A small catheter will curl up in the upper oesophageal pouch and give a false impression of oesophageal continuity. Therefore, a wide-bore catheter, for example, No. 10 gauge, should be used.

confirmed when an orogastric catheter cannot be passed through the mouth and oesophagus into the stomach.

Symptoms soon after birth

Oesophageal atresia should be suspected when a newborn infant appears to be drooling excessively. The infant may have been resuscitated at birth with suction aspiration of mucus using a catheter but then within minutes, develops rattling respirations, tachypnoea or fine frothy white bubbles of mucus in the nostrils or on the lips. This appearance of excessive salivation or of being 'excessively mucousy' is highly suggestive of oesophageal atresia. Often there is a history of maternal polyhydramnios.

Diagnosis before feeding

A firm 10 French catheter should be introduced through the mouth and passed carefully down the oesophagus; if it becomes arrested at about 10 cm from the lips, the diagnosis of oesophageal atresia has been established. A small catheter may curl up in the upper oesophagus and give a false impression of oesophageal continuity [Fig. 6.2]. Ideally, oesophageal atresia should be diagnosed before the infant is fed, because feeding will cause an acute episode of spluttering, coughing and cyanosis, with aspiration of milk into the lungs.

Preoperative investigation

X-ray

An x-ray of the thorax and abdomen is taken to demonstrate the presence of air in the stomach and small bowel, which indicates that there is a fistula between the trachea and the lower segment of the oesophagus [Fig. 6.3]. The

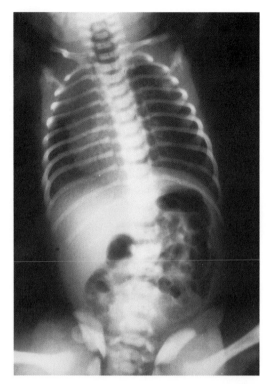

Figure 6.3 Plain x-ray of the chest and abdomen shows air in the oesophageal pouch, stomach and small bowel, indicating that there is a distal tracheo-oesophageal fistula.

x-ray also provides information on the state of the lungs and the presence of vertebral and rib anomalies. It may show evidence of a right-sided aortic arch.

Echocardiography

Nearly 25% of infants with oesophageal atresia have congenital heart disease. It is important to identify cardiac lesions preoperatively because a prostaglandin E_1 infusion will need to be commenced before repair of the oesophagus if the lesion is 'duct-dependent'. In most babies, the cardiac defect does not delay the oesophageal surgery, and oesophageal repair takes precedence over surgery to the heart. An echocardiograph may identify a right aortic arch and influence the surgical approach to the oesophagus.

Renal ultrasonography

If the infant has not passed urine, a renal ultrasound examination must be performed to exclude bilateral renal agenesis. If the infant has no kidneys or has severely dysplastic kidneys, as it occurs in 3% of the cases, no surgery is justified.

Table 6.2 Multiple malformation associations seen with oesophageal atresia

VATER (VACTERL)	CHARGE
Vertebral	Coloboma
Anorectal	Heart
Cardiac	Atresia choanae
Tracheo-oesophageal	Retarded growth
Renal	Genital hypoplasia
Limb (including radial)	Ear

Genetic consultation

If the infant has dysmorphic facies and other features suggestive of a major chromosomal abnormality, early genetic consultation is mandatory. The two most common chromosomal abnormalities are Trisomy 18 and Trisomy 21. In some cases, treatment may be delayed until after the results of chromosomal analysis are known. There are a number of malformation clusters, such as the VATER (or VACTERL) and CHARGE associations, which are well known to occur with oesophageal atresia [Table 6.2].

Treatment

The condition is treated by early complete correction. This involves division of the tracheo-oesophageal fistula and reconstruction of an end-to-end oesophageal anastomosis. In preparation for surgery, the upper pouch should be kept empty by frequent suction. The infant should be placed in an incubator or under an overhead heater to avoid heat loss. Vitamin K is given intramuscularly and intravenous fluids commenced. Antibiotics are given during surgery.

The operation is performed usually within 12 h of admission to hospital. The fistula is closed through a right posterolateral extrapleural thoracotomy. The direct end-to-end anastomosis of the upper and lower segments of the oesophagus establishes oesophageal continuity. In some centres, thoracoscopic repair of oesophageal atresia is performed. Postoperatively, oral feeds can be commenced after 3 or 4 days.

Anatomical variations

Oesophageal atresia without a fistula

In this variant, the blind-ending oesophageal segments have no connection with the respiratory tree. On the initial x-ray, these babies have no gas below the diaphragm [Fig. 6.4]. Typically, the gap between the two segments of the oesophagus may be so great that a primary anastomosis is impossible at birth. A gastrostomy is fashioned to allow enteral feeding and the overflow of saliva from the upper pouch is controlled by frequent suction. At about 6 weeks of age an oesophageal anastomosis is performed. Occasionally, this fails and oesophageal replacement is required. In a further variant of oesophageal atresia, there may be a fistula between the blind upper oesophageal segment and the trachea ('proximal tracheo-oesophageal fistula'): this variant also presents with no gas below the diaphragm on x-ray.

'H' fistula

Sometimes the oesophagus is intact but there is an abnormal fistulous communication between the trachea and

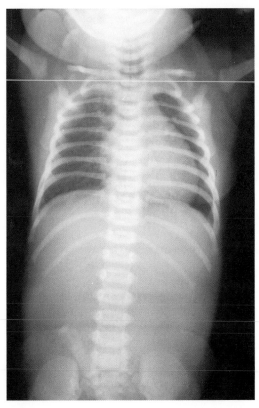

Figure 6.4 In oesophageal atresia without a distal tracheo-oesophageal fistula, there is no air below the diaphragm. Most of these infants have no fistula, while a few have a proximal tracheo-oesophageal fistula.

oesophagus, usually at the level of C7 or T1. These infants present in the first week or so of life with episodes of coughing, cyanosis during feeding, and pulmonary complications. Sometimes they present later with a history of recurrent pulmonary infections or abdominal distension mimicking a bowel obstruction. The diagnosis is made on bronchoscopy or by performing a barium swallow or mid-oesophageal contrast study and observing contrast to pass through the fistula into the trachea. Treatment is by operative division of the fistula, usually through a cervical approach.

Special problems

Effect of prematurity

Prematurity is common in these infants. Provided facilities are available, these infants should have their oesophageal atresia repaired early, before the expected respiratory distress of hyaline membrane disease becomes severe. Failure to divide the tracheo-oesophageal fistula early in these babies may lead to severe problems with ventilation because air escapes preferentially through the fistula into the stomach and may even cause gastric perforation and tension pneumoperitoneum.

Gastro-oesophageal reflux

Gastro-oesophageal reflux is common in oesophageal atresia, and in conjunction with delayed oesophageal clearance may contribute to the development of an oesophageal stricture. The child may require treatment with a proton pump inhibitor or a fundoplication.

Tracheomalacia

Tracheomalacia is a structural weakness of the trachea that commonly occurs in association with oesophageal atresia. It is responsible for the 'seal bark' brassy cough characteristic of oesophageal atresia patients. It tends to improve with time but in the neonatal period may cause breathing difficulties. Occasionally, splinting of the trachea (tracheopexy, aortopexy) is required to prevent collapse of the trachea.

Complications of surgery

There are three main complications:
1 leak from the oesophageal anastomosis;
2 oesophageal stricture;
3 recurrent tracheo-oesophageal fistula.

The majority of anastomotic leaks are minor and are treated by withholding oral feeds, and commencing antibiotics and total parenteral nutrition. They usually seal spontaneously and surgery is required only if uncontrolled mediastinitis or empyema develops. Oesophageal stricture may present with dysphagia or choking on feeds. Gastro-oesophageal reflux is frequently a contributing factor. Treatment usually involves radial balloon dilatation of the oesophagus under fluoroscopic control. Sometimes fundoplication is required if there is coexisting gastro-oesophageal reflux. A recurrent tracheo-oesophageal fistula rarely closes spontaneously and requires re-exploration and division.

Prognosis

In the absence of associated congenital abnormalities or severe prematurity, survival in oesophageal atresia is virtually assured. Most patients have a good quality of life into adulthood.

Key Points

- Excessive salivation or drooling in a neonate suggests oesophageal atresia.
- Diagnosis is confirmed by gentle passage, through the mouth, of a 10 French catheter, which stops at 9–11 cm (distance to stomach is 20–25 cm).
- Babies with oesophageal atresia have a high chance of having other anomalies.
- The prognosis is good in most children with transfer to a tertiary neonatal centre.

Further reading

Beasley SW, Chetchuti PAJ, Puntis JWL (2006) Esophageal atresia. In: Stringer MD, Oldham KT, Mouriquand PDE, (eds) *Pediatric Surgery and Urology: Long term outcomes*, 2nd Edn. Cambridge University Press, Cambridge, pp. 192–216.

Beasley SW, Hutson JM, Auldist AW (1996) Oesophageal atresia. In: *Essential Paediatric Surgery*, Arnold, London, pp. 3–6.

Beasley SW, Myers NA, Auldist AW (1991) *Oesophageal Atresia*. Chapman & Hall, London.

7 Bowel Obstruction

Case 1

A newborn baby develops abdominal distension with bile-stained vomiting and does not pass meconium.
Q 1.1 List three possible diagnoses.
Q 1.2 How would you arrange transport to a neonatal surgical centre?
Q 1.3 Discuss the principles of resuscitation in this circumstance.

Case 2

A diagnosis of Hirschsprung disease is made on a newborn baby.
Q 2.1 What is the definitive diagnostic test for Hirschsprung disease?
Q 2.2 Discuss the surgical treatment.
Q 2.3 Discuss the prognosis.

Case 3

A 1-day-old baby presents with bile-stained vomiting but no abdominal distension.
Q 3.1 List the causes of high-level neonatal bowel obstruction.
Q 3.2 How do you distinguish between these on investigation?
Q 3.3 Discuss the urgency of diagnosis and treatment.

Neonatal bowel obstruction presents with the triad of bile-stained vomiting, abdominal distension and failure to pass meconium. A wide range of congenital anomalies of the gut can cause neonatal bowel obstruction, which causes problems related to the special metabolism of the neonate.

Antenatal diagnosis

Dilated fluid-filled loops of gut may be seen on antenatal ultrasound, indicating bowel obstruction. Sometimes the nature of the obstruction may be characteristic with the 'double bubble' of duodenal atresia; but more often, the findings do not indicate a specific diagnosis. There is considerable variability in the normal appearance of the fetal gut and antenatal diagnosis of bowel obstruction should be reserved for those cases with gross gut dilatation. Polyhydramnios may be associated with intrauterine bowel obstruction, particularly with the more proximal level of

Jones' Clinical Paediatric Surgery, 6th edition. By Hutson, O'Brien, Woodward and Beasley. Published 2008 by Blackwell Publishing, ISBN: 978-1-4051-6267-8.

obstruction. Most pregnancies are now checked with ultrasound at 17–18-weeks' gestation, but this may be too early to diagnose many cases of neonatal bowel obstruction. Intrauterine segmental volvulus or intussusception in later pregnancy is the cause of many gut atresias but ultrasound examination is not routinely performed at this time.

Clinical findings

Bile-stained vomiting in the neonatal period always is significant and must be evaluated carefully as it is indicative of bowel obstruction.

Abdominal distension is a less specific finding as gaseous distension may occur without bowel obstruction. Furthermore, some high bowel obstructions, such as malrotation with volvulus or duodenal atresia, may not have abdominal distension.

The normal neonate passes meconium within 24 h after birth. Neonates with bowel obstruction do not pass meconium, with three notable exceptions: (1) babies with Hirschsprung disease may pass meconium, especially after rectal examination; (2) some sticky meconium pellets may be passed in meconium ileus and (3) onset of symptoms in malrotation with volvulus may be delayed for some time after birth.

Imaging

The plain x-ray is the most important test and will show distension of the gut with fluid levels. The level of the obstruction may be related to the number of fluid levels, for example, a double bubble in duodenal atresia, three or four fluid levels in upper jejunal atresia and many fluid levels in ileal atresia or Hirschsprung disease. Fine calcification indicates prenatal gut perforation with meconium peritonitis. Free gas in the peritoneal cavity is seen when perforation occurs after birth.

Contrast studies are useful in some patients. Incomplete high obstructions are assessed with a barium meal, which will demonstrate a malrotation with volvulus or a duodenal web. A contrast enema is a suitable test for low obstructions, such as Hirschsprung disease or meconium ileus.

Metabolic complications

Neonatal bowel obstruction can lead to rapid and serious metabolic derangement. This is especially so if gut ischaemia occurs. Many of these metabolic problems are related to the neonatal period of development. These problems must be corrected before undertaking transport. Surgical correction cannot be contemplated until the baby has been fully resuscitated. The particular metabolic problems related to bowel obstruction are the following:

1 Fluid loss from lack of fluid intake, vomiting and sequestration of fluid in the gut and peritoneal cavity leads to diminished circulating fluid volume and poor tissue perfusion. This contributes to hypothermia and acidosis.

2 Tissue glucose stores in the neonate are low. If oral intake is blocked and metabolism is stressed by bowel obstruction and poor tissue perfusion, glucose stores will be rapidly exhausted and the baby will switch to anaerobic metabolism with consequent hypoglycaemic acidosis. The acidosis has an adverse effect on cardiovascular activity exacerbating the problem. Hypoglycaemia can cause cerebral damage.

3 The sick neonate is particularly sensitive to hypothermia. Inadequate warming during examination, resuscitation and imaging of the neonate compound the problems.

Much of the preparation of the sick neonate for transport is spent in correcting and maintaining body temperature.

4 Respiratory distress is seen in many babies with bowel obstruction owing to abdominal distension. Inhalation of vomitus may produce pneumonitis and atelectasis.

5 Sepsis from gut organisms (due to transmigration of organisms through the ischaemic or perforated gut wall), causes a rapid deterioration in all metabolic factors. Septicaemia with virulent gut organisms may lead to the rapid demise of the neonate.

General treatment

Transport
The neonatal emergency transport service should come to the sick neonate with a bowel obstruction. Sick neonates do not tolerate handling and movement well. Transport is a particularly stressful time and the metabolic problems should be corrected before transfer.

Nasogastric tube
The passage of a nasogastric tube to aspirate gut content relieves respiratory distress from abdominal distension and helps to measure the fluid losses. It is mandatory in all cases of bowel obstruction.

Resuscitation
Fluid replacement
An intravenous line is established while using an overhead heater to prevent heat loss. Rapid resuscitation with 10 mL/kg boluses of Hartmann's solution is given over 15 min for each bolus. The state of hydration of the baby is assessed in terms of peripheral circulation and urine output. Most babies would require 10–30 mL/kg of resuscitation fluid as a preparation before surgery.

Glucose replacement
Blood glucose levels should be monitored during resuscitation and glucose solution should be given as well as Hartmann's solution. Lack of glucose exacerbates acidosis and can cause fitting.

Correction of acidosis
Acid–base measurement is an important part of neonatal resuscitation. Correction of hypothermia, fluid and glucose replacement will help to correct any acidosis. Sodium bicarbonate given intravenously may sometimes be necessary.

Hypothermia

Hypothermia is a major risk to the sick neonate. A neonatal overhead heater with monitoring of the baby's temperature is used during resuscitation with the establishment of intravenous lines. X-ray imaging is another time of risk for hypothermia. Much of the expertise involved in neonatal transport services is directed to preventing hypothermia during transfer to a neonatal surgical centre.

Sepsis

There is a risk of sepsis with neonatal bowel obstruction and intravenous antibiotics are commenced after cultures are taken.

Hirschsprung disease

In 1887, Hirschsprung described two infants who died with gross abdominal distension due to a severely dilated colon containing masses of faeces. Hirschsprung assumed that the disease affected the megacolon. However, the disease was later shown to be in the narrow distal bowel where there is a lack of ganglion cells (the intrinsic nerves of the gut) in the submucosal and myenteric plexus. In addition, thickened abnormal (extrinsic) cholinergic nerve fibres are found in the affected segment. The affected gut is in a constant state of spasm and will not relax. It is a functional obstruction.

Hirschsprung disease occurs in 1:5000 births, and genetically there are different types:
1 A larger group (80%), in which males are affected five times as often as females, and there is a relatively short aganglionic segment, usually involving the sigmoid colon, rectum and anal canal.
2 A smaller group with a long aganglionic segment, equally common in boys and girls, with a higher degree of 'penetrance' and more likely to affect subsequent siblings.
3 Specific genetic abnormalities (e.g. *GDNF-ret* oncogene; endothelin–endothelin B receptor system) are being described in Hirschsprung disease and these genetic markers will become increasingly important in the understanding of the basis of this disease.

The affected segment begins at the anus and extends proximally for a variable distance – in most cases as far as the sigmoid colon – but sometimes as high as the ascending colon. In a few cases, the affected segment extends into the small bowel, and in rare instances, the entire alimentary canal is devoid of ganglia, excluding hope of survival.

The most common presentation is with complete bowel obstruction in the neonatal period. In some cases, the baby may present at a few months of age with chronic constipation and failure to thrive. Paradoxically, these late-presenting cases may have long segment disease.

The three classic signs are (1) delay in the passage of meconium; (i.e. beyond 24 h after birth); (2) vomitus containing bile and (3) abdominal distension.

Clinical features

Abdominal examination will reveal marked gaseous distension. Rectal stimulation with a probe may cause explosive decompression of meconium and faeces through the tight anal sphincters. A nasogastric tube will drain bile-stained fluid.

Investigation

Plain x-rays will show marked gaseous distension of the gut with air-fluid levels. A contrast enema will show constriction of the segment of bowel affected by Hirschsprung disease tapering through a transition zone to a distended megacolon above the functional blockage of the affected segment [Fig. 7.1].

The diagnosis is made by rectal suction biopsy. The biopsy is processed to examine for absence of ganglion cells by standard microscopy and histochemical preparations are made for acetylcholinesterase staining of overgrowth of extrinsic cholinergic submucosal nerve fibres.

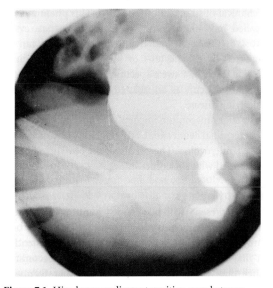

Figure 7.1 Hirschsprung disease transition zone between dilated proximal colon and narrow distal bowel as seen on barium enema.

Acute obstruction develops in the neonatal period, but signs may be delayed for a day or so while the secretions accumulate in the distended stomach and proximal duodenum.

X-rays of the abdomen show a 'double bubble' pattern: two large air bubbles (one in stomach and the other in the dilated proximal duodenum) each with a fluid level and no aeration of the more distal bowel [Fig. 7.4].

A duodenal septum with a hole in the centre may form an incomplete obstruction with episodic vomiting that may be bile-stained. Babies may present this symptom in the neonatal period or at a later age if the obstruction is not so severe. The diagnosis is made on a barium meal study.

Treatment

In atresia of the duodenum, with or without an annular pancreas, the obstruction is repaired by duodeno-duodenostomy. The surgical treatment for duodenal septum is duodenoplasty, but the bile ducts may pose a special problem because they open very close to or actually into the edge of the septum.

Small bowel atresia

Atresia of the bowel beyond the duodenum can occur at any point [Fig. 7.5], most frequently in the distal ileum [Fig. 7.6], but is rare in the colon. There is often only one atresia, although there may be several close together or widely scattered.

The cause may be interruption of the mesenteric arcades by a vascular accident *in utero*, a theory supported by experimental surgery on fetal animals.

The form of the atresia may be a very tight stenosis with no functional orifice, or a thick septum with the bowel in continuity, or a missing segment with a gap of a centimetre or more between the closed ends. The adjacent vascular

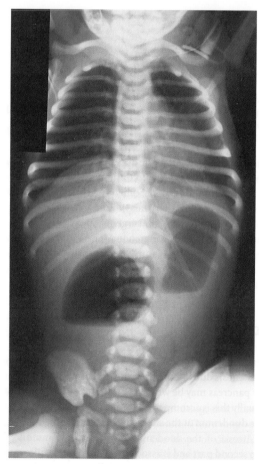

Figure 7.4 Duodenal atresia. Plain x-ray shows a 'double bubble', one in the stomach and the other in the dilated proximal duodenum.

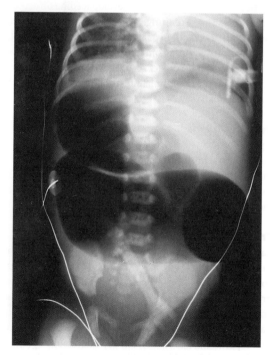

Figure 7.5 Intestinal atresia: plain x-ray showing obstruction of the jejunum. Infant also has *situs inversus*.

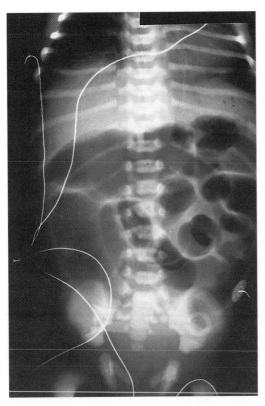

Figure 7.6 Ileal atresia.

arcades are distorted and their terminal branches may be very small or absent. The entire bowel distal to the atresia is collapsed. A barium enema may demonstrate a microcolon.

Duplications of the alimentary tract

These are rare developmental anomalies in which a length of bowel is duplicated in such a way that the two segments share the same blood supply and a common wall, while the mucosal linings are separate. They can arise at any point from the mouth to the anus, and involve any length from 1 to 2 cm to the whole length of the large bowel. A duplication may or may not communicate with the main alimentary channel.

There are two basic types:

1 Short, closed cystic segments. The segment forms a cyst that bulges into the lumen or compresses and angulates the adjoining small bowel, causing obstruction. A small intraluminal cyst may cause obstruction in the neonatal period, but larger ones less intimately connected with the common wall usually cause progressive obstruction later in infancy or in early childhood. Occasionally, a large tense cyst is palpable as a very mobile mass in a child without obstructive symptoms.

2 Long tubular communicating duplications are much less common and more likely to be lined by ectopic (gastric) mucosa, which may cause a peptic ulcer (Chapter 23). If the diagnosis of a duplication containing ectopic gastric mucosa is suspected, it may be demonstrable by means of a technetium 99-m scan. The resection of a long duplication involves the removal of an equivalent length of bowel, and when this is unacceptable because of the inadequate length of bowel remaining, a practical alternative is to remove the lining alone.

Neonatal necrotising enterocolitis

Necrotising enterocolitis is a disease with combined ischaemia and infection of the bowel wall. Although not strictly a 'cause' of intestinal obstruction, it typically presents with abdominal distension and bile-stained vomiting, resembling obstruction. The passage of blood per rectum and a characteristic appearance on abdominal x-ray help to distinguish necrotising enterocolitis from neonatal bowel obstruction. A greater awareness of the entity may have contributed to the increased incidence in recent years, but there has been an absolute increase in the number of cases reported in developed countries.

Predisposing factors

Sick premature neonates can develop necrotising enterocolitis as a further complication of the predisposing factors listed in Table 7.1.

Aetiology

The mechanism has not been elucidated fully. The most widely held theory to explain the intestinal ischaemia is that in a stressed, hypoxic state, blood is preferentially distributed to the heart and brain, at the expense of the splanchnic circulation, skin and muscle.

Local vascular changes have been implicated, for example, a catheter in the umbilical vein, if badly positioned, alters the portal haemodynamics; a catheter in the umbilical artery may have a similar effect on the arterial supply if advanced too far up the aorta, and also has the potential to produce emboli.

Certain bacteria appear to be important; *Klebsiella* species resistant to the commonly used antibiotics are found

Table 7.1 Predisposing factors and observed associations in neonatal necrotising enterocolitis

Prematurity
Respiratory distress:
  Atelectasis
  Hyaline membrane disease
Birth asphyxia
Fetal distress during labour
Prolonged antepartum rupture of membranes
Twins
Caesarean section
Congenital heart disease
Jaundice
Catheterisation of the umbilical vessels
Hyperosmolar feeds
Sepsis

in a significant number of infants who develop necrotising enterocolitis. Other enteropathogens (e.g. *Escherichia coli*, *Clostridium difficile* and *Streptococcus faecalis*) and *Pseudomonas* species also have been isolated.

The type of feed and when it is commenced may have some relevance, for example, the disease appears to occur more frequently in infants who were fed early with artificial milk formulae. Breast milk may afford some protection against the disease in the 'at risk' infant.

Pathology

Necrotising enterocolitis may be generalised and involve most of the small and large intestine or be segmental in distribution. The ileum and colon commonly are affected. There is histological evidence of impaired perfusion, resulting in tissue anoxia and necrosis. The mucosa is affected most, because of a shunting mechanism, but the process may involve the entire thickness of the bowel wall.

When the mucosa is damaged, production of mucus is impaired and the bacteria normally present in the lumen can invade the intestinal wall, further damaging the bowel and entering the bloodstream to produce bacteraemia or septicaemia. The damaged mucosa bleeds into the lumen, and gas collects in the bowel wall [pneumatosis intestinalis] due to the activity of gas-forming organisms or by diffusion of intraluminal gas through breaches in the damaged mucosa.

The consequent pathological course is variable
1 Perforation with general peritonitis;
2 Perforation with local abscess formation;
3 Healing with return of normal function;
4 Healing with stricture formation.

Clinical picture

The typical baby at risk of necrotising enterocolitis is a baby who already has complications from prematurity. The onset of symptoms is between 2 and 14 days after birth. The infant is ill, lethargic, febrile and not interested in feeds. Abdominal distension and bile-stained vomiting occur, and there may be passage of loose stools containing a variable amount of blood.

When complicated by peritonitis, the anterior abdominal wall becomes oedematous and red, with dilated veins, and palpation causes pain. A mass may be palpable if a localised intraperitoneal abscess has formed or if there is a persistently dilated loop of bowel.

Investigations

The radiological findings are typical. Plain films of the abdomen show dilated loops of bowel in which there are intramural bubbles of gas (pneumastosis intestinalis; Fig. 7.7). Gas outlining the portal vein and/or its radicles may be visible. Free gas in the peritoneal cavity, best seen under the diaphragm, is present if the intestine has perforated. Separation of adjacent loops of bowel suggests appreciable amounts of intraperitoneal exudate, an indication of peritonitis, with or without a perforation.

Bacteriological specimens, for example, blood culture and rectal swabs, should be taken before antibiotics are commenced or altered. The nose, throat and umbilicus also are swabbed.

Biochemistry, haematology, electrolytes, acid–base and bilirubin are monitored. The haemoglobin level may fall progressively as a result of sepsis and haemorrhage and serial measurements are required. The platelet and white cell counts are depressed in severe disease. The infants are acidotic.

Management

Initially this consists of stopping oral feeds, decompression of the intestine by suction through a nasogastric tube and parenteral administration of fluids and appropriate antibiotics.

Intensive measures listed in the section on the pre- and postoperative care of the neonate and adequate respiratory management also may be required.

Frequent clinical and radiological reassessment is essential, for it may show the need for surgery.

The indications for operation are
1 Clinical deterioration despite intensive resuscitation.
2 Evidence of bowel necrosis and perforation.

Features that are useful in determining the need for operation include free gas on x-ray, progressive signs of

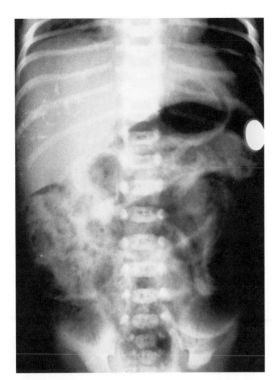

Figure 7.7 Necrotising enterocolitis. Intramural gas.

peritonitis (distended, red and tender abdomen), persistent acidosis despite attempted correction, and a sudden and profound fall in the platelet count.

Operation is confined to the resection of perforated or necrotic bowel and drainage of any intraperitoneal abscesses. The mortality rate until recently was high, but with earlier diagnosis and more effective treatment the outlook is improving.

> ### Key Points
> - Bile-stained vomiting in the neonate is always serious.
> - Abdominal distension, bile-stained vomitus and failure to pass meconium indicates bowed obstruction.
> - Bile-stained vomiting in a normal baby suggests possible malrotation with volvulus, and is an emergency.
> - Neonates with bowel obstruction need special transport to the surgical centre.

Further reading

Applebaum H, Lee SL, Puapong DP (2006) Duodenal atresia and stenosis – annular pancreas. In: Grosfeld JL, O'Neill JA Jr., Fonkalsrud EW, Coran AG (eds) *Pediatric Surgery*, 6th Edn. Mosby Jr., Elsevier, Philadelphia, pp. 1260–1268.

Grosfeld JL (2006) Jejunoileal atresia and stenosis. In: Grosfeld JL, O'Neill JA Jr., Fonkalsrud EW, Coran AG (eds) *Pediatric Surgery*, 6th Edn. Mosby Elsevier, Philadelphia, pp. 1269–1288.

Teitelbaum DH, Coran AG, Martucciello G, Baban A, Jibri N, Jasonni V (2006) Hirschsprung's disease and related neuro-transmusclar disorders of the intestine. In: Grosfeld JL, O'Neill JA Jr., Fonkalsrud EW, Coran AG (eds) *Pediatric Surgery*, 6th Edn. Mosby Elsevier, Philadelphia, pp. 1514–1559.

8 Abdominal Wall Defects

Case 1

Ultrasonography at 18 weeks of gestation showed that the unborn baby had bowel loops within an expanded umbilical cord. Careful scan of the rest of the baby showed no other abnormality, although the mother was warned of the possibility. Amniocentesis and karyotyping failed to show trisomy 13 or 18, and it was elected to continue the pregnancy. A paediatric surgeon was consulted for advice about treatment at birth.

Q 1.1. What is the abnormality?
Q 1.2 Why did it occur?
Q 1.3 What 'first aid' treatment is needed – if transfer is required to the surgical centre?
Q 1.4 What is the management and prognosis?

Case 2

Jody was 17, and did not want her parents to know she was pregnant. She presented in labour with no previous antenatal visits. A vigorous infant was delivered, but the midwife was horrified to see most of the small bowel hanging out through a small hole in the abdominal wall, just to the right of the umbilicus.

Q 2.1 Will the baby live?
Q 2.2 Why is the baby's life at risk?
Q 2.3 Is the baby likely to have multiple congenital anomalies?

Case 3

Frank was born without trouble, at term. Antenatally, there had been some concern about no urine being visible in the bladder on ultrasound. At birth the attachment of the cord was low, and adjacent to an ugly defect with wet, pouting mucosa. The penis was found to be bifid and one testis was undescended.

Q 3.1 What is the embryological defect?
Q 3.2 Can this abnormality be treated?
Q 3.3 Why is the penis split into two halves and what is the likely outcome for sexual function and urinary control?

Exomphalos and gastroschisis

These two developmental abnormalities in the region of the umbilicus are diagnosed on antenatal ultrasonography or present at birth as neonatal emergencies, and require urgent treatment.

Currently, the prevalence of exomphalos (omphalocele) and gastroschisis is relatively similar, although the incidence of gastroschisis is increasing in most regions for reasons that are unclear. The relatively high incidence of coexisting abnormalities in a fetus with exomphalos (35%)

may be a reason for termination, particularly if amniocentesis identifies a major chromosomal abnormality.

First aid at birth

A baby with an anterior abdominal wall defect is at great risk of heat and water loss from evaporation because of the moist exposed viscera. For this reason, the baby should be placed in a humidicrib, with the entire torso wrapped, including the exposed viscera, in fresh plastic 'kitchen wrap' or aluminium foil. Care must be taken to ensure that the exposed bowel is not twisted at the level of the opening in the abdominal wall [Fig. 8.1]. Do not use hot wet packs as these cool too quickly with evaporative heat

Jones' Clinical Paediatric Surgery, 6th edition. By Hutson, O'Brien, Woodward and Beasley. Published 2008 by Blackwell Publishing, ISBN: 978-1-4051-6267-8.

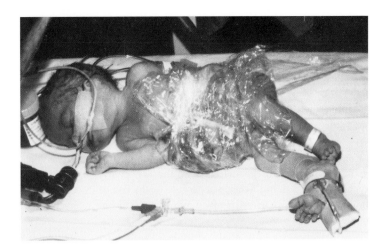

Figure 8.1 First aid management of gastroschisis. The torso is wrapped in plastic 'kitchen wrap' to reduce heat loss from evaporation. A nasogastric tube keeps the bowel decompressed that facilitates operative reduction of the eviscerated bowel. An intravenous line has been inserted.

Table 8.1 Immediate 'first aid' for abdominal wall defect

- Wrap exposed viscera in fresh kitchen wrap (ensure prolapsed bowel is not twisted)
- Careful examination for other anomalies
- Place infant in Humidicrib
- Nil orally
- IV line with 10% dextrose + N/5 saline for exomphalos
- IV Nasogastric tube with aspiration to keep bowel deflated
- If born outside the tertiary paediatric surgical centre:
    Call Neonatal Emergency Transport Service (NETS)
    Call Surgical Registrar at tertiary hospital
- Explain management plan to parents
- Get consent for surgery

---

loss and chill the infant. The main objective is to prevent excessive fluid and heat loss during transfer to the receiving neonatal surgical unit.

Insert a nasogastric tube to keep the bowel empty and do not feed the baby: minimising the gut volume facilitates operative reduction of the herniated bowel.

Commence an intravenous fluid infusion of 10% dextrose + N/5 saline to prevent hypoglycaemia during transport, particularly if the baby has Beckwith–Wiedemann syndrome (organomegaly, exomphalos and hypoglycaemia secondary to excess fetal insulin-like growth factor production).

Transport

The infant with an abdominal wall defect should be referred to a fully equipped paediatric surgical centre without delay. Transport should be arranged through a specialised neonatal transport service, if available. If the diagnosis has been made on antenatal ultrasonography, the delivery should be undertaken in a tertiary obstetric centre with paediatric surgeons standing by [Table 8.1].

Exomphalos

This congenital hernia into the base of the umbilical cord is caused by incomplete folding of the embryonic disc and failure of the umbilical ring to form normally. The hernia is covered by fused amniotic membrane and peritoneum.

Occasionally, the membrane ruptures before birth and the eviscerated bowel becomes matted and indurated with dense adhesions, so that the bowel appears to be shorter than normal. The inflammation is believed to be caused by chemical irritation from faeces and urine in the amniotic fluid. Rupture also may occur during delivery, in which case the bowel appears normal.

The size of the defect in the abdominal wall and the volume of the sac are variable. An intact sac is shiny and translucent but lacks a blood supply and begins to dry out and deteriorate after birth. Within 12 h it becomes opaque and yellowish; later, it becomes black, inelastic and desiccated.

The diagnosis at birth is obvious [Fig. 8.2]; the only difficulty may be in distinguishing a ruptured exomphalos from a gastroschisis. In the latter, there are no sac remnants and the defect is small and separate from the umbilical cord (see below).

Coexisting abnormalities are common in exomphalos, particularly cardiac and renal malformations. Malrotation occurs in 12–20% of cases, but seldom causes volvulus, probably because of adhesions between loops and 'secondary' fixation to the parietes.

Beckwith–Wiedemann syndrome must be recognised early, because of the severe hypoglycaemia that requires immediate correction. These babies produce excess insulin-like growth factor during gestation, which leads to organomegaly, exomphalos and excess bodyweight. A large baby (e.g. 4 kg) with exomphalos and macroglossia is suggestive of the diagnosis. The exomphalos may be secondary to the enlarged viscera, which cannot be accommodated inside the abdomen. Postnatal hypoglycaemia is transient but dangerous because of the risk of brain damage, which may occur if an immediate infusion of glucose is not provided.

Investigations

Chest x-ray and echocardiogram are required to exclude a cardiac lesion and intercurrent pulmonary conditions, such as atelectasis or meconium inhalation. The kidneys can be examined by ultrasonography. Careful physical examination may suggest other serious anomalies, for example, chromosomal aberrations, confirmation of which may modify or even preclude treatment.

Treatment

First aid and the method of transport to the tertiary centre are crucial for optimal outcomes, and are discussed at the end of this chapter. The aim of treatment is to reduce the contents of the exomphalos and repair the defect of the abdominal wall. The method of treatment depends on
1 the general condition of the infant (size, birth weight, maturity, suitability for anaesthesia);
2 presence of other anomalies;
3 whether the sac is intact or ruptured;

4 the size of the umbilical ring;
5 whether part of the liver has herniated into the sac.

Immediate operation and complete repair is the best course when the defect is less than 5 cm in diameter, the infant is fit for surgery, and closure can be obtained.

Excision of the sac (or remnants, if ruptured), and construction of a cylindrical tube (a 'silo') can be used for larger defects. A sheet of silastic or teflon is sewn to the edge of the defect. Alternatively, "Op Site" can be attached to the skin around and over the defect, and is used to serially reduce the volume of the exomphalos over 7–10 days by imbrication, so that the viscera are returned progressively to the abdomen. The prosthesis or Op Site is then removed and the defect repaired surgically. Use of a silo is indicated when the sac has ruptured with massive evisceration, but it is not without problems, such as infection around the sutures that anchor the prosthesis to the edge of the defect.

Rarely, non-operative management may be required when anaesthesia is contra-indicated because of the poor condition of the infant (extreme prematurity, cardiac anomaly, meconium inhalation) or when the defect is extremely large (>8 cm in diameter) and contains herniated liver. The sac is painted with an astringent solution to make it a tough, dry eschar which separates when new skin has covered the area beneath it, after 8–12 weeks. Any substance applied to the exomphalos sac may be absorbed by the baby and care should be taken to use non-toxic substances sparingly. Subsequent wound contraction reduces the hernia progressively over 4–8 months and makes the definitive repair easier. Once the eschar has formed, and normal feeding and stools are established, the infant can be managed safely at home, avoiding prolonged, costly and risky (because of cross-infection) hospitalisation. The appearance of the hernia and eschar may be intimidating to the parents, who need support and encouragement to achieve satisfactory bonding.

Gastroschisis

Recent antenatal ultrasound observations suggest that gastroschisis may result from rupture of a physiological hernia in the cord at 6–10-weeks' gestation. The fetus usually is normal genetically but has had an 'accident' affecting the umbilical cord. The defect in the abdominal wall is small (1–3 cm in diameter) and is nearly always to the right of the umbilicus.

The evisceration may involve most of the small and large bowel, which become densely matted and adherent with

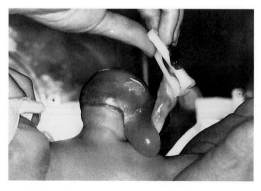

Figure 8.2 Exomphalos.

amniotic (chemical) peritonitis and fibrin from defecation and micturition *in utero* [Fig. 8.3], particularly during the last trimester.

It differs from a ruptured exomphalos in that there is
1 a greater risk of hypothermia;
2 a smaller abdominal wall defect and no covering sac;
3 lower incidence of serious coexisting malformations;
4 a greater (but still small) incidence of a small bowel atresias but these may be 'occult' or hidden by the matted fibrin surface of the exposed bowel.

Treatment

Only two methods are available: (1) immediate operative reduction of the viscera and primary repair; and (2) a prosthetic 'silo' as described earlier, reducing the viscera over 7–10 days, followed by definitive ('secondary') repair. Immediate surgical repair is the method of choice, and where the bowel looks normal and is not thickened or matted, it can be reduced in the neonatal unit without general anaesthesia. In all other cases, success depends on a series of complementary adjuvant steps, and requires expert intensive care and nursing. The method involves the following:
1 correction of any physiological disturbances (temperature, hydration, etc.);
2 anorectal digital dilatation under anaesthesia to decompress the colon;
3 nasogastric suction to minimise bowel gas;
4 enlargement of the defect and intraperitoneal 'milking' of the bowel to evacuate as much meconium as possible through the anus;
5 stretching of the scaphoid anterior abdominal wall to enlarge the capacity of the abdomen;
6 postoperative mechanical ventilation to counteract splinting of the diaphragm caused by high intra-abdominal pressure when the viscera are 'reduced';
7 total parenteral alimentation until effective peristalsis has been restored, sometimes after many weeks;
8 careful examination of the bowel at laparotomy to detect an 'occult' atresia.

High standards of neonatal transport and neonatal surgery lead to a good prognosis for babies born with gastroschisis.

Bladder exstrophy (ectopia vesicae)

Failure of fusion of the lower abdominal wall during embryonic development leaves the bladder exposed as a flat plaque on the lower abdomen [Fig. 8.4]. There is no covering muscle or skin. The pubic rami do not fuse in the midline and remain widely separated. The ureters protrude from the exposed bladder and dribble urine. The urethra is exposed as a flat strip and the bladder outlet sphincters are not functional. Bladder exstrophy, also known as 'ectopia vesicae', is rare, with an incidence of

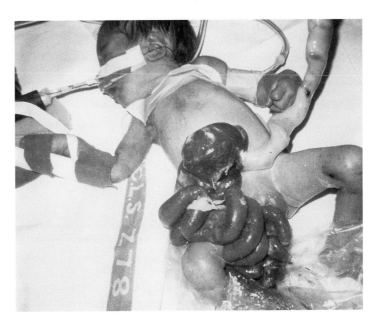

Figure 8.3 Gastroschisis.

1:40,000 births. Reconstructive surgery to close the bladder and abdominal wall with restoration of bladder sphincters is one of the greatest challenges of paediatric urology.

An even rarer variant of bladder exstrophy is known as cloacal exstrophy. In this condition, the shortened proximal colon is fused onto the bladder exstrophy, and there may be an imperforate anus.

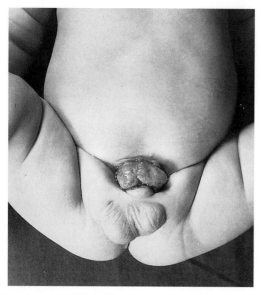

Figure 8.4 Bladder exstrophy.

Key Points

- Defects in the anterior abdominal wall are a neonatal emergency because of risk of heat and water loss, and need immediate first aid.
- Exomphalos is associated with a high risk (35%) of serious anomalies.
- Big babies with exomphalos are at risk of hypoglycaemia, and need immediate IV 10% Dextrose.

Further reading

Brock JW, DeMarco RT, O'Neill JA (2006) Bladder and cloacal exstrophy. In: Grosfeld JL, O'Neill JA Jr., Fonkalsrud EW, Coran AG (eds) *Pediatric Surgery*, 6th Edn. Mosby Elsevier, Philadelphia, pp. 1841–1869.

Bruch SW, Langer JC (2003) Omphalocele and gastroschisis. In: Puri P (ed) *Newborn Surgery*, 2nd Edn. Arnold, London, pp. 605–614.

Tracy TF (1997) Abdominal wall defects. In: Oldham KT, Colombani PM, Foglia RF (eds) *Surgery of Infants and Children: Scientific Principles and Practice*, Lippincott-Raven, Philadelphia, pp. 1083–1093.

9

Spina Bifida

Case 1

Jeannie H was a regular drug-user and shared an apartment with several friends. She became pregnant at 18, avoided antenatal care and presented in labour. The baby had a red, cystic mass over the lumbar spine and no spontaneous leg movement.

Q 1.1 What physical signs are important to note at birth?

Q 1.2 Will the baby have hydrocephalus?

Q 1.3 What is the prognosis for (a) intellect; (b) walking?

Case 2

Antenatal alpha-fetoprotein and midgestation ultrasonography did not reveal any fetal anomaly. At birth, the infant had a small, skin-covered cystic mass over the sacrum. Leg movements were good, but the bladder was palpable.

Q 2.1 What are the urinary tract problems in spina bifida?

Q 2.2 How are urinary and faecal incontinence managed?

Spina bifida is one of the most crippling congenital anomalies. The primary abnormality is incomplete fusion of the neural tube and overlying ectoderm leading to a defect between the vertebral arches. There is protrusion and dysplasia of the spinal cord and its membranes. The resulting nerve deficit may cause paraplegia, urinary and faecal incontinence and multiple orthopaedic deformities. Hydrocephalus is a frequent associated anomaly.

The severity of this anomaly has led to widespread antenatal screening with maternal alpha-fetoprotein levels and ultrasonography in midgestation. In many centres, termination of pregnancy is offered when screening reveals a myelomeningocele. Treatment with high doses of folic acid before conception and during early pregnancy will lower the risk of spina bifida. As a result of these two factors, the incidence in Western countries of live-born infants with spina bifida has decreased dramatically in recent years.

Embryology

Spina bifida and anencephaly are neural tube defects. The fusion of the neural folds should be completed by the fourth week of embryonic development. The mesoderm

around the neural tube forms the meninges, vertebral column and muscles. The less severe anomalies involve failure of vertebral arch fusion and protrusion of the meninges to form a meningocele. More severe anomalies involve the neuro-ectoderm with protrusion of the neural tube itself to form a myelomeningocele. Failure of fusion of the brain causes an encephalocele (see Chapter 12) or anencephaly.

Aetiology and antenatal diagnosis

Spina bifida has been linked to folate metabolism in the maternal diet. There is a earlier history of hydrocephalus, anencephaly or spina bifida in 6–8% of cases: in these, the risk of spina bifida in subsequent pregnancies is 1:20. With two affected children, the risk is 1:8. Prenatal diagnosis in spina bifida is well established. Antenatal ultrasonography may detect the sac and the vertebral defect. The open sac weeps fetal cerebrospinal fluid (CSF) into the amniotic fluid and this can be detected by alpha-fetoprotein estimation of maternal blood or of amniotic fluid obtained by amniocentesis.

Myelomeningocele

This consists of a bifid spine with protrusion and dysplasia of the meninges and spinal cord. The dysplastic spinal

Jones' Clinical Paediatric Surgery, 6th edition. By Hutson, O'Brien, Woodward and Beasley. Published 2008 by Blackwell Publishing, ISBN: 978-1-4051-6267-8.

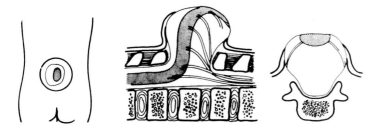

Figure 9.1 Myelomeningocele: tissue of the spinal cord forms part of the wall of the sac, as well as its contents.

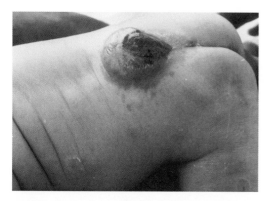

Figure 9.2 Lumbar myelomeningocele: a moderately large sac with well-developed skin at its periphery. The glistening arachnoid membrane and nervous tissue is exposed on the apex of the sac.

cord is splayed over a meningeal sac filled with CSF and is associated with severe nerve deficits below the level of the lesion. This accounts for most of neonates with spina bifida. There is a slight predominance of females. The incidence varies widely from one region to another and there are significant annual variations.

Clinical features

The sac is in the midline, usually in the lumbosacral region [Figs 9.1 and 9.2]. The size of the sac is variable; there is an area of well-developed skin at the periphery but this is thin at the apex, which is covered by the delicate glistening arachnoid membrane with nervous tissue visible on the surface.

The central area becomes ulcerated and infected, and if left untreated there is a risk of meningitis. Epithelialisation occurs slowly, leaving a puckered scar covered with poor quality skin that is liable to ulceration. The coverings may rupture before, during or after birth, with escape of CSF. Rachischisis is the most severe form of spina bifida.

The neural tube lies open, no sac is present, and the spinal cord is a flattened, red, velvet-like ribbon down the centre of back [Fig. 9.3].

Motor loss

There is a flaccid paralysis of the lower motor neurone type, the extent depending on the level of the neurological lesion. In some patients, upper motor neurone spastic paralysis is also present and is due to either isolated normal sections of the cord below the lesion, or to cerebral or spinal cord damage from hydrocephalus or meningitis.

Children can be grouped according to the level of the lesion. The motor loss can be assessed by observing the infant's voluntary (not reflex) movements, and determination of the level is helpful in assessing the probable extent of eventual disability [Table 9.1].

Sensory loss

Sensory loss corresponds closely to the level of motor loss, although the lower level of normal sensation is usually about one segment higher than the lower level of normal motor power. Loss of sensation is most important in the feet, the buttocks and the perineum, because of the risk of pressure sores in these areas.

Meningocele

This is a simple meningeal sac lined by arachnoid membrane and dura, containing CSF and only occasionally nervous tissue [Fig. 9.4]. It is relatively uncommon (6% of cases of spina bifida cystica) and it may be associated with overlying cutaneous lesions including abnormal pigmentation and hair growth.

The sac may be of any size from a small bulge to an enormous protrusion. It may be tense, but more often is soft and fluctuant; some become tense when the baby cries or when pressure is applied to the fontanelle. The skin over the sac is generally intact, although it may ulcerate occasionally.

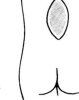 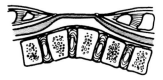 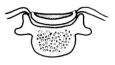

Figure 9.3 Rachischisis: there is no sac and the central canal of the spinal cord lies wide open on the broad deficiency in the posterior vertebral laminae.

Table 9.1 Assessment of level of paralysis

Level of lesion	Incidence (%)	Motor function
Cervical/upper thoracic	1	Paralysis of legs and trunk
Lower thoracic	27	Complete paraplegia, including psoas
Upper lumbar	23	Hip flexion and adduction present
Lower lumbar/upper sacral	45	Hip movements, knee extension, foot dorsiflexion
Lower sacral	4	All normal movement

Hydrocephalus has been reported, but is rare in children with a simple meningocele. The mental state of the child is normal and there are no neurological abnormalities. Deaths are rare and usually are due to meningitis developing before or after operative repair.

Treatment consists of repair of the sac, and when the skin is sound there is no urgency; the repair can be done at any convenient time during infancy. If the sac is ulcerated, it should be repaired immediately after birth, but if this opportunity is missed, epithelium should be allowed to cover the sac, which is then excised at a convenient time later in infancy.

Variants of spina bifida

The vertebrae may be bifid without a meningocele or myelomeningocele sac. This may be a normal variant of spinal arch fusion or represent 'spina bifida occulta', which is more serious. Dysplasia of the skin over the spine is a sign of a potentially serious spina bifida: a hairy patch, pigmented naevus, haemangioma, lipoma or a sinus may be present. A dermal sinus over the spine may link with an intraspinal dermoid cyst. If this becomes infected, an intraspinal abscess may form with destruction of adjacent spinal cord.

A spinal lipoma may be indicated by a bulge over the lumbosacral region. The lower lumbar and sacral nerves run through the fibrolipomatous tissue and progressive nerve damage may occur through spinal cord tethering. These lesions are best demonstrated on magnetic resonance imaging.

Associated anomalies and sequelae of spina bifida

Hydrocephalus

Hydrocephalus is the most important associated anomaly, and is present to some degree in almost all cases of myelomeningocele in early infancy. It needs investigation and treatment in about 70% of the cases . Hydrocephalus is relatively more common when the myelomeningocele is in the lower thoracic and upper lumbar areas, but it may occur with a myelomeningocele at any level. It is an important factor which influences the child's survival and subsequent mental state. The three most common causes of hydrocephalus are the Arnold–Chiari malformation, stricture of the aqueduct of Sylvius and failure of the subarachnoid space to open up at the level of the tentorium.

Orthopaedic deformities

Orthopaedic deformities are common and greatly complicate management of the paraplegia. They include kyphosis, lordosis, scoliosis, paralytic dislocation of the

Figure 9.4 Meningocele: the sac contains CSF only, and the spinal cord is normal.

hips, flexion contractures of the hips and knees, and deformities of the feet. They are caused by inequality of muscular action and bony immobility leading to inadequate growth stimulus to the skeleton.

Urinary tract abnormalities

About 95% of the children with myelomeningocele have a neuropathic bladder. The kidneys are usually normal at birth, but there is a high incidence of progressive renal damage during the first few years of life if the problems of a high pressure, noncompliant bladder, vesicoureteric reflux and chronic pyelonephritis are not treated effectively.

Other anomalies

Many of the other anomalies that are associated with spina bifida are potentially lethal; for example, severe congenital heart disease and visceral malformations.

Complications

Meningitis

Meningitis accounts for approximately one-third of all deaths from spina bifida cystica; it arises either from infection of the ulcerated sac (especially if ruptured) or after surgical repair.

Mental retardation

Mental retardation is related to hydrocephalus, although separate cerebral deficiencies may occur also. Less than 10% of children without clinical hydrocephalus are retarded, and with ventriculoperitoneal shunts, 66% have normal intelligence. Overall, children with myelomeningocele who survive to school age have normal intelligence in approximately 77% of cases; 21% have cerebral damage with disability and 2% have severe cerebral damage.

Pressure sores

These may develop on the feet, sacrum and perineum; in the latter two sites the problem is accentuated by urinary and faecal soiling. Prevention and treatment of pressure sores is of great importance. Full-thickness skin grafts may be helpful to prevent recurrent breakdown for deep, extensive sores in the buttock and sacral area.

Special senses

Paralytic squint (i.e. sixth nerve palsy) is a common complication of hydrocephalus, and optic atrophy with blindness occasionally occuring from raised intracranial pressure, usually in older children. Deafness may also occur, apparently unrelated to the hydrocephalus.

Urinary infection

Stasis in the neurogenic bladder predisposes to urinary tract infection and leads to chronic pyelonephritis which, if untreated, causes progressive renal scarring. Long-term low-dose antibiotics and regular drainage of the bladder by intermittent catheterisation may prevent or limit these problems.

Intermittent catheterisation can be started shortly after birth. The parents pass a 'clean' catheter four to five times a day. In 80% of cases, the child wets a little between catheterisation. In 10%, there is marked wetting and the bladder storage capacity may be increased by using alpha-adrenergic or anticholinergic drugs.

In many children with spina bifida, the neurogenic bladder pattern is that of retention leading to overflow incontinence; the rationale of 'clean intermittent catheterisation' is to empty the bladder frequently, before overflow incontinence occurs. Paradoxically, catheterisation usually lowers the incidence of urinary tract infections by removing stagnant residual urine. Some children in this regimen will also need daily low-dose antibiotics, such as nitrofurantoin or Co-trimoxazole.

As children grow older, wetting becomes less accepta-ble. The main two causes of failure of intermittent cathe-terisation are

1 poor urine storage due to deficiency in the function of the bladder outlet sphincter;

2 a small bladder capacity with a thick-walled, low com-pliance bladder.

When these children reach school age, the bladder storage can be improved by surgery to tighten the blad-der sphincters. The bladder capacity may be increased by endoscopic injection of Botulinus toxin into the detrusor muscle or by the more radical surgery of bladder augmentation using bowel. However, the sur-gery has many complications such as bladder stone, bladder rupture and a small incidence of bladder cancer. Consequently, a patient needs careful counselling prior to surgery and life-long urological follow-up after surgery.

Faecal incontinence

'Accidents' are common during early childhood; normal toilet training should be offered to these children, and the child is taught to evacuate the stool by contraction of the abdominal muscles. Most children are constipated, and the aim is to produce a firm stool that is not soft enough to leak out and not so hard that it will become impacted. This is achieved by diet, laxatives and bulking agents. After adolescence, most patients are clean and regular and evacuate a firm or hard stool. A few patients require a daily suppository or enema. Gross impaction with over-flow is cleared by bowel washouts. The most effective means of achieving this is by performing a laparoscopic appendicostomy that allows regular antegrade irrigation of the colon. This procedure significantly improves the quality of life of these children. Biofeedback techniques are useful for some children.

Psychological and social management

Many children show psychological disturbances as a result of their disabilities, especially in adolescence, although only a few are seriously disturbed. The distur-bances are not directly proportional to the degree of disa-bility or to the level of intellectual functioning; nor are they specific to children with spina bifida. Generally, counselling is sufficient, but some children require addi-tional psychiatric treatment.

Many parents need help to enable them to accept their child's disability. This aspect presents relatively few prob-lems if they have been given a full picture of the condition on antenatal diagnosis or soon after birth if they have been directly involved in treatment, but it can be difficult with parents with earlier psychiatric or marital problems.

Assessment in the newborn

Careful assessment by a specialist team is essential in the neonatal period. A treatment plan should be formu-lated as early as possible and the following points should be noted:

1 The presence of other congenital abnormalities, espe-cially those likely to lead to death in infancy or childhood.

2 The type of spina bifida, that is, myelomeningocele or meningocele.

3 The level, size and state of the sac.

4 The presence of hydrocephalus and the degree of cere-bral dysplasia.

5 The presence of meningitis.

6 The severity of the orthopaedic disability, recorded by charting muscle activity, especially that of the psoas major, quadriceps and the dorsiflexors and plantar flexors of the ankle.

7 The presence of a neurogenic bladder and bowel, as shown by dribbling urine, a patulous anus, perineal anaesthesia and an expressible bladder.

8 The presence of other urinary tract abnormalities, especially of the upper urinary tract; and of urinary tract infection.

9 The dynamics of the family. Special problems exist with families who are unable to cope with the considera-ble strains imposed.

Most of the above points can be evaluated in the neo-natal period, and the predicted disabilities should be fully discussed with the parents as soon as possible.

Treatment

The aim is to produce an ambulant patient, dry and free of the smell of urine and faeces, who is able to function at optimal intellectual and physical level, is educable and capable of employment and independent living. The severity of the disease in some children precludes the attainment of all these objectives. Adverse factors that carry a high mortality or poor potential of life include

1 high-level lesions associated with complete paraplegia (especially if associated with spinal kyphosis);

2 hydrocephalus clinically present at birth;

3 rapidly developing and progressive hydrocephalus after birth;

4 meningitis or ventriculitis;

5 other severe congenital abnormalities;

6 other life-threatening diseases;

7 major renal impairment.

Initial examination and regular supervision in a special clinic are required for accurate assessment and optimal results.

The sac

Early operation reduces the incidence of meningitis and shortens the stay in hospital. It encourages acceptance of the child by the parents, but does not affect the development of hydrocephalus. In some children the prognosis is so poor that repair of the sac in these children may be best deferred until the parents have had sufficient time to understand the nature of the problem and give informed consent.

The guidelines for treatment are as follows.

Treatment at birth

Caesarian section and immediate postnatal repair may preserve neurological function in some babies where antenatal ultrasound demonstrates good leg movement. There is some evidence that trauma during delivery may exacerbate the degree of neurological deficit. Immediate repair of the sac is indicated in low lesions in the absence of the adverse factors listed earlier. Initial deferment of sac repair is appropriate in the presence of any of the adverse factors. If the sac is covered with sound skin there is no urgency to repair it.

Hydrocephalus

The ventriculoperitoneal shunt is required for correction of hydrocephalus (Chapter 12) which commonly develops soon after sac closure.

Orthopaedic treatment

This is directed at preserving motor development, which should be as near normal as the degree of paralysis will allow. The child with extensive paralysis is given a supportive chair at the age of 3 or 4 months; physiotherapists and occupational therapists encourage activities appropriate to the child's age but which otherwise would be delayed by the paralysis. Standing and walking are encouraged as soon as the child is mature enough to cooperate; for the severely paralysed child, this will be at an age later than normal. Children with low lesions walk well without orthoses. Children with high lesions (above L3) generally walk in long orthoses with extensions to the lower trunk and with elbow crutches. They tend to develop fixed flexion deformity of the hips and knees that may require surgical release. Few children fail to achieve walking, but many of those with high lesions will later cease walking because their mobility is greater in a wheelchair than with extensive orthoses and crutches.

The presence of an active quadriceps muscle enables the child to stand by extending the knee joint so long callipers are not required. When the muscles acting on the feet are weak or inactive, plastic ankle-foot orthoses (AFO) are used to stabilise the feet.

In a common situation in which the dorsiflexors of the ankle are strong but the calf is paralysed, transfer of the tibialis anterior tendon posteriorly to the Achilles tendon and calcaneum, will prevent progressive deformity.

No orthopaedic treatment is required for children with low sacral lesions.

Other deformities which may require treatment are kyphosis and scoliosis. Correction and fusion of paralytic spinal deformities in spina bifida require surgery on the vertebral bodies from in front and on the intact vertebral arches from behind. Internal fixation devices are inserted through both approaches.

Schooling and employment

Most children with spina bifida have a need for assistance at school. Difficulties with access, mobility and continence need to be overcome. Some children with shunted hydrocephalus have specific learning problems. There are varying degrees of difficulty with concentration span, attention control, fine motor and perceptual functioning.

Almost all children with spina bifida cystica attend normal school. During the early years in secondary school, vocational guidance is required to direct education and training towards suitable employment. Many professional, commercial, clerical and bench-type jobs are suitable for paraplegic patients.

Prognosis

The antenatal and neonatal mortality for severe spina bifida is high and informed consent for complex and prolonged treatment may not be given.

Deaths after one year of age are usually owing to excessive intracranial pressure after failure of a shunt for hydrocephalus, or to urinary complications. Most patients, even with severe disabilities, reach adult life with varying degrees of independence. All patients require life-long medical support from doctors who understand the nature and implications of their congenital deformities.

Key Points

- Neural tube defects are related to folic acid deficiency in maternal diet.
- Many neural tube defects are identified antenatally (Ultrasonography and alpha-fetoprotein screening).
- Management of spina bifida requires a multidisciplinary team.
- Abnormal skin over the lumbar spine suggests occult spina bifida.

Further reading

Hutson JM, Beasley SW (1988) *Spina Bifida. The Surgical Examination of Children.* Heinemann Medical, Oxford.

Kaefer M (2006) Disorders of bladder function. In: Grosfeld JL, O'Neill JA Jr., Fonkalsrud EW, Coran AG (eds) *Pediatric Surgery*, 6th Edn. Mosby Elsevier, Philadelphia, pp. 1805–1816.

Kaufman BA (2006) Myelomeningocele and hydrocephalus. In: Stringer MD, Oldham KT, Mouriquand PDE (eds) *Pediatric Surgery and Urology: Long Term Outcomes*, 2nd Edn. Cambridge University Press, Cambridge, pp. 958–965.

Smith JL (2006) Management of neural tube defects, hydrocephalus and refactory epilepsy, central nervous system infections. In: Grosfeld JL, O'Neill JA Jr., Fonkalsrud EW, Coran AG (eds) *Pediatric Surgery*, 6th Edn. Mosby Elsevier, Philadelphia, pp. 1987–2017.

10 Disorders of Sexual Development

Case 1

After an uneventful second pregnancy, Mrs H went into labour quickly and was delivered by the midwife. The midwife thought the baby was a boy, but when the obstetrician arrived she said it was probably a girl! Confusion among the labour ward staff was not resolved until a paediatrician confirmed ambiguous genitalia, and arranged transfer to the Children's Hospital. The parents were very upset and distraught.

Q 1.1 What are the criteria for diagnosis of a disorder of sexual development?

Q 1.2 What should the parents be told?

Q 1.3 Is this an emergency?

Q 1.4 How is the gender of rearing decided?

Case 2

On routine genital examination, the intern thought the newborn infant had a hypospadiac phallus and bifid scrotum, containing one testis.

Q 2.1 Can you be sure this baby is a boy?

Q2.2 What criteria discriminate babies with a disorder of sexual development?

No part of a newborn infant's anatomy arouses as much interest initially as the external genitalia. Throughout the pregnancy, the parents have contemplated whether their child will be a boy or a girl. The announcement of the gender of the child triggers a set of socially predetermined and gender-related responses, gifts, congratulations and celebrations, giving the parents pride and pleasure.

It is a crisis, therefore, if the infant's genitalia are abnormal, so that the gender is in doubt [Fig. 10.1]. The urgency of the situation is heightened by the fact that a genital malformation in the newborn may be the outward sign of a potentially life-threatening internal disorder of sexual development (DSD), such as congenital adrenal hyperplasia (CAH).

The responsibilities of the attending doctor are to minimise the distress of the parents and family, and to arrange for the immediate diagnosis and treatment of the underlying medical disorder which may accompany genital ambiguity.

Jones' Clinical Paediatric Surgery, 6th edition. By Hutson, O'Brien, Woodward and Beasley. Published 2008 by Blackwell Publishing, ISBN: 978-1-4051-6267-8.

Definition

Genitalia are described as ambiguous when the phallus is larger than a normal clitoris and too small for a penis; the urethral opening is near the labioscrotal (genital) folds but there is no normal female introitus; the genital folds remain unfused, with an appearance in-between labia and cleft scrotum, and the testes may be undescended or impalpable [Fig. 10.1].

The clinical problems

In a newborn baby with ambiguous genitalia, the parents should be told as soon as possible that sexual development is incomplete, that the gender cannot be assigned immediately, and that consultation with the appropriate specialist will be arranged at once. It will be the specialist's role to outline the steps required to obtain the necessary information to determine the cause of the DSD and the sex of rearing.

The investigations of this complex problem are best carried out in the regional referral centre. Two specific types of DSD are the principal source of ambiguity in the newborn: severe hypospadias with a bifid scrotum and/or undescended testes, and congenital adrenal hyperplasia.

Severe hypospadias with undescended testes

'Hypospadias with undescended testis' should be treated initially as a DSD at birth, if either the 'scrotum' is bifid or one or both testes are impalpable. Only a fused scrotum containing two descended testes confirms normal androgenic function, allowing a hypospadiac phallus to be treated as a local anatomical anomaly of penile development in a boy. Once a DSD has been excluded, males with hypospadias and cryptorchidism can be treated by urethroplasty and orchidopexy at 6–12 months.

Congenital adrenal hyperplasia

This life-threatening condition occurs in 1:8000 live births and is the most important condition to be excluded in the management of a DSD causing ambiguous genitalia.

When CAH occurs in females, the appearance of the external genitalia may make the gender difficult to determine [Fig. 10.2]. The ambiguous appearance results from an autosomal recessive defect causing a deficiency of adrenocortical enzymes, especially 21-hydroxylase. This enzyme is necessary for the biosynthesis of both cortisol and aldosterone. Cortisol levels are low, and this allows a marked increase in the secretion of pituitary adrenocorticotrophic hormone (ACTH), resulting in adrenal hyperplasia. Only androgens are produced, and in a female, these cause virilisation. Low aldosterone levels allow excessive sodium loss in the urine.

The degree of virilisation is often mild [Fig. 10.3]. If the clitoral enlargement is only minor, the diagnosis may be overlooked – a potentially dangerous situation if the associated biochemical defect produces a 'salt-losing' situation, with sudden vomiting and collapse a few weeks after birth.

Investigations

1 The serum electrolytes and blood glucose should be obtained with utmost urgency – within the hour. They

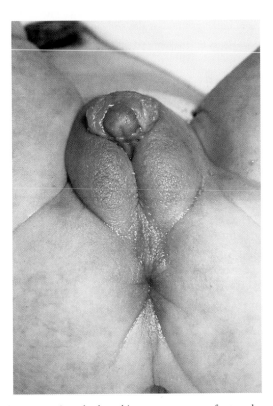

Figure 10.1 Completely ambiguous appearance of external genitalia. Is it a boy or a girl?

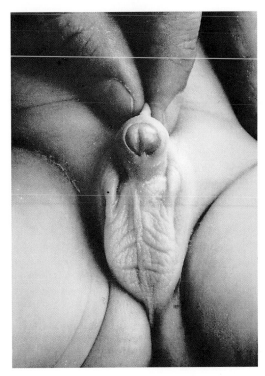

Figure 10.2 Apparent hypospadias and impalpable testes (actually a female with CAH). (Reproduced with permission from Scheffer IE, Hutson JM, Warne GL, Ennis G [1988] *Pediatr Surg Int* **3**: 165–168.)

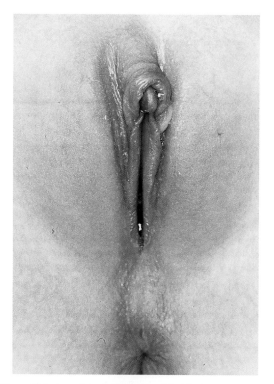

Figure 10.3 An enlarged clitoris in a girl with CAH.

are likely to reveal low sodium, high potassium and hypoglycaemia.

2 Serum 17 hydroxy-progesterone is estimated and the result is obtained in 12–24 h. This metabolite is high in all except rare forms of CAH.

3 Chromosomal analysis is arranged but the result may take between 3 days and 3 weeks.

4 A 24 h urine specimen is collected for estimation of pregnanetriol and to obtain a gas–liquid chromatography steroid profile. The result is obtainable in 5 days.

5 A urogenital sinugram (where x-ray contrast medium is instilled into the external opening) shows a masculinised urethra but the presence of a vagina and cervix.

6 A pelvic ultrasound confirms the presence of a uterus and Fallopian tubes.

Treatment

1 Intravenous rehydration, initially with normal (0.9%) saline.

2 Hypoglycaemia is monitored and corrected with intravenous glucose–saline solution.

3 Cortisone acetate or hydrocortisone are given as soon as blood and urine have been collected for examination.

The anatomy should be established as soon as the biochemical status is stabilised, but is less urgent. The anatomical information confirms the diagnosis, but it is also required to enable planning of the subsequent surgical correction that involves clitoroplasty and vaginoplasty. It is important to realise, and to inform the parents, that females with CAH have normal reproductive potential.

Other disorders of sexual development

Table 10.1 provides examples of the range of disorders of sexual development, but detailed discussion of this complex subject is beyond the scope of this chapter. Instead, the background is summarised in the following sections.

Internal genitalia

Gonadal differentiation is determined by the karyotype with the Y chromosome being essential for testicular development. Other internal organs develop as persistent parts of the paired embryonic ducts, the Wolffian (mesonephric) and Mullerian (paramesonephric) ducts that are present initially in both males and females.

The testes *in utero* secrete three hormones: testosterone, Mullerian inhibitory substance (MIS; also known as anti-Mullerian hormone) and Insulin-like hormone 3 (Insl3). MIS is a protein that promotes regression of the Mullerian ducts. Absence of the Mullerian structures (uterus, fallopian tubes and upper vagina) is evidence that MIS must have been secreted and that a testis must be present. Insl3 stimulates growth of the gubernaculum (or genitoinguinal ligament) during the first phase of testicular descent.

Development of Wolffian ducts requires local stimulation by testosterone, without which the Wolffian ducts atrophy, with failure of development of their derivatives: the epididymis, vas deferens and seminal vesicle.

Chromosomal regulation of sexual differentiation

The X, Y and autosomal chromosomes are responsible for sexual differentiation: the Y chromosome triggers development of the testis via the SRY gene, although the other genes involved remain unknown.

Normal development of the ovaries requires two X chromosomes, and the gene encoding for androgen receptors is also located on the X chromosome. The enzymes required for the synthesis of testosterone are regulated

Table 10.1 Examples of disorders of sexual development

Sex chromosome DSD	46XY DSD	46XX DSD	Others
45X0 (Turner Syndrome)	Androgen insensitivity syndromes	Congenital adrenal hyperplasia	Cloacal exstrophy
47XXY (Klinefelter Syndrome)	Persistent Mullerian duct syndrome		Vaginal atresia
45X/46XY (Mixed gonadal dysgenesis	5 alpha-reductase deficiency Complete gonadal dysgenesis (Swyer syndrome)		Ovopesticular DSD

by autosomal genes, as is the enzyme 5 alpha-reductase. Testosterone and dihydrotestosterone are responsible for masculinising the external genitalia and controlling the inguinoscrotal phase of testicular descent.

Practical decisions in management

Three aspects are important in the management of infants with a DSD causing ambiguous genitalia

1 the specific diagnosis;

2 the sex of rearing;

3 the explanation and counselling given to the parents.

Referral to a regional centre with expertise in managing DSD's is advisable to ensure optimal anatomical and functional outcomes.

Diagnosis

To reach a specific diagnosis, the advice of a paediatric endocrinologist, and detailed biochemical and anatomical investigation, are required because

1 there may be genetic implications affecting counselling;

2 the potential fertility of the infant should be established;

3 urgent medical treatment may be required, as in CAH;

4 a plan for surgical management is necessary.

However, in many children no specific diagnosis is possible.

Sex of rearing

The sex of rearing is determined by (1) the underlying diagnosis (e.g. CAH patients are normally raised as girls, despite virilisation); (2) the size of the male versus female genitalia (e.g. a child with a microphallus and large vagina may be better raised as a girl, despite XY chromosomes). Correct determination of the appropriate sex of rearing

maximises the patient's prospects of fertility and minimises the risk of psychological damage.

Fertility in the male depends upon testes capable of spermatogenesis, a patent pathway and a penis with sufficient erectile tissue for erection and insemination. A good-sized phallus is rarely present in male infants with a DSD causing ambiguous genitalia, and fertility is usually impossible. However, with assistance of reproductive technology (sperm aspiration from epididymis and injection into ova) fertility may be possible in some cases.

In the female, ovulation and a pathway to the uterus are required, but developments in *in vitro* fertilisation, using donor gametes and transplantation of an embryo, now permit pregnancy in a female with a uterus and vagina but no ovaries or Fallopian tubes. There are opportunities, therefore, for active participation in the reproductive process in those raised as females, provided a uterus is present.

Psychological damage is common in both sexes. In a patient raised unsuccessfully as a male, embarrassment due to a microphallus, inability to void standing and a phallus inadequate for intercourse, all create major problems.

Counselling parents

Parents should be told frankly, when the gender is unclear, that tests will be carried out urgently, and how long it will take to fully understand the child's pathology.

The gender is the sex of rearing, and once decided, should be reinforced at every opportunity by referring to the infant as 'he' or 'she', and never 'it'. It is important to reassure parents that genital ambiguity and malformations do not lead to homosexuality, a fear many parents experience, but few express. It is helpful to explain to parents that the genitalia go through an undifferentiated stage in both sexes and that differentiation is extremely complex and not always complete at birth.

> **Key Points**
> - Disorders of sexual development (DSDs) require urgent assessment at birth and often need referral to a regional centre.
> - In babies with 'hypospadias' and undescended testes +/or bifid scrotum, full investigation for DSD is required.

Reference and further reading

Donahoe PK, Schnitzer JJ, Pieretti R (2006) Ambiguous genitalia. In: Grosfeld JL, O'Neill JA Jr., Fonkalsrud EW, Coran AG (eds) *Pediatric Surgery*, 6th Edn. Mosby Elsevier, Philadelphia, pp. 1911–1934.

Grumbach MM, Conte FA (1992) Disorders of sexual differentiation. In: Wilson JD, Foster DW (eds) *Williams Textbook of Endocrinology*, 8th Edn. WB Saunders, Philadelphia, p. 853.

Houk CP, Hughes IA, Ahmed F, Lee PA (2006) Summary of consensus statement on intersex disorders and their management. *Pediatrics* **118**(2): 753–757.

Hutson JM (1995) Endocrine-related urological surgery. In: Brook CGD (ed) *Clinical Paediatric Endocrinology*, 3rd Edn. Blackwell Science, Oxford, pp. 371–382.

Hutson JM, Beasley SW (1988) Ambiguous genitalia: Is it a boy or girl? In: *The Surgical Examination of Children*, Heinemann Medical, Oxford, pp. 257–266.

Scheffer IE Hutson JM, Warne GL, Ennis G (1988) Extreme virilisation in patients with congenital adrenal hyperplasia fails to induce descent of the ovary. *Pediatr Surg Int* **3**: 165–168.

Warne GL, Hughes IA (1995) The clinical management of ambiguous genitalia. In: Brook CGD (ed) *Clinical Paediatric Endocrinology*, 3rd Edn. Blackwell Science, Oxford, pp. 53–68.

11　Anorectal Anomalies

Case 1

A baby boy is delivered in a country hospital. He is found to have an absent anal opening and has passed meconium per urethra.

Q 1.1 How would you arrange referral and transport?

Q 1.2 What will you tell the parents about the management of imperforate anus in the first few weeks of life?

Q 1.3 What is the long-term outlook for the baby?

Case 2

A child with imperforate anus has had an anorectal reconstruction, but at the age of 5 years he is soiling frequently and is about to start school.

Q 2.1 Which method of imaging would give the best visualisation of the relationship of the bowel to the anorectal sphincters?

Q 2.2 If no fault is found with the reconstructive surgery how is this problem managed?

Anorectal malformations are becoming less common. Although imperforate anus is the name given to this condition, in many cases there is a fistulous opening into the urinary tract in the male or the genital tract in the female. There are many different subtypes of anorectal anomalies and these anomalies are also associated with other syndromes such as the VATER association (Vertebral; Anal; Tracheo-oEsophageal; Radial/Renal). Surgical correction of these anomalies is difficult as the rectum and anus have lost their relationship to the sphincter muscles and these muscles may be abnormal in their development and nerve supply.

Classification

There are a number of variations seen in the anatomy of the perineum in infants with anorectal malformations [Table 11.1 and Fig. 11.1]. The key difference between the different types of anomaly lies in the relationship of the terminal bowel to the pelvic floor muscles and the levator ani muscle in particular. In addition, anorectal anomalies are divided into those with or without a fistula to the uro-

Jones' Clinical Paediatric Surgery, 6th edition. By Hutson, O'Brien, Woodward and Beasley. Published 2008 by Blackwell Publishing, ISBN: 978-1-4051-6267-8.

genital tract or the skin. More severe anomalies have arrested development of the bowel above the pelvic floor muscles; these are relatively difficult to treat and the long-term prognosis for normal continence is not good. In lesions where the developing bowel passes down through the pelvic floor muscles and anal sphincters the surgical correction is relatively easy and the long-term prognosis is better, but not always for normal continence. Lesions where the bowel passes down into the levator ani muscle but does not reach the anal canal sphincters have an intermediate prognosis.

Associated anomalies

The mortality and morbidity of imperforate anus is influenced as much by the associated anomalies as the anorectal lesion itself. About 60% of infants with an anorectal malformation have a second abnormality. The commonest of these are genitourinary (30%), vertebral (30%), alimentary (10%) or in the central nervous system (20%). In the alimentary tract, oesophageal atresia and duodenal atresia may be seen. Cardiac and major chromosomal abnormalities may be life threatening. A wide range of urinary tract abnormalities, including neuropathic bladder, vesico-ureteric reflux, duplication of the ureter and ureterocele are common with imperforate anus and may increase the long-term morbidity. The

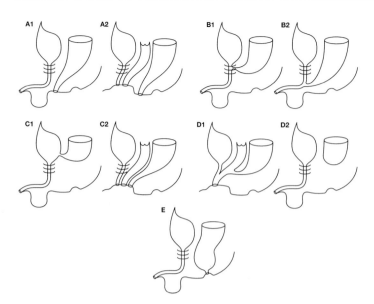

Figure 11.1 A schema of the more common varieties of anorectal malformations. (A1) Male perineal fistula (A2) Female perineal fistula (B1) Rectoprostatic fistula (B2) Rectobulbar fistula (C1) Rectovesical fistula (C2) Rectovestibular fistula (D1) Cloacal anomaly (D2) No fistula (E) Anal stenosis.

Table 11.1 International classification

Major clinical groups	Perineal (cutaneous) fistula
	Recto-urethral fistula
	Bulbar
	Prostatic
	Rectovesical fistula
	Vestibular fistula
	Cloaca
	No fistula
	Anal stenosis
Rare/Regional regional variants	Pouch colon
	Rectal atresia/stenosis
	Rectovaginal fistula
	H-type fistula
Others	

Source: Holschneider and Hutson (2006).

vertebral anomalies may be associated with deficiency of the spinal cord and pelvic nerves which contributes to the anorectal sphincteric dysfunction.

Incidence

Anorectal malformations occur in 1:3000 to 1:5000 births with a slight preponderance in males. Males have high lesions more frequently whereas females tend to have less severe lesions. Most cases of imperforate anus are sporadic and the risk of this problem occurring in a future pregnancy is very small. There are, however, occasional families with a high incidence of anorectal anomalies, which follow an autosomal dominant inheritance pattern.

Clinical features

The newborn baby with a supralevator lesion has no visible anus [Fig. 11.2]. In females, the bowel opening into the genital tract is usually wide enough to decompress the bowel adequately. In males, a fistula to the urinary tract may lead to the appearance of meconium in the urine, an important diagnostic observation [Table 11.2], but this fistula is too narrow, and the infant develops features of a distal bowel obstruction. A fistula opening on the perineal skin is easily visible when it is filled with meconium, but can be very minute and requires a careful search with good illumination [Fig. 11.3].

In females, a detailed search of each perineal orifice is essential, and the internal anatomy can be predicted when the site of the external opening has been located. For example, faeces may be described as coming from the vagina, yet rectovaginal fistulas are relatively uncommon, and a more careful examination will usually reveal a small orifice tucked into the vestibule just outside the vaginal orifice (a rectovestibular fistula) [Fig. 11.4].

The most severe anomaly seen in the female is the cloaca, where there is only one opening in the perineum: the urethra, vagina and bowel all open into the vault of this

Table 11.2 Clinical evaluation of anorectal anomalies

MALE

- A fistula opening on to the skin of the perineum or penis indicates a low lesion. [Fig. 11.3].
- Meconium in the urine indicates a high lesion with a fistula to the urinary tract (urethra or bladder).
- If there is no perineal skin fistula, imaging is required to diagnose the level where the bowel stops and confirm whether there is a fistula to the urinary tract.

FEMALE

- 3 openings on to the perineum indicate low lesion.
- 2 openings on to perineum (urethra and vagina) with no visible fistula indicate high lesion – the rectum opens directly into the vestibule or vagina.
- 1 opening on to the perineum (cloaca) indicates a severe complex cloacal anomaly.

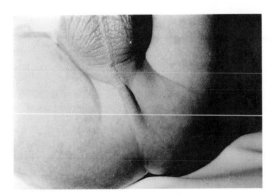

Figure 11.2 The featureless perineum of a male baby with a rectourethral fistula.

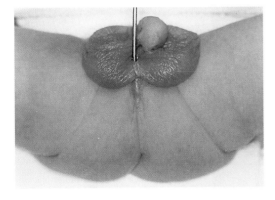

Figure 11.3 A perineal (cutaneous) fistula in a male, with a probe in the fistula in the scrotal raphe.

common cloacal channel. This is the most difficult of all the anorectal malformations to treat.

A careful and complete physical examination of all babies with imperforate anus must be conducted to detect any associated spinal, gastrointestinal and cardiac anomalies. This includes the passage of a stiff nasogastric tube to exclude oesophageal atresia (see Chapter 6). Chromosomal abnormalities such as Down syndrome may also occur.

Imaging

The newborn baby with an anorectal anomaly will need extensive imaging to determine the relationship of the rectum and anus to the anorectal sphincter muscles and also to demonstrate associated anomalies in the spine, urinary tract, cardiovascular and gastrointestinal systems.

1 X-rays of the spine and chest will demonstrate any associated 'VATER' anomalies. Sacral agenesis is of particular importance as loss of the pelvic nerves leaves a poor outlook for continence.

2 The lateral decubitus x-ray uses bowel gas as contrast to measure the position of the terminal bowel against the bony landmarks, to determine its relation to the sphincter muscles [Fig 11.5].

3 Magnetic resonance imaging provides the best evaluation of the state of the sphincter muscles and their relationship with the rectum and anus.

4 Ultrasonography in the first few weeks of life will reveal if there is any deficiency or tethering of the lower spinal cord, and will detect any structural abnormalities of the urinary tract. An echocardiograph is also performed.

5 A micturating cystourethrogram [Fig. 11.6] will show any fistula into the urinary tract (e.g. rectourethral fistula) and demonstrate other associated urinary tract problems (e.g. vesico-ureteric reflux).

Treatment and prognosis

Certain generalisations can be made
- The identification of a fistulous opening in the perineum indicates that there is a low anomaly and the prognosis is good.
- In males, meconium in the urine, indicates a high lesion and will often need a preliminary colostomy.

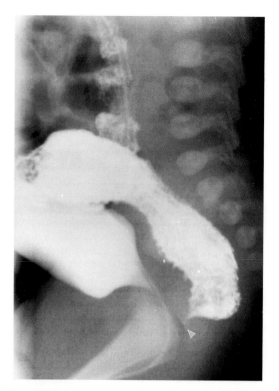

Figure 11.6 A micturating cystourethrogram showing contrast in a rectourethral fistula outlining the distal colon as well as the bladder.

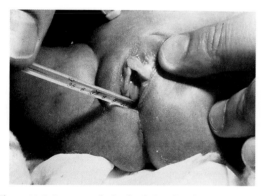

Figure 11.4 A rectovestibular fistula in a female with the thermometer passing cranially up the fistula behind the vagina.

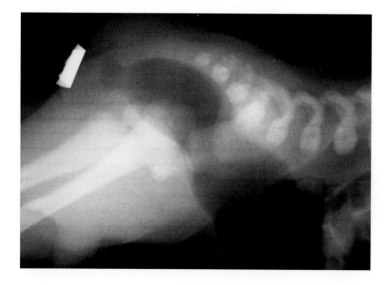

Figure 11.5 Prone, cross-table lateral radiograph in a baby with ano fistula, but an imperforate anal membrane, with gas-filled bowel extending nearly to the marker on the skin.

- In females, a fistula should be expected and a thorough search made for it. In those without a fistula, a colostomy is required. In most of those with an identifiable fistula, immediate local surgery is simple and the prognosis is good.
- An expressible bladder with perineal anaesthesia and sacral agenesis indicates major nerve disruption to the bladder and anorectal sphincters. The prognosis for normal continence is poor.

Low lesions with a perineal fistula

The long-term outlook for continence is good, apart from occasional smearing, staining of underwear, and a tendency to constipation with faecal accumulation.

An anocutaneous fistula in either sex, or anovestibular and anovulvar fistulas in females, require a perineal operation to repair the anus. Imperforate anal membrane and anal stenosis require simple incision and dilatation.

High lesions (usually without a perineal fistula)

In most cases, a colostomy is performed at birth. At the age of 3–4 months, definitive surgery is undertaken. This is done using a midline perineal approach or laparoscopically. A muscle stimulator is used to identify the anal sphincter and pelvic floor muscles forming the levator ani sling. The terminal bowel is identified and any rectourinary fistula is closed. The bowel is brought down through the sphincters to the normal site of the anus. This 'pull through' operation provides the best anatomical reconstruction of the anorectal anomaly, yet despite this accurate reconstruction, the results for normal faecal continence are still not good. Although the anorectal sphincter complexes are present in more severe anomalies, the muscles are often poorly developed or the nerve supply is deficient. Recurrent faecal impaction, major soiling or less severe, but distressing, minor soiling are still common problems. A carefully controlled diet to avoid diarrhoea along with a programme of enemas or home bowel washouts can give quite good 'assisted continence' in well-organised families. An occasional child needs antegrade colonic irrigation via an appendicostomy (Malone operation).

Imperforate anus is a difficult condition to diagnose and treat. Associated anomalies such as the VATER association can cause as much morbidity as the anorectal anomaly. Lesions with a perineal fistula do reasonably well with minimal surgery, but high lesions require extensive reconstructive surgery and the results for continence in these depend as much on the long-term support and care of the family with bowel management as on the skill of the surgeon.

> **Key Points**
> - Babies with anorectal malformations need careful investigation for other anomalies.
> - At birth, immediate transfer to a neonatal surgical centre is optimal.
> - Surgical management and prognosis depend on the type of anomaly and whether or not a fistula joins the colon to the skin or urogenital tracts.

References and further reading

Davies MRQ (1997) Anatomy of the nerve supply of the rectum, bladder, and internal genitalia in anorectal dysgenesis in the male. *J Pediatr Surg* **32**: 536–541.

Holschneider AM, Hutson JM (eds) (2006) *Anorectal Malformations in Children. Embryology, Diagnosis, Surgical Treatment, Follow-Up.* Springer, Berlin Heidelberg New York.

Head and Neck

12   The Scalp, Skull and Brain

Case 1

A 3-month-old, ex-prem infant presents with a big head.
Q 1.1 When should you be concerned about enlargement of an infant's head?

Case 2

A 4-year-old boy presents with early morning headaches, vomiting and ataxia.
Q 2.1 When does a child with headaches need investigation?
Q 2.2 Can we be optimistic about the outcome of children with brain tumours?

Case 3

A 7-year-old girl with a V-P shunt is complaining of vomiting and drowsiness.
Q 3.1 Does the absence of ventricular dilatation on CT or MRI scan exclude shunt dysfunction?

Case 4

You are called to the postnatal ward to see a baby, just born, with a lump at the glabella.
Q 4.1 What do you say to the parents of a newborn child with an encephalocele?

Case 5

A 4-month-old infant has a flattened occiput on one side.
Q 5.1 What could the diagnosis be, and what treatment is required?

The infant with a large head

Measurement of head circumference is an essential component of the routine examination of the young child. The growth curve of head circumference must be interpreted along with the weight and height curves. This is done using standard percentile charts. When suspicion arises that an infant's head is enlarging too rapidly, measurements must be repeated over a period of weeks or months, and compared with the normal curve for this dimension. Deviations from normal [Fig. 12.1] are grouped as follows:
1 A steadily increasing divergence from the normal curve, commencing at birth.
2 A normal curve interrupted by some event, for example a subdural haemorrhage or an infection, with subsequent increase greater than normal.

3 An accelerated rate of growth initially, followed by less rapid growth which continues at a high level but parallel to the normal curve.
4 The head circumference commences at a high level and remains high but grows at the appropriate rate.

The first two groups need treatment, but in the third, unless the accelerated growth in the initial period is very great, operation may be deferred, and surgery is not usually required for the fourth.

An enlarging head may be the result of factors other than the accumulation of CSF, although these are uncommon. The infant's head may enlarge because of thickening of the skull bones, as in diffuse fibrous dysplasia, and be readily recognisable in x-rays. The brain itself may be large, without any increase in the size of the ventricles. Intelligence in these children is often subnormal. One cerebral hemisphere may be larger (hemimegalencephaly) and is associated with cortical dysplasia, developmental delay, epilepsy and hemihypertrophy of the body. Localised expanding lesions, for example, subdural haematoma, simple intracerebral or arachnoid cysts or, very occasionally, a cystic neoplasm, may also cause enlargement of the head.

Jones' Clinical Paediatric Surgery, 6th edition. By Hutson, O'Brien, Woodward and Beasley. Published 2008 by Blackwell Publishing, ISBN: 978-1-4051-6267-8.

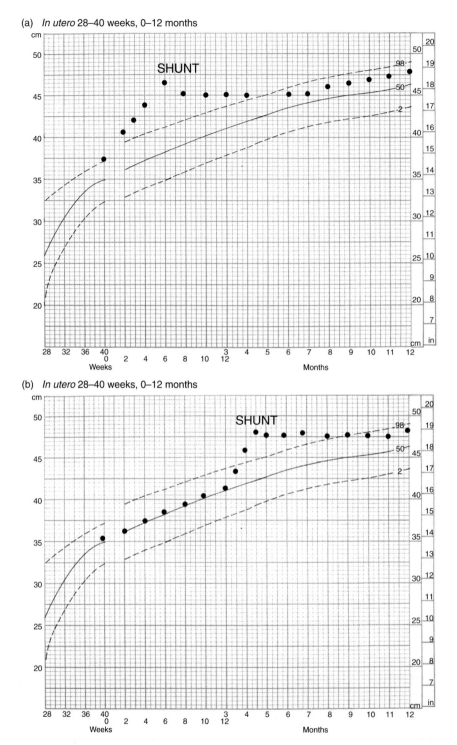

(a) *In utero* 28–40 weeks, 0–12 months

SHUNT

Weeks
Months

(b) *In utero* 28–40 weeks, 0–12 months

SHUNT

Weeks
Months

Figure 12.1 Variations in the growth curve of the infant head, showing the mean, 98th and 2nd percentiles. The additional curves represent (a) hydrocephalus present from birth; (b) acquired hydrocephalus after meningitis at 3 months. In each case, insertion of a shunt is followed by a return towards normal.

Benign enlargement of the subarachnoid space is a cause of macrocephaly. It is due to widening of the subarachnoid spaces and must be distinguished from chronic subdural haematoma. It is more common in male infants with a family history of macrocephaly. The head will usually grow at an accelerated rate within the first year of life but settles to grow at a normal rate although at or above the 98th percentile. The fontanelle may be full in these children. No treatment is required unless the plateau of growth rate is not reached.

Hydrocephalus

Most infants with a large head suffer from excess CSF caused by (1) excessive production; (2) obstruction along the CSF pathway or (3) impaired absorption into the veins.

Increased production of CSF causing hydrocephalus is rare and is caused by papilloma, hypertophy or carcinoma of the choroid plexus.

Obstruction to the flow of CSF is the commonest cause of hydrocephalus, and is further subdivided as follows:

1 *Non-communicating or obstructive hydrocephalus* in which there is no communication between the ventricles and the subarachnoid space. The ventricles are greatly enlarged without distension of the basal cisterns or cerebral sulci [Fig. 12.2].

The most frequent causes of obstruction are

a Primary developmental anomalies such as aqueduct stenosis or a congenital cyst; for example, suprasellar arachnoid cyst, or posterior fossa cyst with hypoplasia of the vermis (Dandy-Walker syndrome).

b Haemorrhage or infection. Intracerebral and intraventricular haemorrhage in premature babies is common.

c Tumours may obstruct the ventricular system in the older child, but only 5% of cases of hydrocephalus in infancy are caused by a neoplasm.

2 *Communicating hydrocephalus* in which the ventricles communicate with the basal cisterns, but there is an obstruction in the subarachnoid spaces or in the arachnoid villi/sagittal sinus.

Failure of absorption of the CSF may occur temporarily, as a result of inflammatory exudate around the basal cisterns and arachnoidal villi following meningitis, or as a result of haemorrhage in the subarachnoid space. Permanent and severe derangement follows thrombosis of the sagittal or lateral sinuses in the newborn as a result of dehydration; the result is a sudden enlargement of the head. Inadequate absorption of CSF also may occur rarely when the intracranial venous pressure is raised, for example an arteriovenous malformation involving the venous sinuses.

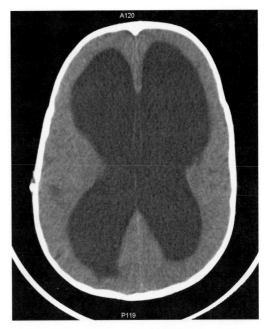

Figure 12.2 Non-communicating hydrocephalus. CT scans showing massive dilatation of the ventricles.

The history, physical signs, a chart of the rate of head growth [Fig. 12.1] and special investigations such as ultrasound, CT or MR are all considered to determine a cause [Table 12.1], plan the treatment and estimate the prognosis of the child with a large head.

Clinical signs

A head circumference which is increasing faster than the normal increments for the age of the infant is the main clinical feature and the indication for investigation and treatment. The deviation is depicted by plotting the measurements of the circumference obtained at regular intervals on a graph of the normal curve [Fig. 12.1]. Auscultation for a bruit is a useful clinical sign for an underlying vascular malformation.

The shape of the head becomes abnormal. The frontal region is prominent in all types, but in stricture of the aqueduct, expansion of the lateral ventricles produces an 'occipital overhang' above the small posterior fossa as well. The opposite occurs when the fourth ventricle is expanded as a result of occlusion of its foramina; the external occipital protuberance is pushed upwards. Raised intracranial pressure produces a wide anterior fontanelle, palpable separation of the cranial sutures, and a raised or drum-like note on percussion of the skull.

Table 12.1 Causes of childhood hydrocephalus

(i) Communicating hydrocephalus
    Increased production
        Choriod plexus papilloma
    Decreased absorption
        Haemorrhage
        Infection
        Venous hypertension
           Sinus thrombosis
(ii) Non-communicating hydrocephalus
    Congenital
        Stenosis of the Aqueduct of Sylvius
        Dandy-Walker malformation
        Suprasellar arachnoid cysts
    Acquired
        Tumours
        Cysts
        Haemorrhage

Abnormal neurological signs from hydrocephalus alone are unusual. The sixth cranial nerve is vulnerable because of its long course and, a lateral rectus palsy causing internal strabismus may occur. Persistent downward deviation of the eyes ('setting sun' sign) is present with advanced hydrocephalus causing pressure on the quadrigeminal plate. There may be brainstem signs when the obstruction is acute and hydrocephalus develops rapidly, with increased extensor tone, rigidly extended lower limbs and clenched hands with the fingers over the infolded thumb. False localising signs may be present, that is, a fourth or sixth cranial nerve palsy. Retraction of the head and opisthotonus also may be present.

Transillumination of an infant's head by a beam of bright light in a darkened room often will show characteristic patterns. General transillumination indicates a gross and uniform dilatation of the ventricles. Unilateral translucency may indicate a subdural collection of fluid, and other localised bright areas may indicate large cysts or a large dilated fourth ventricle.

Investigations

Ultrasound imaging is a non-invasive means of diagnosing hydrocephalus in infancy and is done by placing the ultrasound probe on the anterior fontanelle. Little or no special preparation is required; the procedure is risk free and can be repeated as often as necessary. Once closure of the fontanelle occurs, the technique is no longer applicable.

Computed tomography (CT) or magnetic resonance (MR) are used in the older child, and in infants if more detail is required. These provide a clear image of the intracranial anatomy and a precise means of detecting the presence of hydrocephalus, determining its extent and frequently demonstrate the site and cause of obstruction. MRI, despite the obligatory need for a general anaesthetic in a younger child, is becoming the modality of choice due to the lack of irradiation, the higher resolution of cerebral anatomy and the ability to analyse CSF flow.

The CSF dynamic scan involves the injection of a radionuclide tracer into the CSF pathway. Its passage through the ventricles and subarachnoid space is followed. Obstructions and abnormalities in the passage of CSF, from production to final absorption, can be recorded. With the advent of MRI radionuclide studies are infrequently used.

In more complex cases, intracranial pressure monitoring may help to determine the need, or otherwise, for treatment.

Plain x-rays are generally of no great value but may be used to confirm a diagnosis of raised intracranial pressure.

Treatment

Not all infants with enlargement of the head require operation, but if there is evidence of a continued deviation from the normal curve and/or signs of raised intracranial pressure the child should be investigated. Operation is indicated when there is sustained deviation from the normal curve in infants without obvious evidence of severe brain damage.

There are various methods of controlling an expanding head, which depend on three principles:
1 Reduction of CSF production. Production of CSF can be reduced by a drug that acts directly on the choroid plexus (carbonic anhydrase inhibitor) or by an osmotic agent. Control is frequently incomplete and of short-term benefit only.
2 Reconstitution of CSF pathways within the cranium. Removal of a mass may allow CSF to return to a normal flow pattern. Tumours in the posterior fossa frequently cause hydrocephalus and excision of the tumour leads to a rapid resolution in most cases. The placement of an endoscope into the ventricles via a burr hole (*neuro-endoscopy*), is an important technique for inspection, biopsy and therapeutic manoeuvres such as fenestration of a cyst into the ventricle, or the creation of an opening in the floor of the third ventricle (*third ventriculostomy*), which may correct an obstructive hydrocephalus.
3 Diversion of CSF to a site outside the cranium. External removal of CSF is the usual method of treating this

disorder. In communicating hydrocephalus, particularly in premature infants, removal may be undertaken intermittently, through lumbar puncture or through a ventricular reservoir; this controls the hydrocephalus until normal pathways are re-established.

A *ventriculo-peritoneal shunt* is usually the definitive operation of choice in children of all ages. This shunt comprises a ventricular catheter, a valve or flushing device beneath the scalp, and a long kink-resistant tube passing along the chest wall to enter the peritoneal cavity. A long length of tube is placed within the peritoneal cavity to allow for subsequent growth of the patient. Less frequently, a ventriculo-atrial shunt to divert the CSF into the right atrium is performed.

Complications of shunts

Most children with shunts are 'shunt dependent' and they will not tolerate malfunction of these devices.

1 *Obstruction*. Most frequently the ventricular catheter becomes occluded with choroid plexus or cerebral tissue. The lower end may be obstructed by the growth of the child that displaces the lower end into an unsuitable position, by adherence to the greater omentum or by fracture of the tube. Rarely, the valve may malfunction. Revision of the shunt is required.

2 *Infection*. The shunt system becomes colonised by pathogenic organisms that requires removal of the shunt, temporary external drainage of the CSF until it is sterilised with antibiotics, then replacement of the shunt.

3 *Disconnection*.

4 *Overdrainage*. The ventricles become small and the child may develop chronic headache due to low intracranial pressure. The opening pressure of the valve may need to be raised.

A child with a shunt must be reviewed at regular intervals during the growing years. In general, if the diagnosis is established before hydrocephalus is advanced, if there are no other significant brain anomalies, and if the treatment is appropriate and maintained, then the patient has every chance of developing normally. A child with a shunt is not restricted in activities.

Congenital abnormalities of the cranium

Errors in the development of the scalp, skull and brain are not as common as those of the spinal cord, but they present the same variety of abnormalities. Only the more common or important ones are described here.

Dermoid sinus

This is found most frequently in the mid-occipital region and may communicate with a more deeply situated dermoid cyst containing sebaceous material and hairs. The sinus may have some fine hairs (often a different colour) protruding from it and usually discharges sebaceous material. The deeper component can cause all the signs of an intracranial tumour with cerebellar signs predominating; it may also become infected.

An intracranial dermoid can occur without an external sinus. Infection is uncommon and the cyst presents by causing local pressure or obstruction of the CSF. Rarely, the cyst ruptures, leading to aseptic meningitis.

Dermoid cysts of the scalp are common over the anterior fontanelle and near the orbital margin and are described in Chapter 16.

Craniosynostosis

Premature closure of the cranial sutures, which act as lines of growth, restricts development of the region, with compensatory growth occurring at other suture lines. The subsequent distortion in the shape of the skull results in severe cosmetic deformities, but only occasionally does it cause sufficient diminution of the intracranial capacity to limit the growth of the brain. A description of the different deformities is given in Chapter 15 (craniofacial anomalies).

Treatment

The abnormal appearance and the risk of developmental delay are the two indications for surgery. Developmental delay probably occurs in only 10% of these children, and its likelihood is to be suspected when radiographs show signs of increased intracranial pressure, that is increased cerebral convolutional markings ('copper beating') and separation of the unfused sutures. Headache, vomiting and papilloedema are rare, but exophthalmos and ophthalmoplegia are not infrequent.

Early operation, before 3 months of age, results in a head of almost normal size and shape. Operative correction ranges from simple linear craniectomy (excision of a strip of bone along the fused suture) to radical removal and repositioning of the vault bones (Chapter 15).

Plagiocephaly

This is a common deformity which skews the entire skull. One frontal region and the opposite occipital region are flat and the contralateral areas are full and rounded. The effect is that the longest diameter is displaced from the sagittal axis towards the side with the prominent frontal contour.

Congenital plagiocephaly may be caused by contact of the fetal head with the maternal pelvis or with irregularity of the uterine wall, for example fibroids. Acquired plagio-cephaly in the first 3–4 months after birth has become common probably because mothers are advised to ensure their babies are put to sleep in a supine position. There may also be a torticollis causing one occipital area to bear the weight of the cranium and the brain, which deter-mines the shape of the thin and largely membranous cal-varium [Chapter 16]. X-rays may show sclerosis along the lambdoid suture line without fusion. This is the 'sticky' lambdoid suture. The deformity can be minimised by placing babies with postural or sternomastoid torticollis in such a way that they sleep on each side alternately and never directly supine.

The deformity tends to improve after the age of 6 months and continues to correct until puberty. A minor degree probably persists indefinitely, though this is not readily detected when hair obscures the contours of the skull. Surgery generally is not indicated except in infants with a significant cosmetic deformity.

Premature fusion of the lambdoid suture is an uncom-mon cause of plagiocephaly. Operative repair is required.

Cranium bifidum (including encephalocele)

Defects at the cephalic end of the neural tube of the embryo are much less common than in the thoraco-lumbar region. The same basic deformities occur, mostly in the occipital region, but in some countries, for example, Thailand, they are more common in the frontal (sincipi-tal) area.

The herniations are in the midline [Fig. 12.3], well covered with skin and lined by meninges, and may con-tain CSF alone (meningocele) or, more frequently, brain (encephalocele). Occasionally, the herniation occurs into the nasal cavity, and the sac is then covered by mucosa, not skin.

Other intracranial abnormalities also may be present, and imaging is necessary to detect these before surgical repair.

Simple excision of the sac, replacement of viable her-niated cerebral contents, and sound closure of the dura and the bone defect usually can be effected. Occipital encephaloceles may cause severe brain dysfunction (mental retardation, visual defects, hydrocephalus), which may preclude treatment. The sincipital encephalo-celes are repaired using craniofacial techniques with good cosmetic results and usually a good neurological outcome [Chapter 15].

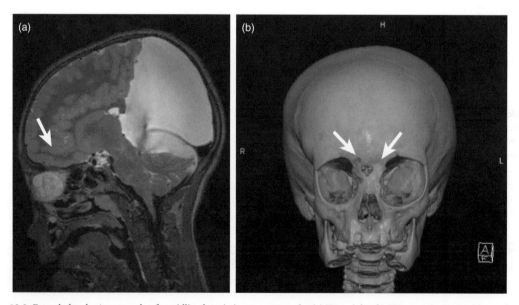

Figure 12.3 Encephalocele. An example of a midline herniation as seen on the (a) T2 weighted MRI scans (arrow) with cranium bifidum as seen on the (b) CT scan (arrow). This is an example of a neural tube defect.

Intracranial tumours

Tumours of the central nervous system are the largest group of malignancies, excluding leukaemia, in childhood. Radical surgery and adjuvant chemotherapy or radiotherapy in selected cases may produce long-term survival. There are also many benign and slowly growing intracranial tumours which may be cured following surgery.

Mode of presentation

The mode of presentation in children differs in many ways from that seen in adults
1 The common types of tumour and their sites of origin are different; for example, the preponderance of tumours in the posterior fossa in childhood [Table 12.2].
2 Young children adapt better to an expanding intracranial lesion because of the expansion of the skull; accommodation for weeks or even months is possible, but once this fails, the final decline is often rapid and catastrophic.
3 Many tumours arise close to the CSF pathways in relatively 'silent' areas, so neurological signs are few or absent until the flow of CSF is obstructed, when signs of raised intracranial pressure; for example, headache, vomiting and papilloedema, develop with alarming suddenness.
4 Early signs often affect the vision, but loss of acuity or diplopia are not appreciated in early childhood and never arise as symptoms in infants.
5 Neurological signs may present early, while evidence of raised intracranial pressure appears much later. In infants and younger children, the dramatic development of raised intracranial pressure may initiate a search for localizing signs that only then are recognised.

Intracranial tumours can be divided into three main groups, each of which produces a more or less typical clinical pattern.

Group 1: Glial tumours of the cerebral hemispheres

These are less common than those in the posterior fossa and cover the full spectrum of gliomas varying from benign to highly malignant, although histology is a much less reliable guide to prognosis than in adult gliomas.

The clinical picture is similar to that of adults and diagnosis and management follow the same lines. The tumour is surgically excised as far as possible without causing deficit.

Group 2: Tumours in the region of the third ventricle

These form a very important group in childhood. Their progress is often insidious until there are signs of ventricular obstruction but localizing neurological signs may be detected early. Those situated anteriorly produce defects in vision, and endocrine disturbance; and those posteriorly cause hydrocephalus, disturbances in ocular movements, and rarely precocious puberty.

Gliomas of the optic chiasm

Gliomas of the optic chiasm and optic nerves are associated with neurofibromatosis in 30–50% of cases. They cause bizarre field defects, loss of visual acuity, optic atrophy, squint and sometimes proptosis, before obstructing the third ventricle. Infants may present with hydrocephalus or with involvement of the hypothalamus causing wasting and anorexia known as the 'diencephalic syndrome', and a similar lesion in older children may cause precocious puberty.

They usually behave in a very indolent manner, but a large or progressively enlarging tumour may be surgically debulked and many are sensitive to chemotherapy. Shunts to relieve ventricular obstruction are sometimes necessary. Long-term survivals are not uncommon.

Craniopharyngioma

The craniopharyngioma grows insidiously. It arises in, above or behind the sella turcica from a remnant of the

Table 12.2 Cerebral tumours. Percentage distribution of 300 consecutive tumours at Royal Children's Hospital, Melbourne

Group 1	Cerebral hemispheres	18%
Group 2	Third ventricle	17%
	Optic chiasm 5%	
	Craniopharyngioma 5%	
	Pineal tumour 5%	
	Glial tumours 2%	
Group 3	Posterior fossa	53%
	Medulloblastoma	
	Solid/cystic astrocytoma	
	Brainstem glioma	
	Spinal tumours	12%

primitive Rathke's pouch and compresses the pituitary gland, pituitary stalk or hypothalamus, slowing growth and development and gradually depressing vision. It is variably comprised of solid epithelial components and cysts filled with brown turbid fluid described as 'machine oil'. The tumour is usually not suspected until the child has had defective sight for years, growth and development have lagged behind or the child tires easily and is unable to keep up with his peers.

Small craniopharyngiomas can be removed totally without damage to the adjacent optic nerve or the pituitary gland. Large craniopharyngiomas are one of the most challenging problems for the paediatric neurosurgeon. There is controversy over whether to attempt a complete excision, with chance of cure but risking serious morbidity. Morbidity includes visual pathway injury and persistent pituitary deficiency. Hormone replacement therapy and DDAVP (arginine vasopressin) have improved the outlook for these patients. Radiotherapy is used for recurrent tumours and as an adjunct for those tumours whose excision is deliberately incomplete.

Pineal region tumours

The main types of pineal tumours are
1 Germ cell origin – germinoma, embryonal carcinoma, yolk sac tumour, choriocarcinoma and teratoma.
2 Pineal cell tumours – pineocytoma, pineoblastoma.
3 Glial tumours.

Pineal tumours often obstruct the aqueduct before local signs develop so that headache, vomiting, papilloedema and impaired consciousness are the presenting features. Later, pressure on the upper brainstem causes a loss of upward gaze, a distinctive localizing sign. Precocious puberty is an uncommon feature. These tumours range from highly malignant to benign. Diagnosis is based on radiological appearances and CSF and blood markers. Surgical treatment varies according to pathology with hydrocephalus often requiring independent treatment. Chemotherapy and radiotherapy are often employed as adjuvant or primary therapy. The prognosis depends on the histology and tumour burden following the primary treatment. Even though germinomas are malignant, they may be cured with chemotherapy or radiotherapy.

Group 3: Tumours of the posterior fossa

These form about 50% of all intracranial tumours in childhood, but only 25% in adulthood, and those in the cerebellum cause ventricular obstruction early, so that headache and vomiting – characteristically in the early morning – appear before neurological signs such as incoordination, ataxia, hypotonia and tremor. In brainstem gliomas, gross incoordination, ataxia and cranial nerve palsies precede signs of increased intracranial pressure. There are four common tumours in this region.

Medulloblastoma

This is a malignant tumour of the vermis forming a large mass that blocks the fourth ventricle [Fig. 12.4]. It may spread out into the basal cisterns and characteristically disseminates widely throughout the CSF pathways, particularly in the spinal canal.

The tumour occurs more often in males at about 2 years of age, with a typical history of morning headaches and vomiting, change in personality and clumsiness of gait. Papilloedema and truncal ataxia are the common neurological signs and there may be tilting of the head when the child sits up. The tumour may recur locally and disseminate unless it responds to adjuvant chemotherapy and craniospinal radiotherapy in children over the age of 3 years. Children under 3 years of age require aggressive adjuvant chemotherapy. The overall 5-year survival is 60–80%.

Astrocytoma of the cerebellum

An astrocytoma may be solid tumour, a nodule of tumour in the wall of a cyst or even form the lining of a simple cyst. Children are older (about 5 years) than those with a medulloblastoma; the length of the history is 3–6 months rather than weeks, beginning with morning headaches and vomiting. Much later, usually in the 2–3 weeks before diagnosis, squint, incoordination and ataxia appear. The clinical signs are fairly constant: papilloedema, squint, mild ataxia and incoordination of hand movements.

There is usually a localised tumour, in one lateral lobe, which is often completely excised. Radiotherapy is reserved for tumours with more aggressive histological grades that have recurred. There is a high rate of cure of the benign (pilocytic) astrocytomas following surgery alone.

Brainstem glioma

This usually causes diffuse brainstem enlargement without much evidence of a localised tumour. The age incidence is wide and the signs are caused by cranial nerve palsies and involvement of the long tracts passing through the brainstem: gross strabismus, facial weakness, difficulty in swallowing, hemiparesis and ataxia occur. The child is miserable and pathetic, quite different from those with other types of posterior fossa tumours. Hydrocephalus is uncommon.

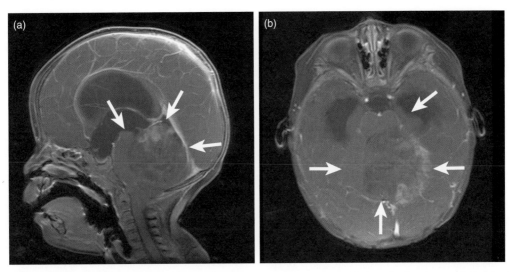

Figure 12.4 Medulloblastoma. An MRI scan showing a massive posterior fossa tumour blocking the fourth ventricle in (a) sagittal section and (b) transverse section. The tumour is arrowed.

The diagnosis is confirmed by MR scan, and surgery is usually not indicated. Radiotherapy and chemotherapy are used. In most patients, the signs resolve rapidly during treatment but recur within 3–6 months. The prognosis of the diffuse malignant brainstem glioma is very poor despite this therapy. A few patients with less aggressive tumours achieve a longer period of survival. There are some focal and benign tumours of the brainstem that can be largely excised with a good prognosis.

Ependymoma

The mode of presentation is similar to medulloblastoma. At operation, the tumour frequently is attached to the floor of the fourth ventricle and, like the medulloblastoma, the tumour has the same tendency to metastasise in the CSF pathways. The overall prognosis is worse than medulloblastoma particularly in those with incomplete excision with 5-year overall survival rates of 50–65%.

Tumours in the spinal canal

In infancy, neuroblastoma is the commonest. Primary vertebral and intrathecal tumours are uncommon. In the first 2–3 years of life the commonest lesion is a metastasis from a medulloblastoma. These lesions may present following a short history of poor limb movement and general malaise.

In later childhood other intrathecal tumours appear, for example, neurofibromas of the nerve roots and astrocytomas and ependymomas of the spinal cord. The child presents variably with chronic spine pain that may be severe and unremitting, scoliosis, slowly progressive weakness of the limbs, with abnormal reflexes and sphincter disturbance. The diagnosis is established by MR. Surgical decompression, biopsy and excision of the tumour are performed. The child with a spinal tumour may also present acutely with spine pain and signs of spinal cord compression: paralysis, sensory loss and sphincter disturbance. This is a surgical emergency.

Intracranial vascular disorders

Arteriovenous malformations

Arteriovenous malformations (AVMs) are congenital developmental vascular lesions of the brain, which comprise abnormal arteriovenous fistulas, which subsequently lead to dilated arteriolised veins, multiple tortuous feeding arteries and a central nidus of capillary-like fistulous vessels. Aneurysms may develop on the feeding vessels due to the high flow rates and the lesions may vary in size considerably. The presentation is often rupture with intracerebral and sometimes subarachnoid haemorrhage [Table 12.3]. This is the commonest cause of spontaneous intracranial haemorrhage in children. The children present

Table 12.3 Presentation of intracranial A–V malformations

1 Rupture with intracranial (or subarachnoid) haemorrhage
2 Epilepsy
3 Chronic headache
4 Focal neurological signs (rarely) (adjacent brain ischaemia)

with sudden severe headache, focal neurological signs, epileptic seizure and rapid obtundation, if the clot enlarges sufficiently. The treatment involves evacuation of clot and excision of the AVM. Elective excision of an unruptured AVM is complex. It may involve surgical excision, preceded by embolisation. Some small deep-seated AVMs may be treated with focused radiotherapy (stereotactic radiosurgery).

Intracranial aneurysms

Intracranial aneurysms occur at all ages, but are generally rare in children. The causes are (1) Congenital 'Berry' aneurysms – these occur at branch points of the major basal cerebral arteries at the Circle of Willis, and in children, often reach giant proportions. (2) Related to connective tissue disorders. For example, Ehlers-Danlos syndrome; (3) Post-traumatic, 'false' aneurysms either from blunt or penetrating trauma; (4) Mycotic aneurysms, which result from infected emboli. For example, following endocarditis subarachnoid haemorrhage results from aneurysm rupture and craniotomy and clipping of the aneurysm is the definitive treatment.

Vein of Galen malformations

Vein of Galen malformations are rare. Congenital arteriovenous fistulas arising in the region of the Vein of Galen may result in a large dilatation of this vein, the straight sinus and the posterior venous sinuses. These high flow fistulae may cause congestive heart failure in newborn infants, or may present later with enlarging head, hydrocephalus, failure to thrive and epilepsy. Their management

is complex, but there is an increased trend to neuro-radiological embolisation of the feeding vessels, or of the vein of Galen aneurysm itself. Surgical division of major feeders may also be required. The outlook for the child depends on the completeness of fistula obliteration and how much ischaemic damage is present in the surrounding brain.

Key Points

- A big head requires investigation if circumference is crossing the percentiles or if it is an abnormal shape.
- Frequent, 'different' or early morning headaches need investigation.
- Ventriculo-peritoneal shunts are life saving for hydrocephalus and allow normal activity. Recognition of shunt blockage is based on clinical diagnosis.
- Encephalocele is a complex neural tube defect.
- Brain tumours have a variable prognosis, depending on cell type, site of origin and whether there are secondary neurological deficits or hydrocephalus.

Further reading

Albright AL, Pollack I, Adelson PD (eds) (2000) *Operative Techniques in Pediatric Neurosurgery*, 1st Edn. Thieme Medical Publishers, New York.

Choux M, Di Rocco C, Walker M, Hockley A (eds) (1999) *Pediatric Neurosurgery*. Churchill Livingstone, London, Edinburgh, New York.

Cinalli G, Maixner W, Sainte-Rose C (eds) (2004) *Paediatric Hydrocephalus*. Springer Verlag, Italia, Milano.

Cohen ME, Duffner PK. (1994) (eds) *Brain Tumours in Children. Principles of Diagnosis and Treatment*, 2nd Edn. Raven Press, New York.

David DJ, Poswillo D, Simpson D (1982) *The Craniosynostoses: Causes, Natural History and Management*. Springer Verlag, Berlin.

Drake JM, Sainte-Rose C (1995) *The Shunt Book*. Blackwell, London.

McLone D (ed) (2001) *Paediatric Neurosurgery: Surgery of the Developing Nervous System*, 4th Edn. WB Saunders, Philadelphia.

13 The Eye

Case 1

A 3-year-old girl is brought to see you because her parents are concerned that her eyes are misaligned.
Q 1.1 Why should this be taken seriously?
Q 1.2 How can you determine if the parents' observations are correct?

Case 2

Parents of a 3-month-old boy are worried that he cannot see properly and that at times his eyes seem to wobble uncontrollably.
Q 2.1 Do the parents have anything to be really worried about?
Q 2.2 What are you going to do with this child?

Case 3

A 6-month-old baby has a sticky eye since the age of about 1 week. Her mother has to clean the affected eye several times a day.
Q 3.1 How are you going to advise this child's parents and what treatments are available?
Q 3.2 Should this child be prescribed topical antibiotic eye drops?

Case 4

A 6-year-old boy is brought to see you with a 3 h history of a painful red eye.
Q 4.1 How are you going to assess this child?

Vision loss may have profound effects on a child's development. A systematic clinical approach allows rapid diagnosis of most conditions affecting a child's eye and vision [Table 13.1]. Timely and appropriate management will then reduce the chance of permanent visual loss.

Accurate diagnosis is dependent on obtaining a good history and appropriate clinical examination (see below) supplemented where necessary by further investigations.

Examination of the child's vision and eye

Measurement of vision in preverbal children is by observation rather than formal testing. Asking the parent, 'How well does your child see?' or 'What do you think your child sees?' will provide useful clues to the level of vision.

At birth, an alert infant can fix on a face briefly. By 6 weeks of age, most infants smile in response to a face, and also will be able to follow a face or light through an arc of 90°. By 6 months of age, an infant can reach for a small object and actively follow moving objects in the environment. By 12 months, a child can pick up tiny objects such as hundreds-and-thousands ('sprinkles') [Table 13.2].

Table 13.1 Common ocular symptoms and signs in children

Suspected poor vision
Misaligned eyes
Wobbly eyes
Inflamed eyes
Droopy eyelids
Watery or sticky eyes
White reflex (leukocoria)
Big or small eye
Injured eye
Headache

Jones' Clinical Paediatric Surgery, 6th edition. By Hutson, O'Brien, Woodward and Beasley. Published 2008 by Blackwell Publishing, ISBN: 978-1-4051-6267-8.

Table 13.2 Measuring vision

Parents' assessment	Any age
Fix on face/light through 90°	6 weeks
Fix on moving objects	6 months
Pick up coloured sprinkles	12 months
Name simple pictures	2 years
Letter/shape matching	3–4 years
Snellen eye chart	5–6 years

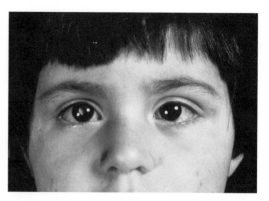

Figure 13.1 The 'white' reflex. The normal red reflex is replaced by a white reflection in the right eye in this child with retinoblastoma.

At 2 years of age, most children can name simple pictures to accurately document visual acuity. Letter- or shape-matching tests of vision are possible at about 3–4 years of age. Formal Snellen measurement of acuity is managed by most children once they reach school age (5–6 years).

Always document the estimate of vision for each eye. For a preverbal child, this may consist of statements like 'Fixes on a face with left eye, but not with right'. If more formal measurement is possible, document the Snellen fraction. For example, 'right eye – 6/9'. This means that at a distance of 6 m, the child can read the '9' line of letters or symbols. Most tests are performed at 3 or 6 m, but if the child's vision is reduced, the chart can be brought closer to the child.

Reduced visual acuity in a child is often the result of amblyopia. Amblyopia arises during development of the visual cortex when 'defective' information is being sent from the eye to the brain. Common causes of amblyopia are strabismus (misaligned eyes or 'squint') and unequal refractive error. To avoid diplopia the immature brain can suppress the information from one eye when strabismus is present. If the two eyes have an unequal refractive error, one will generally have a more blurry retinal image and thus a poor signal will be sent to the visual cortex, resulting in amblyopia. Amblyopia is best treated when the visual cortex is still immature and adaptable: visual cortical maturation occurs by about 7 years of age.

Inspection will provide much useful information. Abnormal pupil reactions, significantly misaligned eyes, abnormal eye movements (such as nystagmus), inflamed eyes, droopy eyelids, red, watery or discharging eyes, will all be obvious on simple inspection.

Examination of pupil reactions is important in objectively assessing the integrity of the anterior visual pathways (eyes and optic nerves). Normal pupils are of equal or very nearly equal size. The pupillomotor (efferent) pathway originates in a common area of the third nerve nucleus. Thus, if one eye is blind the pupils will appear of equal size in ambient light. A difference in pupil reaction and size will become apparent if a bright light source (such as a direct ophthalmoscope) is alternately directed at one eye and then the other (the 'swinging light test'). When the light is shone in the normal eye both pupils will constrict and when the light is switched to the blind eye both pupils will dilate. This abnormality is called a *relative afferent pupil defect* and is an important, objective sign of visual impairment in one eye or optic nerve. The afferent pathway of the pupil response leaves the optic nerves at the chiasm to pass to the third nerve nucleus. Thus, lesions of the visual system posterior to the chiasm will not cause abnormalities of pupil reactions.

Examining the red reflex with a direct ophthalmoscope will reveal much about the internal structure of the eye. The red reflex is examined with a direct ophthalmoscope set to the zero power lens and observing the child's eyes from a distance of about 1 m. A normal red reflex is red to orange and uniform over the pupil, and should be the same in each eye. Children with darker iris pigmentation will tend to have duller red reflexes than those with lightly pigmented eyes.

A white reflex [Fig. 13.1] generally indicates significant pathology within an eye and indicates the need for urgent dilated fundus examination by an ophthalmologist. In children over 1 year of age, the pupils can be safely dilated with cyclopentolate 1% or tropicamide 1%. In children less than one year, 0.25% or 0.5% preparations should be used.

Observing the corneal light reflections will indicate strabismus in a child who is not cooperative with cover testing. When a light is positioned directly in front of a child's face, the corneal light reflections should be symmetric. Asymmetry of the corneal light reflections suggests that the eyes are misaligned.

Cover testing is the method of choice to determine if a child has strabismus (misaligned eyes or squint). The cover test is done by first getting the child to fix on an object while the observer determines which eye appears to be misaligned. The eye that appears to be fixing on the object (and not misaligned) is then covered while the apparently misaligned eye is observed. If strabismus is present, a corrective movement of the misaligned eye will be seen as this eye takes up fixation on the object of regard [Fig. 13.2]. If no movement is seen, the eye is uncovered. The cover test is then repeated but the other eye is covered this time and the eye that is not covered is again observed for a corrective movement, and if present strabismus is confirmed. The test can be repeated as many times as necessary. If no movement is seen following repeated covering of either eye, then no strabismus is present. Care must be taken to let the child fix with both eyes open before covering either eye, otherwise normal binocular control may be disrupted and a small latent squint (phoria) may be detected. Latent squints are normal variants and of no significance.

Eversion of the upper eyelid is helpful if a foreign body is suspected to be the cause of a red irritable eye. The upper eyelid is everted by first asking the child to look down. A cotton-bud is then applied about one centimetre from the lid margin to act as a fulcrum about which the eyelid will be everted. Finally, to evert the eyelid the eyelashes are gently pulled initially downward and then rotated upward. The subtarsal conjunctiva can then be inspected and any foreign body removed with a second moistened cotton-bud.

Refractive errors (focusing problems)

A basic understanding of refractive errors helps a great deal in making sense of ophthalmology. There are three principal refractive errors. These are hypermetropia (long-sightedness), myopia (short-sightedness) and astigmatism. The easiest way to understand refractive errors is to consider the eye in a relaxed state.

When relaxed, a hypermetropic eye focuses light from a distant object behind the retina. To bring such an image into clear focus on the retina, accommodative effort has to be used or a converging (plus) lens placed in front of the eye (i.e. the focal length of the eye has to be changed) [Fig. 13.3]. Conversely, a myopic eye, when relaxed, focuses light from a distant object in front of the retina. No amount of further relaxing will enable the eye to lessen its focal length to bring such an image into clear focus. A diverging (or minus) lens will do this, thus a myopic eye can only 'see' a distant object clearly with the aid of some type of lens [Fig. 13.4]. Astigmatism is more complex but can be thought of as a regular distortion of the image on the retina by an eye that has different focal lengths in different axes.

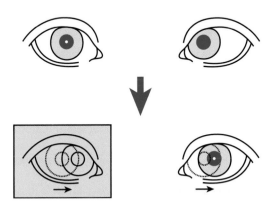

Figure 13.2 Cover test. The child's attention is attracted with a toy or light (top). Once the eye that appears to be looking directly at the toy is covered, the other eye is observed for a refixation movement (bottom). In convergent squint, there is outward movement of uncovered eye (pictured). In divergent squint, the eye moves inward. If no movement is seen repeat the cover test covering the other eye.

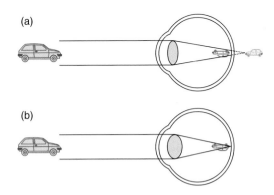

Figure 13.3 Hypermetropia (long-sightedness).
(a) When the eye is relaxed the image of a distant object is 'focused behind' the retina, producing a blurred retinal image.
(b) By accommodation (changing focal length), the image is focused on the retina.

(a)

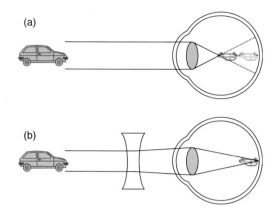

(b)

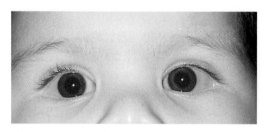

Figure 13.4 Myopia (short-sightedness).
(a) When the eye is relaxed, the image of a distant object is focused in front of the retina, producing a blurred image.
(b) Only by placing a diverging lens in front of the eye can a distant object be focused clearly on the retina.

Figure 13.5 Pseudostrabismus. This infant has prominent epicanthic folds giving the appearance of misaligned eyes. Note that the corneal light reflections are symmetrical. Cover testing failed to reveal misalignment of either eye.

Refractive errors can be compensated for by the use of glasses. In young children, refractive error can be measured accurately with the aid of cycloplegic eye drops and retinoscopy. This method of measuring refractive error is objective, and requires minimal cooperation from the child. It can be done very easily on preverbal children to determine need for glasses. Focusing problems of all types are relatively common in childhood. During primary school years, approximately 5% of children wear glasses.

Most children are born a little hypermetropic, and because of a child's prodigious accommodative capability can easily overcome this to see clearly and hence glasses are not necessary. If a child is excessively hypermetropic, large amounts of accommodative effort will be required

to focus clearly. Such large amounts of accommodation may result in excessive convergence and the child will develop a convergent squint (see Strabismus below).

Strabismus (turned eyes or squint)

Strabismus is one of the commonest eye problems in childhood. An understanding of strabismus is important because a turned eye may, in the rare case, indicate a major problem with one eye (e.g. cataract or retinoblastoma); more commonly, it is associated with reduced vision (amblyopia) in one eye. Thus, a turned eye may be secondary to poor vision or may be the cause of reduced vision (amblyopia). Early diagnosis of squint and appropriate intervention increases the chance of restoring or preserving vision.

The initial assessment of a child suspected of having strabismus involves confirmation of the misalignment (observation, corneal light reflection and cover testing), measurement of vision in each eye and examination of red reflex to detect major structural defects in either eye. All children with confirmed or suspected strabismus should be referred to an ophthalmologist. If a major structural defect is suspected on the basis of an abnormal red reflex, specialist opinion should be obtained urgently.

Infants have relatively broad and flat nasal bridges and if this is associated with prominent epicanthic folds, a very strong impression of convergent strabismus can arise. This is known as pseudostrabismus [Fig. 13.5] and is quite common. Careful assessment, as outlined above, will enable pseudo and true strabismus to be distinguished.

Most children with strabismus have a full range of eye movement and thus the misaligned eyes are not the result of a muscular abnormality or nerve damage. Childhood strabismus is usually the result of failure of development of normal binocular coordination of the eyes. There may be a primary failure of binocular coordination. This is seen with early onset convergent strabismus (known as infantile esotropia).

Strabismus associated with a full range of eye movement is called concomitant strabismus. If the eyes converge excessively it is known as esotropia, and if the eyes diverge, it is called exotropia. Vertical misalignment is called hypertropia if the eye goes up and hypotropia if the eye goes down [see Fig 13.9].

Infantile esotropia is seen before 6 months of age and is generally a large angle convergent strabismus [Fig. 13.6]. These infants seldom have any significant refractive error

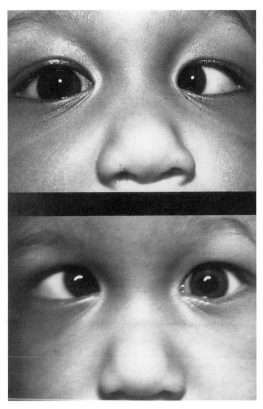

Figure 13.6 Infantile esotropia. This infant has a large angle alternating esotropia. Note the marked asymmetry of the corneal light reflections.

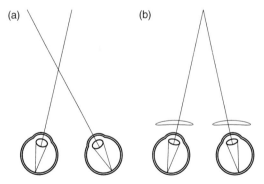

Figure 13.7 Accommodative esotropia. (a) Excessive accommodation of hypermetropic eye may result in excessive convergence and esotropia. (b) By placing corrective (plus) lens in front of the eyes, the amount of accommodation needed to see the object is reduced and so is the convergence; hence, eyes are now correctly aligned.

and surgery is usually required to realign the eyes successfully. Patching may be necessary for the treatment of amblyopia.

Accommodative esotropia usually has its onset between 18 months and 4 years of age and initially is often intermittent. It occurs in children who are excessively hypermetropic (long-sighted). To overcome hypermetropia and focus a clear image on the retina, accommodative effort is used. Accommodation consists of the combination of changing focal length of the lens and converging the eyes (so that both are directed at the nearer object of regard). Thus, in children with excessive hypermetropia there is increased focusing and at times excessive convergence (causing accommodative esotropia) [Fig. 13.7]. This can be corrected by prescribing glasses that compensate for the appropriate amount of hypermetropia. Amblyopia is often seen with accommodative esotropia and requires treatment. If glasses only partly correct the esotropia, surgery may be indicated to obtain optimal alignment.

Intermittent divergent strabismus is unusual before 18 months of age. It is often more noticeable on distance fixation and may be associated with closure of the deviating eye, especially in bright light. Amblyopia is uncommon as the deviation is intermittent, and presumably, when the eyes are straight, normal visual development proceeds. In some cases, the divergence becomes more constant, and in such situations, surgery may be undertaken to improve alignment.

All children with strabismus need review periodically until aged 10 years, to detect any amblyopia and to monitor ocular alignment. Even after successful realignment with surgery or glasses, amblyopia may occur and the eyes may also deviate again.

Children require general anaesthetic (day surgery) for strabismus surgery to be undertaken. The principle of such an operation is to align the eyes correctly by weakening and strengthening extra ocular muscles so as to rotate one eye relative to the other. Simple analgesia, such as paracetamol, is sufficient for post-operative pain management. Post-operative nausea and vomiting is not unusual in older children (over 5 years of age). This is generally self-limited and not a major problem, settling with restriction of oral intake and a little patience.

Wobbly eyes

Nystagmus is to-and-fro movement of the eyes, and is almost always involuntary. In childhood, most nystagmus is a primary defect in the child's ability to keep the eyes still, or the result of early failure of normal development of vision. Nystagmus in childhood is seldom the result of medication, cerebral degeneration, cerebro-vascular disease or cerebral tumour as is the case in adults.

Congenital nystagmus is a primary defect in the mechanism that stabilises the eyes and results in mild to moderate reduced vision (6/9–6/24). It is seldom evident before 6–8 weeks of age, and will often reduce or dampen in a particular direction of gaze (called the null point). Thus, to maximise vision a child may adopt a compensatory head posture to take advantage of the null point. If the compensatory head posture is extreme, surgery may be necessary to manipulate the null point so that it is closer to the primary position of gaze.

Sensory nystagmus is caused by poor vision and is usually obvious by 3 months of age. Causes include bilateral congenital cataracts, albinism and congenital retinal dystrophy (Leber's congenital amaurosis). These conditions are rare, but immediate recognition will result in a better final visual outcome, and early intervention will minimise developmental problems associated with lifelong reduced vision (e.g. in albinism and congenital retinal dystrophy).

Watery (epiphora) and sticky eyes

An eye will become watery and sticky because of failure of tear drainage or an inflammatory response (increased production of tears, mucus and cellular response). Congenital nasolacrimal duct obstruction and bacterial conjunctivitis are typical examples of each cause. It is possible that the two problems may co-exist in the one child. An irritated eye may be painful and erythematous, depending on the cause [Table 13.3].

Congenital nasolacrimal duct obstruction affects about 10% of newborn infants and resolves spontaneously in about 95% by one year. It presents as a watery and sticky eye in the first 2 weeks of life. Despite the persistent discharge, the eye is generally neither red nor inflamed. The differential diagnosis includes trauma, conjunctivitis and infantile glaucoma (see Big and small eyes below). An inflamed eye suggests infective conjunctivitis.

If the obstruction persists, the lower lid will often become red and sometimes slightly scaly as a result of the skin being constantly moist. If obstruction persists beyond 12 months of age, probing under a general anaesthetic is indicated and is generally curative.

Ophthalmia neonatorum presents with copious discharge from the eyes in the first few days of life, and is the result of infection acquired during birth (e.g. *Neisseria gonorrhoea* and *Chlamydia trachomatis*). Gonococcal conjunctivitis is serious because of the risk of spontaneous perforation of the cornea, loss of vision and generalised sepsis. Chlamydial conjunctivitis is important because of the risk of more generalised chlamydial sepsis. For accurate and prompt diagnosis, conjunctival swabs should be directly inoculated on to culture medium plates and conjunctival scrapings taken for Gram staining and immunofluorescent staining. Systemic, as well as topical, antibiotic therapy is indicated.

Bacterial conjunctivitis occurring beyond the first few days of life is generally the result of relatively innocuous organisms (e.g. *Staphylococcal* spp. and *Haemophilus spp.*). Microbiological investigation is not indicated initially and a broad-spectrum topical antibiotic should be prescribed (such as neomycin/polymixin or chloramphenicol). Topical chloramphenicol preparations have an extremely low risk of secondary agranulocytosis.

Viral conjunctivitis is relatively common at all ages, and may be very difficult to differentiate from bacterial conjunctivitis. There may be somewhat less discharge with viral conjunctivitis. When there is uncertainty as to aetiology, topical antibiotics as for bacterial conjunctivitis should be used.

Preseptal cellulitis is a bacterial infection of the skin and soft tissue of the eyelids and will present with redness and swelling. Often there is discharge and watering as well. This infection may respond to oral antibiotics but frequently parenteral antibiotics are needed. In rare cases, an infection spreads to the orbital tissues from the surrounding nasal sinuses. This is orbital cellulitis, a more serious infection than preseptal cellulitis and presenting with proptosis (forward protrusion of the eye), redness of eye and eyelids, and painful limitation of eye movements. If untreated, orbital cellulitis will frequently result in loss of vision because the raised pressure in the orbit will interfere with the blood supply to the globe, which in turn may lead to infarction of the optic nerve or retina. Treatment involves parenteral antibiotics, urgent CT scan to define the extent of any orbital abscess and drainage of any significant collection of pus.

Big and small eyes

A young child's eye will become bigger if the pressure within it is raised, as in infantile glaucoma. Less commonly,

Table 13.3 Watery and sticky eyes: common symptoms, signs and causes

Problem	Symptoms	Signs
Neonatal conjunctivitis (ophthalmia neonatorum)	Severe pain	Moderate epiphora Copious discharge Moderate–severe erythema
Congenital nasolacrimal duct obstruction	Painless	Mild–moderate epiphora Mild–copious discharge Minimal erythema
Infantile glaucoma	Photophobia	Moderate epiphora No discharge Minimal erythema Enlarged and cloudy cornea
Viral conjunctivitis	Moderate discomfort	Moderate epiphora Mild discharge Mild–moderate erythema
Bacterial conjunctivitis	Moderate to severe discomfort	Moderate epiphora Copious discharge Moderate–severe erythema
Allergic conjunctivitis	Itch often prominent	Mild–moderate epiphora Stringy discharge Mild erythema
Chemical conjunctivitis	Intense pain	Severe epiphora Mild discharge Moderate–severe erythema
Corneal abrasion	Intense pain	Moderate epiphora No discharge Variable erythema Fluorescein staining
Foreign body	Intense pain	Moderate epiphora No discharge Variable erythema Variable fluorescein staining
Preseptal cellulitis	Moderate pain	Minimal epiphora Variable discharge Marked erythema and swelling of eyelids – the eye is white
Orbital cellulitis	Severe pain Reduced eye movements	Minimal epiphora Variable discharge Marked erythema – swelling of eyelids – the eye is often inflamed and proptosed

the eye is enlarged as in megalocornea (literally 'big cornea'). Small eyes in children result mainly from defects in growth of the eye, and there may be other major anomalies of the eye.

Infantile glaucoma (buphthalmos, or 'ox eye') is a rare condition with deficient drainage of aqueous fluid from the anterior chamber: The intraocular pressure rises and the infant's sclera and cornea stretch and the eye enlarges. The stretching of the cornea damages the inner corneal layers (Descemet's membrane and associated endothelium).This allows the cornea to become oedematous and opaque. The damaged cornea causes irritation and light sensitivity. Thus, the features of infantile glaucoma are an enlarged, cloudy cornea with watering and photophobia [Fig. 13.8]. There is no significant discharge, which differentiates infantile glaucoma from nasolacrimal obstruction and conjunctivitis.

Treatment for infantile glaucoma is surgery to restore aqueous fluid drainage from the anterior chamber. Such surgery is usually successful, though the stretched cornea will remain and these eyes are often myopic (short-sighted).

An eye that is small but otherwise normal is termed a nanophthalmic eye. If the eye is associated with an ocular anomaly, the eye is microphthalmic. Microphthalmos is frequently associated with a failure of development of part of the uveal coat of the eye (iris and choroid). Such a defect in the iris or choroid is called a coloboma. Microphthalmic eyes often have poor vision that cannot be improved.

Injured eyes

Trauma to the eye can be physical (blunt or sharp), radiation (thermal and electromagnetic) or chemical.

Direct blunt trauma to the eye may disrupt iris blood vessels causing bleeding in the anterior chamber of the eye (hyphema), tear the iris, dislocate the lens, rupture the choroid and (rarely) rupture the eye wall (sclera) if the force is sufficient. Simple inspection of the eye will reveal most of these injuries, and choroid and globe rupture may be suspected on the basis of the nature of the injury and associated poor vision. Referral to an ophthalmologist is

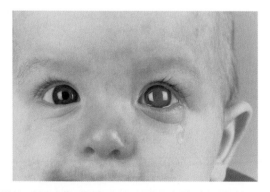

Figure 13.8 Infantile glaucoma presents with photophobia, tearing and on examination the affected eye(s) are enlarged and the cornea is cloudy. Compare the left and right eyes in this illustration.

necessary in these cases for confirmation of the injury and further management. The prognosis for vision is poor with severe injuries.

Blunt trauma to the eye may result in a blow-out fracture of the bones of the orbital wall rather than rupture of the globe: the orbital floor and medial wall are most often fractured, as they are thin bones. The extraocular muscles and their fascial connections may become entrapped in a blow-out fracture, leading to restrictive strabismus. Surgery may be needed to free the entrapped tissue and repair the fracture.

Sharp trauma may result from tiny objects, such as a subtarsal foreign body, causing a corneal abrasion, or fingernail scratches, through to penetration of the eye by sharp objects such as a scissors blade or knife. Surface trauma can be easily diagnosed with the help of fluorescein stain and a cobalt blue light. Areas of epithelial abrasion will fluoresce green. If a round ulcer and/or vertical linear abrasions are seen, a subtarsal foreign body should be suspected and the upper lid should be everted and foreign body removed with a moistened cottonbud. Superficial trauma is treated with antibiotic ointment and a patch, and daily review until the ulcer or abrasion is healed.

In penetrating injuries of the eye (cornea or sclera), the intraocular contents may prolapse out through the wound, the iris and pupil may appear distorted or the anterior chamber may be shallowed. Any suspected penetration of the eye must be referred to an ophthalmologist for further investigation and management. The eye should be protected with a cone that does not exert any pressure on the eye. If vomiting is likely or occurs, an anti-emetic should be given to reduce the chance of further prolapse of intraocular tissue.

Thermal injuries to the eye itself are rare as the eyelids protect the eye. Facial burns may cause scarring that interferes with lid function leading to exposure and drying of the eye's surface. If a primary thermal injury to the eye is suspected, fluorescein dye should be used to detect any ulceration. If ulceration is found, treatment is with antibiotic ointment and a patch.

Radiation injuries to the eye are rare in childhood, and most are the result of intentional irradiation as part of medical therapy for facial and ocular neoplasm. Typical injuries are cataract, dry eye syndrome, radiation retinopathy and optic neuropathy. These changes are seen some considerable time after the irradiation.

Chemical burns to the eye are unusual in childhood, but potentially very serious, especially if the chemical is alkaline. Many domestic cleaning agents are alkaline.

Strong alkali will denature and dissolve protein, and penetrate deeply into the surface of the eye. Acids tend to coagulate surface structures and this often prevents deeper penetration of the acidic chemical into the eye. Immediate first aid consists of copious irrigation with water for at least 10 min. Local anaesthetic eye drops relieve pain while the eye is irrigated. All chemical burns of the eye should be referred to an ophthalmologist.

White pupil

The pupil is normally black because very little light is reflected back out of the eye. Any abnormal reflecting surface in the eye increases reflected light and causes the pupil to appear coloured rather than black. Cataracts, retinal tumours and chorioretinal colobomas are the most common causes of a white pupil [see Fig. 13.1]. These conditions are all rare, but important because of their effect on vision and, in some instances, the importance of early recognition and treatment.

A cataract is any opacity within the lens. Cataracts will frequently present because a white pupil has been noted. Bilateral congenital cataracts cause poor vision in infancy, while unilateral congenital cataract may go unrecognised as one eye has normal vision. Both bilateral and unilateral congenital cataracts are treatable if diagnosed early. Cataracts are readily detected by inspection of the red reflex with the direct ophthalmoscope.

Most cataracts in childhood are congenital and causes include hereditary (dominant, recessive and X-linked), metabolic (e.g. galactosaemia), association with systemic syndrome (e.g. Down syndrome) and congenital infection (e.g. rubella embryopathy). Many, especially unilateral cataracts, are idiopathic.

Management of cataracts in children involves surgical removal of the cataract and visual rehabilitation with glasses or contact lenses. In older children, an intraocular lens can be implanted in the eye but in children under 2 years this is not possible. These children often develop amblyopia and require long-term follow-up.

Retinoblastoma most often presents with a white pupil (the white tumour is seen immediately behind the lens) [see Fig. 13.1]. Other presentations are with strabismus, poor vision or a known family history of retinoblastoma. Prompt recognition and treatment is vital to preserve vision and life.

Sporadic and hereditary forms of retinoblastoma are recognised. The sporadic form is the result of two separate mutations that negate the action of the retinoblastoma gene ('Rb gene') within a single retinoblast cell and thus is always unilateral. The hereditary form arises when the first of these two mutations occurs within a germ cell (most often a sperm). The second mutation occurs within the retinoblast. As all retinoblasts descend from an affected germ cell having the first mutation, more than one retinoblastoma will usually develop and hence the hereditary form is often bilateral.

Treatment of retinoblastoma may involve removal of the eye (enucleation), chemotherapy, freezing of the tumour (cryotherapy), laser heating of the tumour (often combined with chemotherapy (thermochemotherapy) or irradiation (both external beam or a local implanted source of irradiation – plaque brachytherapy). Currently, 5-year survival is about 98%.

Lumpy eyelids

Swellings in the eyelids are common in childhood. Most are the result of minor infections, obstructed oil glands or bruising. Benign tumours occur occasionally and malignant tumours very rarely.

Lid infections are common in children and most arise in the lash follicles (stye or hordeolum externum) and meibomian glands (hordeolum internum). Unless there is significant secondary erythema of the surrounding lid, topical and systemic antibiotics are not indicated. Occasionally, severe preseptal cellulitis will follow a focal lid infection and systemic (often intravenous) antibiotics will be needed.

Chronic inflammation of a meibomian gland (chalazion) is generally chemical inflammation rather than infection, and occurs when the gland contents escape into the lid following blockage of the duct. A chalazion will appear as a lump in the substance of the lid and is often not particularly inflamed in appearance. Topical antibiotics seldom hasten resolution. Warm compresses may give symptomatic relief and help drainage. Chalazia may persist for many months; some will discharge through the conjunctiva or the skin. On occasions, surgical drainage is indicated for a persistently inflamed and large chalazion.

Angular dermoids occur at inner or outer aspects of the upper lid [Fig. 16.8, Chapter 16]. These are benign hamartomas that grow in proportion with the rest of the child. Rarely direct trauma will cause rupture of a dermoid and significant inflammation will ensue. A deep extension necessitating extensive surgery more often occurs with medial angular dermoids. A CT scan should be undertaken before a planned excision if a dermoid is firmly adherent to bone.

Malignant tumours of the eyelid and orbit are rare. Rhabdomyosarcoma is the most frequent, and presents with rapidly progressive (days to weeks) eyelid swelling and proptosis. The overlying skin may appear reddened but other signs of acute inflammation (pain and fever) are absent. Management includes imaging to delineate site and extent of the lesion, incisional biopsy, chemotherapy and often external beam irradiation. This management is multidisciplinary. The overall survival rate for this form of rhabdomyosarcoma is excellent. Metastatic orbital tumours occur, with neuroblastoma being the most common [Fig. 13.9].

Droopy lids

Ptosis (or blepharoptosis) is a droopy upper eyelid and results from innervational or muscular defects of the

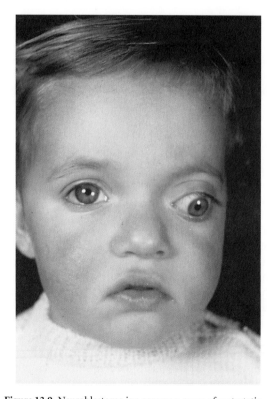

Figure 13.9 Neuroblastoma is a common cause of metastatic tumour of the orbit with proptosis. Note the protrusion and hypotropia (downward direction) of the left eye.

levator superioris or Muller's muscles. Innervational defects include third cranial nerve palsy, Horner syndrome (sympathetic nervous system) and myaesthenia gravis. Most ptosis in childhood is congenital and has no other systemic associations. Acquired ptosis in childhood requires thorough investigation looking for a cause.

Congenital ptosis is usually an isolated abnormality in the function of one or both levator muscles. The affected muscle is often described as being 'dystrophic', but there is, generally, no association with more widespread muscular dystrophies. Congenital ptosis will appear worse when the child is tired or unwell; this is not evidence of ocular myaesthenia gravis. A child with ptotic eyelids will often adopt a compensatory chin-up head posture to look straight ahead or to look up.

Ptosis will cause visual defects if the lid occludes the visual axis or if it induces astigmatism by altering the corneal curvature. Ptosis is also a cosmetic concern, in that it may make an affected child look sleepy or dull. Surgical correction is possible in most cases. Early surgery is indicated when the ptotic eyelid is interfering with the development of vision. If intervention is primarily for reasons of appearance, surgery is usually undertaken just prior to school commencement.

Headache

Headache in children occasionally is caused by an ocular abnormality. Astigmatism and high hypermetropia (longsightedness) are rare causes of childhood headache. Sustained attention to a near object will often cause some visual discomfort and headache. This is really a fatigue or tension headache and in general does not indicate any significant eye problem. These headaches are often described as a tightening around the head and are not associated with other symptoms.

Migraine headaches are common in childhood and may be associated with visual symptoms. The typical visual aura is blurring of central vision with zigzag bright lines (fortification spectra). These headaches are recurrent; they are often associated with nausea and vomiting, photophobia and phonophobia and the child is almost invariably pale during the episode. Most settle with simple analgesia (paracetamol) and rest. A family history of migraine is common.

Eye examination may help in determining the cause of some headaches. Raised intracranial pressure will usually cause headache that is often worse in the morning and after lying down. The pain is often described as dull, pounding and persistent. It may be associated with nausea and vomiting and sometimes transient blurring of vision (visual obscurations). If the intracranial pressure is raised, fundus examination will reveal papilloedema in most cases. The commonest causes of raised intracranial pressure that present with headache are 'benign' intracranial pressure (pseudotumour cerebri) and tumours causing obstructive hydrocephalus.

Abnormal head posture

Children will adopt abnormal head postures for many reasons. Structural abnormalities, hearing loss, visual defects, habit and (rarely) central nervous system tumours can all cause abnormal head posture. Sternocleidomastoid muscle 'tumour' or hemivertebra are examples of structural abnormalities causing abnormal head posture.

If vision is improved with the head held in a particular position, a child will characteristically adopt this position [Fig. 13.10]. Visual stimuli for abnormal head posture include strabismus, where binocular depth perception is improved or diplopia is avoided, loss of vision in one eye, dampening of nystagmus, ptosis and severe photophobia.

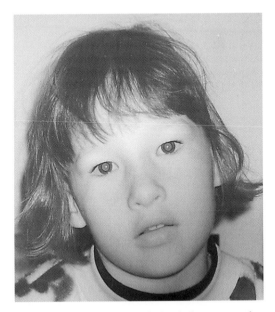

Figure 13.10 This child developed a head-tilt at 5 years of age. Investigation revealed a pineocytoma compressing the quadrigeminal plate.

Postoperative care of the child after eye surgery

The principles of postoperative eye care for children are (1) maintaining general comfort; (2) protecting the eye when necessary, (3) minimising specific complications and (4) returning the child to normal activities as soon as is reasonable.

Pain is usually minimal after paediatric eye surgery. Paracetamol is sufficient for most postoperative pain relief. Immediately after strabismus procedures, children are often distressed and disoriented. This phase may last minutes to an hour or so, and in most instances will settle with comforting alone. More than infants, older children are likely to require postoperative analgesia.

Nausea and vomiting may occur after strabismus procedures. Avoidance of pre- and intra-operative narcotic analgesia and intra-operative anti-emetic will minimise these problems. Limited oral intake in the early postoperative period will lessen the occurrence and severity of nausea and vomiting. Rarely, severe vomiting occurs snecessitating readmission and rehydration.

Patches to protect the eye are generally only needed after intraocular surgery (cataract and glaucoma) and eyelid surgery (ptosis repair and drainage of chalazion). Patches may often annoy a child and should be avoided following strabismus surgery.

Postoperative eye drops (antibiotic and steroid preparations) minimise the risk of infection and inflammation, especially following intraocular surgery. Benefit following strabismus procedures is less evident. Lubricating ointment is used for days to weeks after ptosis repair, to protect the ocular surface during healing.

Swimming should probably be avoided for 1–2 weeks after most eye operations because of the eye irritation from chlorinated or salt water. Care must be taken with face- and hair-washing, as soap or shampoo will be more irritating after an eye operation.

> **Key Points**
> - Amblyopia may develop if squint and/or poor vision is untreated.
> - A white reflex suggests significant pathology and needs urgent referral.
> - Conjunctivitis in the first few days of life results from serious infections acquired during birth.

Further reading

Beasley SW, Hutson JM, Myers NA (1993) *Paediatric Diagnosis.* Chapman & Hall, London, pp. 118–127.

Isenberg SJ (1994) *The Eye in Infancy*, 2nd Edn. Mosby, St. Louis.

Roberton DM, South M (2007) *Practical Paediatrics*, 6th Edn. Churchill Livingstone, Elsevier, Philadelphia.

Taylor D, Hoyt CS (2005) *Pediatric Ophthalmology and Strabismus*, 3rd Edn. WB Saunders, Elsevier, Philadelphia.

Wright KW, Spiegel PH (2003) *Pediatric Ophthalmology and Strabismus*, 2nd Edn. Springer Verlag, Berlin.

14 The Ear, Nose and Throat

Case 1

An 18-month-old girl who has an upper respiratory tract infection for a week has been irritable for the past 2 days, particularly at night. She has had three ear infections over the past 3 months and has not yet developed any speech. She presents to the emergency department with a temperature of 37.8°C and is mildly unwell. Otoscopy reveals opaque tympanic membranes. Mother thinks she has another ear infection.

Q 1.1 Why is the tympanic membrane opaque?
Q 1.2 What is the management?
Q 1.3 Is hearing impaired in this child?

Case 2

A 6-year-old boy presents to his local doctor with yet another episode of acute tonsillitis and has also been snoring heavily at night. His mother wonders whether or not it is time for him to have his tonsils and adenoids removed.

Q 2.1 What advice would you give?

Case 3

A 4-week-old infant presents with a concerned mother giving a history of stridor since birth. The child is noisy but appears well and is thriving.

Q 3.1 How is stridor assessed?
Q 3.2 What are the causes of congenital stridor?

Otitis media

Introduction

The term otitis media implies the presence of a middle ear effusion. Fluid develops because of dysfunction of the eustachian tube, which normally provides ventilation and drainage of the middle ear together with protection of the middle ear from nasopharyngeal contamination. For both infective and structural reasons, otitis media is common in the first 3 years of life, particularly over the winter months.

The tympanic membrane is a window to the middle ear, and is usually translucent against a background of an air-filled middle ear. An opaque tympanic membrane may be due to fluid in the middle ear or simply thickening of the membrane itself [Fig. 14.1]. The diagnosis of otitis media can be confirmed by demonstrating impaired mobility of the tympanic membrane by either pneumatic otoscopy or tympanometry (type B tympanogram).

Otitis media presents clinically as a spectrum of diseases that are all characterised by the presence of a middle ear effusion. At either end of the spectrum, depending on the degree of bacterial infection present, the child may be labelled as having

1 acute suppurative otitis media;
2 otitis media with effusion.

Acute suppurative otitis media (ASOM)

The diagnosis of ASOM is based on the presence of a middle ear effusion associated with features of inflammation that are either local (pain), or systemic (fever, irritability) provided there is no other explanation for the systemic symptoms. Bacteria are cultured in approximately 90% of cases, with the commonest organisms being *Streptococcus pneumoniae,* non-typable *Haemophilus influenzae* and *Branhamella catarrhalis.* Most cases of ASOM will settle spontaneously without antibiotics, and treatment is not required when symptoms are only mild. Antibiotics should be administered in children under 12 months of age or if significant or prolonged symptoms are present. Amoxycillin (40 mg/kg/day in three divided doses for 5 days) is

Jones' Clinical Paediatric Surgery, 6th edition. By Hutson, O'Brien, Woodward and Beasley. Published 2008 by Blackwell Publishing, ISBN: 978-1-4051-6267-8.

(a)   (b)   (c)

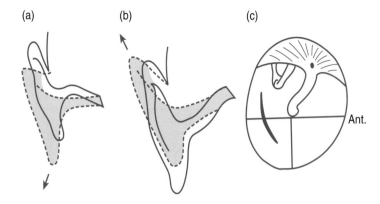

Ant.

Figure 14.1 The tympanic membrane. (a) The direction of the canal in infants and young children: to visualise the membrane, pull the pinna downwards and outwards; (b) in older children and adults the pinna is drawn upwards and backwards; (c) the normal eardrum is transparent, with the incus and stapes visible in the background. The site for the myringotomy or tympanostomy tube is shown.

Table 14.1 Duration of effusion after ASOM

Period after ASOM	Percentage middle ear effusion
2 weeks	70
1 month	40
2 months	20
3 months	10

recommended. Spontaneous perforation may occur, and is usually associated with relief of pain.

Follow-up of ASOM involves review after 48 h if the child remains unwell. Acute drainage of the ear is occasionally required if significant local or systemic symptoms persist despite adequate antibiotic treatment, or if complications occur. Suppurative complications of ASOM are uncommon. Complications within the temporal bone include

• Acute mastoiditis that presents with post-auricular swelling due to a subperiosteal abscess that has spread from the mastoid.

• Sigmoid sinus thrombosis that presents with features of raised intracranial pressure due to impaired venous drainage, particularly with involvement of the right side, the usual side of the dominant sinus.

• Facial paralysis due to inflammation extending to an exposed region of the facial nerve as it traverses the middle ear.

Extra-temporal suppurative complications with CNS involvement are rare.

The middle ear effusion associated with ASOM persists for a variable period of time beyond resolution of the infective features [Table 14.1], and while present, will be associated with impaired hearing in the involved ear.

Otitis media with effusion (OME)

Middle ear effusion is typically associated with mild hearing loss. When bilateral, this may lead to delayed speech development, behavioural problems and educational difficulties. Bacteria can be cultured in 25% of the cases and as a consequence, antibiotic treatment may be of some benefit.

Surgical intervention by way of insertion of tympanostomy tubes provides external ventilation of the middle ear, but does not correct the underlying eustachian tube dysfunction and is therefore only of benefit while the tubes remain in situ. Tympanostomy tubes should be considered where OME is associated with

• significant symptoms related to hearing loss or recurrent ear infections;

• the clinical situation is thought unlikely to improve spontaneously in the near future.

Factors contributing to the likelihood that OME will persist include the length of time the effusions have been present, seasonal factors (OME is associated with upper respiratory tract infections over the winter months) and anatomical factors such as the presence of a cleft palate or other craniofacial anomalies.

Standard tympanostomy tubes usually last between 6 and 9 months; however, tube designs are available that may remain functional for years. Reinsertion of tubes is necessary in 25% of cases. The longer the tubes remain, the higher the rate of tympanic membrane perforation, which is approximately 1% per year. Tubes may discharge intermittently, particularly with upper respiratory tract infections, and infection is best treated by topical antibiotics.

Cholesteatoma

The presence of squamous epithelium (skin) in the middle ear constitutes cholesteatoma. This squamous epithelium may spread throughout the middle ear cleft (middle ear, attic, mastoid) and cause bone destruction due to a combination of enzymatic action and infection. This may result in conductive hearing loss, sensorineural hearing loss, facial paralysis and intracranial infection.

Cholesteatoma may be congenital or acquired. Congenital cholesteatoma may be recognised in the early phase by the presence of a white mass deep to the tympanic membrane usually in the antero-superior quadrant.

Acquired cholesteatoma usually occurs owing to tympanic membrane retraction associated with impaired middle ear ventilation as a result of eustachian tube dysfunction. This may involve the tympanic membrane inferior to the lateral process of the malleus (pars tensa) or superior to it (pars flaccida). Development of a retraction pocket can be observed clinically and cholesteatoma formation prevented by insertion of a tympanostomy tube. Acquired cholesteatoma may also occur because of traumatic or iatrogenic (e.g. tympanostony tube insertion) implantation of squamous epithelium into the middle ear, medial migration of squamous epithelium from the external auditory canal through a tympanic membrane perforation that abuts the external auditory canal, and squamous metaplasia of middle ear mucosa owing to chronic infection. When extensive, removal of cholesteatoma usually requires a combined surgical approach to both the mastoid and middle ear.

Acute tonsillitis

Bacterial tonsillitis is caused by the Group A haemolytic streptococcus. The clinical features include sore throat, fever and systemic upset, inflamed tonsils and cervical lymphadenitis. Bacterial tonsillitis is usually seen in the 4–14-year-old age group. The diagnosis of acute tonsillitis needs to be differentiated from a viral upper respiratory tract infection or pharyngitis and specific viral causes of acute tonsillitis, particularly infectious mononucleosis. Tonsillitis under the age of 4 is usually viral, and a hallmark of this condition is a lack of response to antibiotic treatment.

Bacterial infection can be confirmed by obtaining a throat swab. However, a positive culture must be interpreted in the light of streptococci being cultured from the surface of the tonsil in 10–40% of healthy carriers. Demonstrating a rising streptococcal antibody titre is of no value in acute diagnosis.

Rheumatic carditis and post-streptococcal glomerulonephritis are now rare complications of acute tonsillitis. Treatment of acute tonsillitis generally aims to minimise morbidity and decrease suppurative complications, and is by a 10-day course of penicillin.

Infection may extend beyond the tonsil as cellulitis (peritonsillar cellulitis) or an abscess (quinsy) [Table 14.2]. A peritonsillar abscess requires drainage, which can be performed under local anaesthetic in older children.

Tonsillectomy may be considered for recurrent attacks of acute tonsillitis in children in whom the history of tonsillitis is expected to be one of frequent infections, characterised by significant morbidity, and continuing for a number of years. In short, the cumulative morbidity of acute tonsillitis is anticipated to be far in excess of that caused by tonsillectomy. Pain following tonsillectomy may occur for up to 2 weeks following surgery, and during this period, secondary haemorrhage occurs in 3% of cases. This settles spontaneously in the majority of cases. Immediate postoperative haemorrhage is best treated by return to the operating theatre for haemostasis.

Adenotonsillar hypertrophy (ATH)

Symptomatic enlargement of the adenoids and/or tonsils is commonly seen in children. However, the tonsils and adenoids tend to involute towards the end of the first decade of life. Obstructive symptoms related to ATH may range from simple snoring to severe obstructive sleep apnoea [Table 14.3]. Where parental observation of sleep pattern is uncertain, objective evidence can be obtained by polysomnography (sleep study).

Table 14.2 Signs of quinsy

- Increased systemic symptoms
- Drooling of saliva
- 'Hot potato' speech
- Trismus
- Unilateral bulging tonsil and soft palate
- Fluctuance on palpation

Table 14.3 Symptoms of obstructive sleep apnoea

- Snoring
- Sleep disturbance with laboured breathing and restlessness
- Daytime tiredness
- Episodes of sleep apnoea
- Failure to thrive
- Cor pulmonale

The integrity of the upper airway during sleep, and the severity of obstructive symptoms depend on
- degree of obstruction by the adenoids and tonsils;
- negative pressure generated during inspiration that will collapse the airway;
- neuromuscular tone that serves to prevent airway collapse.

In the presence of ATH, the decision to proceed with adenotonsillectomy depends on the severity and impact of the symptoms, and the likelihood that the ATH will continue in the immediate future. Adenoidectomy alone, which is a significantly lesser procedure, should be sufficient when the tonsils are small and only the adenoids are enlarged. The adenoids can be visualised by flexible nasendoscopy performed under local anaesthetic or by a lateral radiograph of the nasopharynx. Adenoidectomy should not be performed in the presence of a structural or functional abnormality of the palate (e.g. cleft palate), because it may cause velopharyngeal incompetence with hypernasal speech.

Sinusitis

The clinical features of acute sinusitis merge with those of viral upper respiratory tract infection with purulent rhinorrhoea, nasal obstruction, cough and low-grade fever. The diagnosis of acute sinusitis should be reserved for those cases with high fever and purulent rhinorrhoea in excess of 4 days. Sinus CT scans tend to be unhelpful as they are 'abnormal' in up to half of otherwise healthy children.

The organisms causing acute sinusitis are the same as those causing ASOM and a similar antibiotic regime is usually recommended, together with nasal decongestants.

Sinusitis may present with a suppurative complication and be responsible for complications in the orbit and brain. Periorbital and orbital inflammation is usually a complication of acute sinusitis, particularly involving the ethmoids. Periorbital cellulitis is characterised by inflammation of the eyelids and usually settles with antibiotics.

Orbital cellulitis can be distinguished from periorbital cellulitis by the presence of systemic symptoms, chemosis, proptosis, ophthalmoplegia and decreased visual acuity. Spread of infection into the orbit may produce subperiosteal abscess usually along the medial wall of the orbit adjacent to the ethmoid sinus, for which reason a CT scan must be performed in all cases. If there is no abscess, medical treatment should be continued. However, if an abscess is present, surgical drainage is necessary. Central nervous system complications include extradural, subdural and frontal lobe abscesses.

Congenital stridor

In assessing stridor, timing of the stridor is most important. Inspiratory stridor suggests an abnormality at or above the level of the cervical trachea whereas expiratory stridor suggests an abnormality in the thoracic trachea. Severity of the stridor can be judged by the presence of associated laboured breathing and retractions. Long-standing airway obstruction in young children leads to failure to thrive, owing to the increased effort of breathing and poor feeding.

The airway can be examined by transnasal awake flexible laryngoscopy, which provides a view of the upper airway from the nose to the larynx. Radiological imaging by airway fluoroscopy and barium swallow may reveal tracheal collapse or compression. When no diagnosis has been made and the child has significant symptoms, assessment of the upper and lower airway under general anaesthetic by bronchoscopy is required.

The causes of stridor can be classified according to whether they are structural or functional, and by their location [Table 14.4]. Obstruction is usually functional in neonates with the commonest cause of stridor being laryngomalacia, owing to inspiratory collapse of the supraglottis. This presents with low-pitched vibratory inspiratory stridor. Intervention is generally not necessary and the stridor resolves by 2 years. Neonates are obligate nose breathers for the first 3 months of life and nasal obstruction will cause significant upper airway obstruction.

Trauma

Fractured base of skull with temporal bone fracture

A fractured base of skull may present with bleeding from the ear following a head injury. This may also be associated

Table 14.4 Causes of congenital stridor

Nose/nasopharynx	Mucosal congestion
	Nasal stenosis
	Choanal atresia
Oropharynx	Glossoptosis (Pierre Robin sequence)
Supraglottis	Laryngomalacia (neuromuscular disorder)
Glottis	Bilateral vocal cord paralysis
Subglottis	Acquired subglottic stenosis (post intubation)
	Congenital subglottic stenosis
Trachea	Tracheomalacia
	Extrinsic (vascular compression)
	Intrinsic (cartilage softening)
	Tracheal stenosis (complete tracheal rings)

with the leakage of cerebrospinal fluid. Alternatively, blood or cerebrospinal fluid may collect behind an intact tympanic membrane. Temporal bone fractures may cause conductive hearing loss owing to ossicular injury, sensorineural hearing loss and facial paralysis.

Nasal trauma

Nasal trauma, even without a nasal fracture, may cause a septal haematoma that can be recognised as a soft bulge on the septum associated with nasal obstruction. If it is not drained, pain and fever will develop as a septal abscess forms; and the abscess causes destruction of the nasal septum and collapse of the nose.

The nose should be assessed for a cosmetic deformity because of bone displacement once the initial oedema has settled, at around 5 days. Radiology is of no benefit as the decision to reduce the fracture is based on the presence of a cosmetic deformity. Fracture reduction should be performed within 10–14 days of the nasal injury.

Oropharyngeal injury

Oropharyngeal injury typically occurs when a child falls with a stick in the mouth, causing injury to the palate or posterior pharyngeal wall. Initial assessment involves nasal endoscopy under local anaesthetic to assess the integrity of the posterior pharyngeal wall, and lateral neck x-ray to detect any air in the retropharyngeal tissues, the presence of foreign material and any associated cervical spine injury.

Hospital admission is required when there is
- Significant palatal laceration that requires repair.
- Ongoing bleeding.
- Child unable to feed.

- Upper airway obstruction.
- Significant retropharyngeal injury with risk of development of a retropharyngeal abscess.
- Possibility of internal carotid artery damage from an injury immediately posterior to the tonsil. Blunt trauma, which may cause intimal disruption and carotid thrombosis, is as potentially dangerous as penetrating trauma.

Common conditions of the mouth

Mucus retention cysts

Goblet cells in the buccal mucosa may become blocked and form a pale pedunculated retention cyst on the inner aspect of the lip, the gingivo-labial sulcus or the lining of the cheek. They sometimes evacuate spontaneously, but usually annoy the patient, worry the parents and occasionally interfere with feeding. They are best removed if troublesome.

Ranula

A ranula is a larger sessile cyst in the floor of the mouth under the tongue, arising as an extravasation cyst of the sublingual salivary gland. It may become large enough to interfere with speech, swallowing and breathing. It should be deroofed (marsupialised).

Tongue-tie

In tongue-tie, the lingual frenulum is short and may be attached to the very tip of the tongue. Interference with feeding or speech is uncommon, but it may restrict the child's ability to lick ice-cream. When tongue protrusion beyond the lower lip is not possible and is symptomatic, the tight frenulum can be divided under general anaesthesia.

Further reading

Glasziou PP, Del Mar CB, Sanders SL, Hayem M (2004) Antibiotics for acute otitis media in children. *Cochrane Database Syst Rev* 2004, Issue 1, Art. No.: CD000219. DOI: 10.1002/14651858.CD000219.pub2

Lim J, McKean M (2001) Adenotonsillectomy for obstructive sleep apnoea in children. *Cochrane Database Syst Rev* 2001, Issue 3, Art. No.: CD003136. DOI: 10.1002/14651858.CD003136.

Lous J, Burton MJ, Felding JU, Ovesen T, Rovers MM, Williamson I (2005) Grommets (ventilation tubes) for hearing loss associated with otitis media with effusion in children. *Cochrane Database Syst Rev* 2005, Issue 1, Art. No.: CD001801. DOI: 10.1002/14651858.CD001801.pub2

Potsic WP, Wetmore RF (2006) Otolaryngologic disorders. In: Grosfeld JL, O'Neill JA Jnr., Fonkalsrud EW, Coran AG (eds) *Pediatric Surgery*, 6th Edn. Mosby Elsevier, Philadelphia, pp. 813–834.

15 Cleft Lip, Palate and Craniofacial Anomalies

Case 1

A term neonate has a small jaw, wide cleft palate and airway obstruction when supine.
Q 1.1 What is the diagnosis?
Q 1.2 How should this be managed in the next few hours, few days and in the long term?

Case 2

A child is born with a unilateral cleft lip and palate.
Q 2.1 What is the risk of a sibling being born with a similar problem?
Q 2.2 What is the risk if a parent is also affected?

Case 3

An ultrasound at 16 weeks of gestation shows syndactyly of all digits of all limbs and significantly decreased anterior–posterior cranial dimensions.
Q 3.1 What is the most likely cause?
Q 3.2 What are the principles of management?
Q 3.3 Will the I.Q. be normal?

Cleft lip and palate

A cleft lip is a cleft of the 'primary' palate and involves the lip, the alveolus between the lateral incisor and the canine and the anterior portion of the hard palate as far back as the incisive foramen. The cleft results from failure of the mesoderm to merge between the frontonasal process and the maxillary process of the first branchial arch between 4 and 7 weeks of gestation.

The 'secondary' palate forms the hard and soft palate behind the incisive foramen. Palatal clefts are caused by failure of fusion of the two-hemipalatal shelves between 7 and 10 weeks of gestation.

Incidence, aetiology and risk

Congenital clefts of the lip and palate are common malformations. They occur in approximately 1 in 600 live births. A cleft lip, with or without cleft palate (CL ± P) makes up about 70% of patients, and is seen more commonly in boys. CL ± P is more commonly found in Asians and least

Jones' Clinical Paediatric Surgery, 6th edition. By Hutson, O'Brien, Woodward and Beasley. Published 2008 by Blackwell Publishing, ISBN: 978-1-4051-6267-8.

frequently in black races. Cleft palate alone (CP) accounts for 30% of cases, is more common in girls and has no racial differences. CL ± P is a different clinical group from CP. Clefts are inherited in a multifactorial, polygenic way. There is a positive family history in 25% of cases, particularly CL ± P. Where one child already has a cleft, the risk of the second being affected is 2% for cleft palate and 4% for cleft lip and palate. If the parent has a cleft, the risk for their first child is also 4%. The risk increases to 16% if a cleft parent has already had an affected child.

Other associated congenital anomalies may occur in up to 30% of patients and some may be life threatening. One of these is the Pierre Robin sequence that may be present in those with a cleft of the secondary palate. It consists of a small lower jaw (micrognathia), a cleft palate which is usually wide and U-shaped, and the tendency for the base of the tongue to be positioned posteriorly and fall backwards causing obstruction (glossoptosis). The sequence is thought to be caused by early under-development of the mandible causing elevation of the tongue that prevents fusion of the palatal shelves at about 10 weeks of gestation. These patients may have early feeding difficulties, failure to thrive and apnoeic episodes.

A submucous cleft palate is often overlooked. In these patients, the uvula is bifid and the soft palate is grooved in the midline where there is a cleft in the muscle. There is also a palpable notch in the posterior margin of the hard palate. These patients require careful assessment and usually need surgical repair in the same manner as an overt cleft palate. Isolated cleft of the uvula is present in 1 in 80 Caucasians and 1 in 10 Asians and is asymptomatic.

Classification

Clefts of the lip may be incomplete, complete, unilateral or bilateral [Fig. 15.1]. Bilateral clefts need not be symmetrical. Two-thirds also have a cleft of the secondary palate involving both the hard and soft palate posterior to the incisor foramen.

Management

Major clefts of the lip and palate are usually diagnosed prenatally by ultrasound. The parents are usually counselled by an appropriate plastic surgeon and geneticist prior to birth. The proposed management is discussed with the parents as soon as possible and the early explanation and support has made the management far easier than when the diagnosis was only made at birth.

After birth, there is an early neonatal referral to the plastic surgical team who coordinates the patient's cleft care. The deformity affects not only the patient's appearance, but also early feeding, hearing, speech, dental and maxillofacial development. The cleft lip and palate team includes specialists from many disciplines and the care requires coordination.

Children with the Pierre Robin sequence need early careful observation. Difficult feeding, failure to thrive or apnoeic episodes require admission to a neonatal intensive care. Babies who are mildly affected can often be managed conservatively with positional nursing alone until they are more mature. Others may require a nasopharyngeal airway and even nasogastric feeding. More severe cases may need infant mandibular lengthening with distraction osteogenesis surgery. Operations to pull the tongue forward are now rare. Tracheostomies are avoided if at all possible.

Feeding

Sucking is often not difficult for the baby with a small incomplete cleft lip alone. Even though the *Orbicularis Oris* sphincter is incomplete, the babies can often make a lip seal around the nipple. However, babies with clefts involving the palate are unable to close the nasal cavity off from the pharyngeal cavity and cannot generate enough negative intra-oral pressure to gain enough suction. In a majority of cases, these children need to be fed with a squeeze (or gravity feed) bottle [Fig. 15.2] which delivers the milk to the posterior part of the tongue. Once this is done, the babies can swallow normally. There are a number of specially designed teats that deliver milk as they are compressed in the mouth. Parents are educated and helped to find the best feeding regime that suits their particular child.

Cleft lip repair

Repair of the lip is usually performed when the baby is about 2 months old (or 5 kg weight) and the distorted nose repaired at the same time. In patients with severe

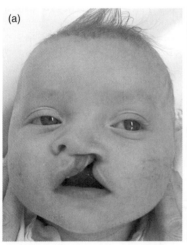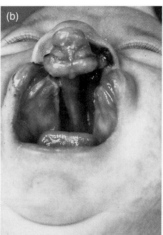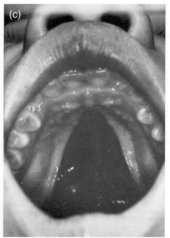

Figure 15.1 Classification of cleft lip and palate. (a) Left unilateral complete cleft lip involving the nose, lip, alveolus and primary palate (b) bilateral complete cleft lip and palate (c) complete cleft of secondary palate.

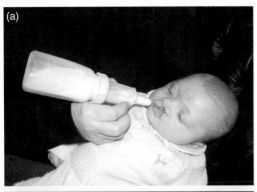

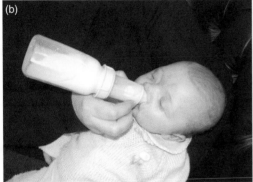

Figure 15.2 Haberman feeding bottle for cleft palate babies.

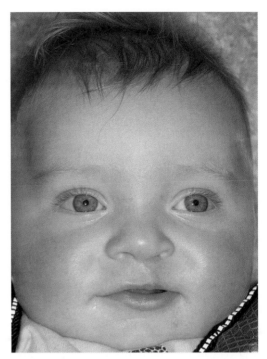

Figure 15.3 Unilateral cleft lip and palate after repair (same patients as in Fig. 15.1a).

bilateral or wide unilateral clefts, presurgical manipulation of the maxillary segments is often attempted by the orthodontist. This makes the surgery easier and often improves the final result. The aim of the lip repair is to obtain a definitive closure of all components of the lip, in particular the *Orbicularis Oris* muscle sphincter. The anterior nasal floor is closed and, if conditions are favourable, the anterior palate may be closed at the initial surgery as well [Fig. 15.3]. With the nose, the distorted lower alar cartilages are properly repositioned.

Cleft palate repair

Clefts of the secondary palate are usually repaired between 6 and 9 months of age (about 8 kg weight) prior to the acquisition of speech. Unnecessary delay in palate repair may affect the prognosis for normal speech as the child develops compensatory speech patterns that are difficult to correct later with speech therapy. The aim of the procedure is to create a palatal mechanism which functions to separate the oral and nasal cavities during speech and swallowing. This usually occurs with a combination of elevation of the soft palate against a constricting posterior pharyngeal wall. The key to the repair is accurate dissection and realignment of the cleft *Levator Palatini* muscles of the soft palate. This usually involves the use of an operating microscope.

Speech

Approximately 90% of patients with cleft palate will achieve normal or acceptable, intelligible speech. Speech should be assessed periodically following surgery. Speech therapy will benefit patients with articulation problems, or those who use compensatory mechanisms to produce certain sounds. Failure of closure of the soft palate to the pharynx (velopharyngeal incompetence) will allow nasal escape of air during speech. Significant velopharyngeal incompetence may require further surgery with lengthening of the palate, posterior repositioning of the Levator muscles and possibly adding local tissue flaps to the posterior palate or the pharyngeal wall (pharyngoplasty). Pharyngoplasty is more likely in patients whose cleft palate repairs were delayed and those who had submucous cleft palates where the diagnosis was initially missed. It is also more likely for children with velopharyngeal incompetence who do not have a cleft but have some form of neuromuscular weakness of the palatopharyngeal sphincter.

Problems in the ear, nose and throat

Children with a cleft palate often have abnormal eustachian tube drainage leading to a high incidence of middle ear mucus build-up and possible otitis media. Some patients will require tympanostomy tubes (Grommets) for middle ear ventilation. The mucus build-up decreases with age and with palate repair. However, hearing may be impaired early on and cleft patients require frequent otoscopic and audiological evaluation.

Tonsils and adenoids occupy a significant space in the pharynx. Their removal is discouraged in cleft patients except when there are severe recurrent infections.

Dental and orthodontic treatment

Virtually all children with cleft lip and palate will require orthodontic treatment in the long term. Early dental care and hygiene is most important. Adult teeth cannot erupt without the presence of bone. The cleft alveolus usually is bone-grafted at some time between 8 and 12 years to allow the proper eruption of the adult canine tooth. Supernumerary or abnormal teeth are seen quite often in cleft patients and may need removal.

When growth is complete, some patients require orthognathic surgery to re-position the hypoplastic maxilla and to obtain a functional and aesthetic dental occlusion.

Secondary surgery

Secondary surgery may be required to repair any bad scars or asymmetries before school. However, with good primary repairs this is now seldom necessary. The nasal deformity has often been dealt with at primary surgery and does not need adjustment for many years.

However, with pubertal growth, the pericleft structures often do not have the same potential for development as the normal opposite side. In addition, with puberty, inherited familial characteristics develop that may accentuate cleft deformities (such as a big nose). At this stage, secondary lip and nose revisions are common. If the central philtrim component of a bilateral cleft appears too short or hypoplastic, it can be rebuilt utilising a tissue flap from the central lower lip (Abbé flap). Orthognathic surgery for final jaw aesthetics and dental occlusion is usually completed after facial growth (about 17 years of age for girls and 19 years for boys).

Craniofacial anomalies

Facial appearance is to a large extent determined by the underlying bony skeleton [Table 15.1]. It is now possible to

Table 15.1 Craniofacial deformity – a classification

CONGENITAL
Clefting disorders
- Cleft lip and palate
- Major craniofacial clefts (Tessier classification including Treacher Collins syndrome)
- Bizarre facial clefts (amniotic bands)
Craniosynostosis (premature fusion of craniofacial bone sutures)
- Non-syndromic (usually a single suture fusion)
- Syndromic (usually autosomal dominant fibroblast growth factor receptor gene mutations. For example, Apert, Crouzon)
Encephaloceles (herniation of the CNS beyond the cranial cavity)
- Failure of anterior neural tube closure
- Some associated with severe major clefting disorders
Microsomias (dysplastic under-development of first and second branchial arch and related structures)
- Usually unilateral; 15% bilateral
Disorders of bone growth
- Fibrous dysplasia; craniometaphyseal dysplasia; neurofibromatosis, etc.

ACQUIRED
Tumour (sarcomas etc)
Trauma
Disorders of growth (e.g. prognathism; condylar hyperplasia)

elevate the soft tissues of the face and orbits in a subperiosteal plane. Similarly, intracranially the dura can be separated from the skull. This then provides a safe method to osteotomise, reshape and reconstruct the craniofacial skeleton. The same techniques can be utilised for congenital deformities, resection of tumours with reconstruction and craniofacial trauma. The principles of exposure and correction are the same but the timing may differ.

Congenital craniofacial deformities
Principles of dysmorphology

Congenital anomalies may result from malformations, deformations or disruptions. Craniofacial *malformations* are the result of intrinsically abnormal development, for example cranial suture synostosis and clefts of the lip and face. *Deformations* are the result of extrinsic compression *in utero*, for example, deformational plagiocephaly. *Disruptions* are the result of an extrinsic disruptive intra-uterine mechanical force, for example, amniotic bands producing bizarre facial clefts (fitting no particular pattern) and constriction ring syndrome.

Cranial growth

The cranial sutures are not centres of growth, but rather 'gaps' that allow the cranial bones to be pushed out by the growing brain. Bony growth occurs secondarily by deposition of bone at the sutures (sutural growth) and at the pericranial surface (appositional growth), as well as absorption of bone from the dural surface. Pathological fusion of a suture restricts growth perpendicular to the suture, with compensatory growth occurring in other non-restricted areas of open sutures.

The growth of the brain and its surrounding cranium is rapid in the first 2 years of life, reaching half-adult size by 9 months and three-quarters by the age of 2 years. In cranial suture synotosis, the ensuing deformity will worsen with ongoing cranial growth in the first 2 years of life. If more than one suture is involved, the volume of the cranium or orbital cavities may be restricted with secondary effects on the brain or eyes. In contrast, in deformational plagiocephaly with an otherwise normal skull and normal sutures, once the deforming force is removed, growth of the brain may be expected to improve the deformity without surgical correction. Disruptions, such as bizarre facial clefts, are not likely to be modified by further growth.

Craniosynostosis

Craniosynostosis is premature fusion of one or more cranial bone sutures [Table 15.2]. The commonest form is fusion of a single suture where there are no features of an associated syndrome. Current genetic testing will not reveal any abnormalities. The suture involved may be unicoronal or bicoronal, metopic, sagittal or rarely lambdoid. With non-syndromic sutural synostosis, there is often some localised pressure on the brain near the suture, but it is uncommon to have generalised raised intracranial pressure (<15%). In general, the more sutures that are fused in the skull, the greater the chance of raised pressure. The aetiology is unknown at this stage but likely to have genetic basis. Rare cases can occur following rapid decompression of hydrocephalus, maternal Epilim ingestion during pregnancy (Fetal Valproate Syndrome), thyrotoxicosis and rickets. If the fused suture is on one side of the head, the head growth tends to be asymmetric leading to plagiocephaly (crooked head). Plagiocephaly can also occur owing to uterine deformational processes without synostosis. Deformational plagiocephaly tends to improve with ongoing cranial growth once the deforming forces are removed [Figs. 15.4 and 15.5].

Table 15.2 Craniofacial deformity – a classification by head shape

Descriptive terminology	Observations	Possible causes
Plagiocephaly	Crooked or twisted head	• Unilateral coronal synostosis • Lambdoid synostosis (rare) • Intra-uterine deformational forces • Torticollis
Scaphocephaly	Long 'boat-shaped' head	Sagittal suture synostosis
Trigonocephaly	Triangular, 'bow-sprit' forehead	Metopic (frontal) suture synostosis
Turricephaly	Tower-like forehead	• Fusion of sutures around the anterior fontanelle (metopic, coronal and sagittal) • Some syndromes; Crouzon, Apert, Pfeiffer
Brachycephaly	Short head (A-P length)	• Bicoronal synostosis (syndromic and non-syndromic)
Kleeblatschadel	Clover-leaf skull	• Multiple cranial suture synostoses (some severe, Pfeiffer, Crouzon, Apert)
Orbital hypertelorism (Tele-orbitism)	Orbits too far apart	• Encephaloceles, median and paramedian • Craniofacial clefts • Some craniosynostoses

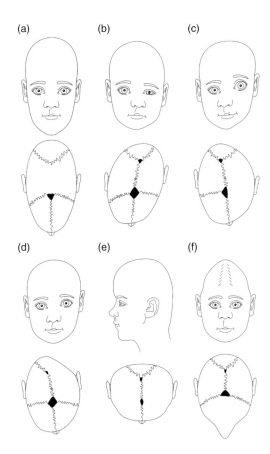

(a)   (b)   (c)

(d)   (e)   (f)

Figure 15.4 Descriptive names are applied to various head-shapes, which do not necessarily reflect the aetiology. (a) Scaphocephaly ('boat-shaped') with fusion of the sagittal suture. (b–d) Plagiocephaly ('crooked head') may be due to deformation (b), unilateral coronal synostosis (c), or unilateral lambdoid synostosis (d). (e) Brachycephaly ('short head') is usually due to bicoronal synostosis, and often seen with Crouzon or Apert syndrome. (f) Trigonocephaly ('triangular forehead') is seen with isolated metopic suture synostosis.

Syndromic craniosynostoses are not so common but are usually autosomal dominant genetic inheritance. The majority of the syndromes have been shown to involve mutations of Fibroblast Growth Factor Receptor genes (*FGFR 1, 2* and *3*). Crouzon, Apert and Muenke syndromes fall into this pattern. Bicoronal synostosis with midface hypoplasia occurs in Crouzon. In Apert syndrome, the synostosis is even more severe and associated with complex syndactyly of the hands and feet. Delays in mental development and the chances of raised intracranial pressure are high. There are many craniosynostosis syndromes and as the knowledge of genetic mutations is increasing, more correlation with the specific phenotypic clinical expressions is expected. A large majority of the syndromic synostoses have associated peripheral limb abnormalities. The incidence of raised intracranial pressure, primary brain anomalies and cervical spine anomalies is also increased.

Craniofacial microsomia

Craniofacial microsomia is the most common encompassing term to describe a spectrum of conditions such as hemifacial microsomia, first and second branchial arch syndrome, Goldenhaar syndrome, oral-mandibular-auricular syndrome, oculoauriculovertebral syndrome and soforth.

Common to all these conditions, there is variable hypoplasia or dysplasia of structures embryologically derived from the first and second branchial arches. Usually there is under-development of the maxilla, mandible and temporo-mandibular joint. In more severe cases, this can be associated with cleft lip and palate and even lateral macrostomia. Epibulbar dermoids may occur with Goldenhaar syndrome and there may be cranial nerve weaknesses, especially the facial nerve. Pre-auricular skin tags, sinuses and external ear deformities are a common manifestation and severe cases may have plagiocephaly and orbital dystopia. Craniofacial microsomias are usually unilateral, but 15% are bilateral.

Encephaloceles

Encephaloceles are congenital herniations of the central nervous system beyond the cranial cavity (see Chapter 12). Sincipital (anterior) encephaloceles usually exit the skull between cranial bone junctions (e.g. fronto-ethmoidal) and are subclassified by where they exit onto the face. A second group can occur in association with severe major facial clefting. Encephaloceles may cause secondary craniofacial deformities such as hypertelorism of the orbits, trigonocephaly and orbital dystopia. About 25% of children with encephalocele have other central nervous system abnormalities.

Facial clefts

Facial clefting is basically classified into three categories: cleft lip and palate (the major group), major Tessier Clefts (relatively rare) and bizarre facial clefting (extremely rare).

The clefting process may range from some mild notching to a complete absence of tissue with an associated encephalocele. Very mild clefts may show subtle signs such

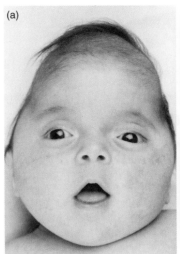
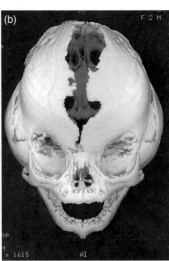

Figure 15.5 An infant with Kleeblatschadel deformity, or 'clover-leaf skull' due to multiple sutural synostosis. This may occur in several craniofacial syndromes, the commonest being Crouzon and Pfeiffer. (a) Preoperative, age 3 months. (b) 3-D CT scan.

as defects in the eyebrows or a widow's peak in the hairline. Tessier's classification [Fig. 15.6] is very useful and the clefts are numbered anticlockwise around the orbit and clockwise around the mouth. The commonest Tessier cleft is midline (0–14 type). This can vary from a mild bifidity of the nose to a complete facial cleft with an encephalocele.

Bizarre facial clefts fit no particular pattern and are thought to be due to amniotic bands in the uterus.

Craniofacial neoplasia

Neoplasia is rare in the craniofacial region in infants. Benign lesions include fibro-osseous lesions and dermoids. Neoplasms are best treated with a wide resection and reconstruction to prevent local recurrence and secondary growth deforming effects. Utilising craniofacial principles, this can be achieved with little deformity to the patient. Ewing's Sarcoma, for example, is treated with induction chemotherapy until maximum reduction in tumour size is achieved. This is followed by craniofacial resection of the remaining tumour mass and reconstruction, prior to maintenance chemotherapy, usually with excellent results. Radiotherapy is avoided in children where possible; it is frequently associated with deforming growth restriction, as well as possible late induction of new tumours.

Trauma

Extensive craniofacial trauma can occur in children. It often results from horse-kick injuries, falls from balconies, bungy-jumping injuries and motor vehicle accidents. Complex fractures are best treated primarily utilising craniofacial techniques, with accurate reduction of fractures, rigid fixation and primary bone grafts as required; the soft tissues are then meticulously repaired and re-suspended to the repaired framework. Secondary deformities, such as enophthalmos, orbital dystopia and subsequent deformities relating to growth (e.g. failure to develop a frontal sinus unilaterally due to a fracture of the fronto-orbital region in childhood) are also best addressed later with craniofacial techniques.

Management of craniofacial anomalies
Conservative management

Children with deformational craniofacial malformations usually improve slowly after birth when the deforming stimuli cease (e.g. deformational plagiocephaly and torticollis). However, the spontaneous improvement is often slow and diagnostic difficulties may arise. Often x-rays and an expertise opinion are necessary to exclude synostosis. With deformational plagiocephaly, mild cases will usually return to normal during childhood. More severe cases will take until puberty to improve. Helmet moulding therapy can speed up the process in early infancy (before 9 months). In rare cases, extremely severe cases of deformational plagiocephaly may require surgery.

Operative management

Patients with craniosynostosis require surgery. This is usually undertaken in the first year of life so that the continuing rapid growth of the brain can be utilised to help attain a normal long-term head shape. The principle of the surgery is to remove the fused suture (s) and to rebuild the affected area of the cranial vault to where it should have

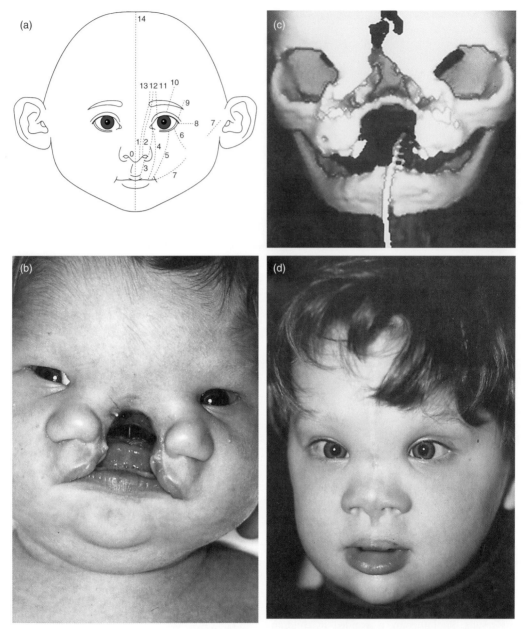

Figure 15.6 (a) The Tessier classification of craniofacial clefts; (b) A patient with a severe 0–14 midline Tessier cleft. (c) 3-D CT scan of the patient (with endotracheal tube *in situ*). The bony cleft continues in the 14 position and hypertelorism of the orbits is demonstrated. (d) Postoperative appearance after complete mobilisation of the orbits and maxillae with midline closure.

been, had the synostosis not occurred. If the craniosynostosis is severe and associated with raised intracranial pressure, then the surgery is urgent. Children with tumours and encephaloceles are often operated on early so as to remove the expanding force of the lesions and return the craniofacial skeleton to a normal configuration.

Most children with craniofacial deformities require monitoring and treatment until their growth ceases as late teenagers. Periodic adjustment surgery may be required during that time and not finalised until adulthood.

Key Points

- Clefts of lip and palate are usually diagnosed antenatally, but if not, need immediate neonatal referral to the plastic surgical team who coordinates management.
- Babies with cleft lip alone can usually breast feed.
- Cleft lip is repaired about 2 months of age (5 kg).
- Cleft palate is repaired about 6–9 months of age (8 kg), before speech develops.
- Cleft lip and palate require team management throughout childhood for ENT, dental, orthodontic, speech and cosmetic management.
- Craniofacial anomalies need early referral to the tertiary centre for multidisciplinary team management, and often early surgery in the first year.

Further reading

Holmes AD, Klug GL, Breidahl AF (1997) The surgical management of osseous cranial base tumours in children. *Aust NZ J Surg* **67**: 722–730.

Holmes AD, Meara JG, Kolker AR, Rosenfeld JV, Klug GL (2001) Frontoethmoidal encephaloceles: reconstruction and refinements. *J Craniofac Surg* **12**(1): 6–18.

Mathes SJ (ed) (2006) Cleft lip and craniofacial anomalies. In: *Plastic Surgery, Pediatric Plastic Surgery*, Vol. IV, Saunders Elsevier, Philadelphia, Ch. 85, pp. 87–88, 90–95.

Mathes SJ (ed) (2006) Pediatric facial fractures. In: *Plastic Surgery, The Head and Neck*, Part II, Vol. III, Saunders Elsevier, Philadelphia, Ch. 67, pp. 381–462.

Thorne CH (ed in chief) (2006) *Grabb & Smith's Plastic Surgery*, 6th Edn. Lippincott Williams & Wilkins, Philadelphia, Ch. 21, pp. 23–26, 28–29.

16   Abnormalities of the Neck and Face

Case 1

Thomas is 2 years old, and was well until 2 days ago when he developed fever and a tender lump under the right side of his jaw.
Q 1.1 What is the differential diagnosis?
Q 1.2 Is surgery required, and if so, when?

Case 2

Anita was first noticed to have a small, hard lump on her eyebrow at 6 months of age. Since then it has grown gradually larger.
Q 2.1 What is the lesion and how is it treated?

Case 3

Ahmed (18/12) is noticed to have a lump under his chin in the midline. It varies in size a little and recently became red and sore.
Q 3.1 What is the differential diagnosis of midline neck lumps?
Q 3.2 What treatment does Ahmed need?

The neck is one of the commonest sites for cystic and solid swellings during childhood. Lesions are either 'developmental anomalies' arising from remnants of the branchial arches, the thyroglossal tract, the jugular lymphatics or the skin; or 'acquired', as in diseases in the lymph nodes, salivary glands or the thyroid gland [Table 16.1].

Branchial cysts, sinuses, fistulae and other remnants

These arise from the branchial arch system. Persisting branchial clefts give rise to an epithelial-lined branchial cyst, branchial sinus (blind-ending tract) or branchial fistula (communication between two epithelial-lined surfaces). The branchial arch itself may give rise to mesodermal remnants, usually cartilaginous, lying along the line of development of the arch.

Sinuses and fistulae most commonly arise from the second branchial cleft, occasionally from the first and

rarely from the third branchial cleft. In second branchial cleft defects, the tract commences in the tonsillar fossa and passes with the glossopharyngeal nerve between the internal and external carotid arteries to end in the skin at the anterior border of the lower third of the sternomastoid muscle. First cleft fistulae run from the external auditory canal to the skin below the lower border of the mandible. The rare third branchial cleft fistula opens internally into the piriform sinus and externally on the skin overlying the lower end of the sternomastoid muscle.

Branchial fistulae usually present in early childhood when a drop of mucus is observed leaking from the external orifice or when a persisting damp patch is noticed on the clothing. Sinuses may be present at any time during childhood and sometimes may be complicated by infection. The treatment for both is surgical excision.

Branchial cysts are uncommon in childhood. They usually arise from the second cleft and emerge from beneath the anterior border of the sternomastoid in the upper third of the neck. They may extend upwards behind the angle of the jaw to the base of the skull or antero-inferiorly towards the midline, lying on the carotid sheath. The fluid contents are milky and contain cholesterol crystals. They may become infected and these cysts should be excised.

Jones' Clinical Paediatric Surgery, 6th edition. By Hutson, O'Brien, Woodward and Beasley. Published 2008 by Blackwell Publishing, ISBN: 978-1-4051-6267-8.

Table 16.1 Swellings in the neck

Developmental anomalies
Branchial cleft: cyst, sinus or fistula
Branchial arch: cartilage
Thyroglossal cyst
Ectopic thyroid
Cystic hygroma
Epidermal cyst
Acquired lesions
Inflammation of cervical lymphatics:
   Acute lymphadenitis
   Atypical mycobacterial lymphadenitis
   Acute lymph node abscess
Lymph node tumours:
   Primary neoplasia
   Secondary (neuroblastoma)
Submandibular gland: calculus
Parotid gland: sialectasis
Thyroid gland: goitre

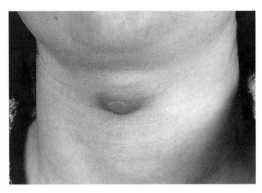

Figure 16.1 Thyroglossal cyst which has become infected.

Branchial arch remnants usually arise from the second branchial arch and present as a skin tag at the anterior border of the lower third of the sternomastoid. These lesions are excised for cosmetic reasons.

Thyroglossal cyst

The descent of the thyroid anlage from the floor of the fetal mouth leaves a track from the foramen caecum of the tongue to the thyroid isthmus. A cyst lined by respiratory epithelium may arise anywhere along the track, but is usually close to and adherent to the hyoid bone (75%). Typically, there is a tense rounded cyst in the midline or just to one side, which moves on swallowing and on protrusion of the tongue. The cysts also may be submental (15%), lingual (2%) and suprasternal (8%) in position. Infection may supervene [Fig. 16.1] and an infected thyroglossal cyst may be mistaken for acute bacterial lymphadenitis in the submental lymph nodes. The thyroglossal cyst and the entire thyroglossal track should be excised, preferably before infection occurs; this excision should include the middle third of the hyoid bone to minimise the risk of recurrence (Sistrunk operation).

Ectopic thyroid

Ectopic thyroid is now a rare cause of midline neck swelling, as it presents as 'low-thyroid function' on neonatal

screening. The swelling tends to be softer than that of a thyroglossal cyst but the diagnosis may not be apparent until at operation, when the lesion is found to be solid and vascular. If this lesion is suspected preoperatively, a thyroid isotope scan should be performed to determine the distribution of all functioning thyroid, because the ectopic thyroid may be the only functioning thyroid tissue present. In this situation, it is not excised: the mass is divided in the midline and rotated on its vascular pedicle laterally to lie behind the strap muscles. Other thyroid swellings in children are rare. Neonatal goitre may result from excessive maternal iodine ingestion. Thyrotoxicosis is rare in young children. Adenoma and papillary carcinoma are seen occasionally in older children.

Cystic hygroma

A cystic hygroma is a hamartoma of the jugular lymph sacs. It presents in infancy and is more common in boys than girls [Fig. 16.2]. Cystic hygromas are of two types: either a simple or multicystic lesion merely compressing adjacent structures; or a complex lesion which infiltrates other structures including the mouth, pharynx, larynx or mediastinum, and which may contain cavernous haemangiomatous elements. This type resembles lymphangiomas found elsewhere in the body.

Simple cystic hygromas are more common, and are usually found as unilateral fluctuant, transilluminable swellings centred on the anterior triangle. The cysts are of varying sizes and contain clear fluid (lymph). They may enlarge suddenly and rapidly owing to viral or bacterial infection or haemorrhage. The effect of this will depend on the site and size of the cysts. A clinical emergency may arise if the increased swelling compromises the airways.

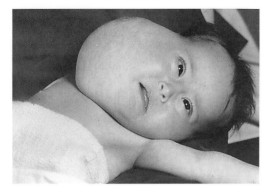

Figure 16.2 Cystic hygroma in a baby with Down syndrome.

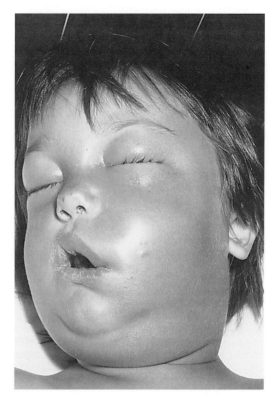

Figure 16.3 Periorbital cellulitis: sinusitis is the common source of infection.

In the absence of these complications, surgical excision or injection of sclerosant is undertaken for cosmetic reasons and the prognosis is good.

Complex cystic hygromas are less common, and complications arise because of extensive soft-tissue involvement. These malformations may involve either the oropharynx, leading to difficulty with speech and swallowing, or the larynx and trachea, leading to a life-threatening respiratory obstruction. Involvement of the mediastinum and pleural cavity similarly may lead to respiratory embarrassment. They present on the first day of life and emergency care may necessitate insertion of an endotracheal tube, and sometimes a tracheostomy. The baby should be referred for assessment by a multidisciplinary team (Vascular Anomalies Clinic). Surgical excision may be undertaken relatively early, and involves debulking the extensive lesion. Injection of sclerosing agents is useful in some cases.

Epidermoid cysts

Inclusion dermoids arise from ectodermal cells detached during fetal growth. They are often in the midline or along lines of fusion, for example, the midline cervical dermoid that may be mistaken for a thyroglossal cyst. They contain sebaceous 'cheesy' material surrounded by squamous epithelium. They enlarge slowly and should be removed. The commonest inclusion dermoid is the external angular dermoid at the orbital margin (see below).

Less common varieties include the sublingual dermoid which lies between the mylohyoid and genioglossus muscles in the floor of the mouth. It may interfere with speech and swallowing and can be excised through a

submental incision. It may be confused with a ranula or mucocele of the floor of the mouth, a lesion which contains mucus.

A rare developmental anomaly found in this region is the midline cervical cleft, a vertical open groove that results from failure of fusion of the branchial arches. Surgical repair should be undertaken.

Periorbital cellulitis

Infection in the soft tissues and sinuses around the eye can cause periorbital cellulitis with rapid extension across the face [Fig. 16.3]. The danger with this infection is that it may spread to the cavernous sinus, which is potentially lethal. Children with periorbital cellulitis should be admitted to hospital for ophthalmology assessment and treatment with intravenous antibiotics (see Chapter 13), and may need ENT opinion regarding drainage of pus from the orbital cavity (see Chapter 14).

Diseases of the lymph nodes

Infection is the commonest cause of lymph node enlargement in childhood. It may be caused by bacteria, viruses or non-tuberculous mycobacteria. In many cases, the lymph nodes are reacting to an upper respiratory tract or ear infection; this is known as non-specific reactive hyperplasia. Lymph nodes also may become enlarged because of primary or secondary malignancy. A surgical biopsy is indicated when the diagnosis is in doubt or if persistently enlarged lymph nodes (>3 cm) are present for longer than 4–6 weeks.

Reactive hyperplasia

Persistently, enlarged lymph nodes are seen in many children with frequent upper respiratory tract infections. These nodes are not painful and are a normal response to infection. Occasionally, a markedly enlarged hyperplastic node (>3 cm) may come to excision biopsy to exclude tumour or other diagnoses.

Acute lymphadenitis

Acutely tender enlarged lymph glands are commonly seen during upper respiratory tract infections. Lymphadenitis usually settles with rest, analgesia and – if bacterial infection is suspected – antibiotics.

Acute lymph node abscess

Lymphadenitis may progress to an abscess, particularly in children aged 6 months to 3 years. The swelling enlarges over 3 or 4 days and may become fluctuant. An abscess in deeper nodes may not exhibit fluctuation. The overlying skin eventually becomes red and, if untreated, the abscess will finally point and discharge. The management of an abscess in a child is incision and drainage under general anaesthesia. Damage to the mandibular branch of the facial nerve must be avoided when submandibular abscesses are incised.

Atypical mycobacterial adenitis

M.avium-intracellulare, *M. scrofulaceum*, *M. fortuitum* and *M. chelonei* cause chronic cervical lymphadenitis and 'collar stud' abscesses in children. In most Western countries, Human TB and Bovine TB strains have been nearly eradicated. However, mycobacterial lymphadenitis is still a problem in the preschool children. The atypical mycobacteria are found in the soil and infection is from the child's dirty hand to the mouth and then to the tonsillar or parotid lymph node. Initially the node is enlarged and

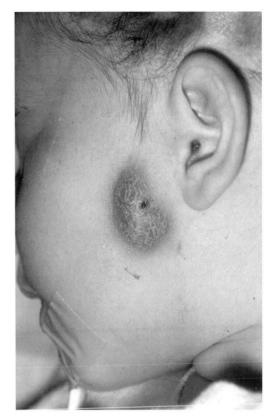

Figure 16.4 Atypical mycobacterial 'cold' abscess.

firm, but non-tender. Over a period of 4–6 weeks, the node produces a collar stud abscess in the subcutaneous tissue causing the overlying skin to become a characteristic blue-purple colour [Fig. 16.4]. Untreated, the collarstud 'cold' abscess will ulcerate through the skin and lead to multiple discharging sinuses. Atypical mycobacteria respond poorly to antibiotics and require surgical excision to remove the infected lymph nodes. The mandibular branch of the facial nerve may be at risk during excision of an affected jugulodigastric lymph node. The diagnosis of atypical lymphadenitis is confirmed by histological examination of the lymph node and culture of the pus and lymph node tissue.

Lymph node tumours
Primary neoplasia

Hodgkin's and non-Hodgkin's lymphomas may occur in cervical lymph nodes in older children.

Secondary neoplasia

Nasopharyngeal and thyroid tumours and neuroblastoma may present with cervical node enlargement. In most cases, the marked enlargement and rocky hardness of the lymph nodes makes the diagnosis of neoplasia obvious. In other circumstances, the differential diagnosis between a large hyperplastic lymph node and a neoplastic node is difficult and necessitates excision biopsy.

The submandibular gland

The commonest cause of enlargement is a small calculus in the submandibular duct. It produces rapid and painful enlargement of the gland during eating. The gland becomes hard and tender and fluctuates in size. The submucous part of the duct in the floor of the mouth should be inspected for a tiny calculus impacted near the orifice under the tongue. An x-ray of the floor of the mouth may show an opaque calculus which is too small or too proximal to be seen with the naked eye. The submandibular calculus can be removed by simple incision of the duct.

The parotid gland

Recurrent enlargement is common in the parotid gland and is due to recurrent parotitis associated with sialectasis, a condition analogous to bronchiectasis, which affects the lesser ducts and their tributaries. Parotid calculi are extremely rare.

Symptoms of sialectasis usually commence at 2–4 years of age, and the first attack may be misdiagnosed as mumps, although both sides are seldom swollen at the same time. One or both parotids are affected and the attacks are unilateral or alternate from side to side. The gland becomes generally enlarged and mildly tender: fever and malaise are mild or absent.

Purulent fluid issues from the orifice when the duct is compressed, and *Streptococcus viridans* or other weakly pathogenic organisms may be found on culture. The attacks are self-limiting and last 3–4 days, but the symptoms may persist intermittently for several years.

The diagnosis is clinical and with ultrasonography. However, if a sialogram is performed, it will show a snowstorm of sacculations 2–4 mm in diameter along the radicles of the gland [Fig. 16.5] but no duct obstruction. The changes are often present in both glands, even when the symptoms have been confined to one side.

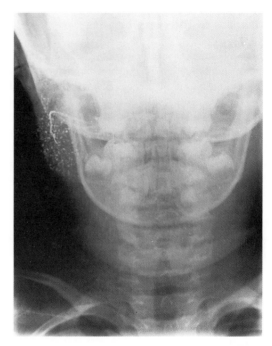

Figure 16.5 Sialogram showing sialectasis. A contrast x-ray of the parotid duct showing a 'snowstorm' of saccular dilatations of the lesser ducts in the enlarged parotid.

The condition is self-limiting and treated by massage of the parotid, tart drinks to promote the flow of saliva and chewing gum. Most children improve by about 10 years of age, and sialograms during adolescence often show that the sialectasis has disappeared. Parotidectomy is not necessary.

Torticollis

The common causes of torticollis in infants and children are, in order of frequency:

1 fibrosis in the sternomastoid muscle;
2 postural torticollis (a legacy of the position *in utero*);
3 cervical hemivertebrae;
4 imbalance of the ocular muscles.

Postural torticollis is present from birth and disappears in a few months. Similarly, the associated plagiocephaly (Chapters 12 and 15) and scoliosis, do not require treatment, for they are caused by intra-uterine moulding.

Cervical hemivertebrae produce a mild angulation of the head and neck. The cause is readily seen in x-rays, which should be taken in all cases of torticollis where the sternomastoid muscle is not tight. No treatment is necessary, for the degree of torticollis is mild and the course is not progressive.

Ocular torticollis is not detectable until the age of 6 months and is usually not noticed until the child is at least 1 or 2 years old. Strabismus suggests that this is the cause, but it is not always obvious and may be latent or intermittent. An ocular imbalance is the most likely cause of torticollis in a child without hemivertebrae, with normal sternomastoid muscles and a full normal range of passive rotation (i.e. the chin can be made to touch each acromion). Treatment is the correction of the imbalance by adjusting the attachment of the eye muscles to the globe.

Sternomastoid fibrosis

This is found in two groups of patients:
1 Infants 2–3 weeks old present with a localised swelling in one sternomastoid muscle, that is, a sternomastoid 'tumour' [Fig. 16.6].
2 Older children present with torticollis and a tight, short fibrous sternomastoid muscle. Rotation of the head towards the affected side is limited, growth of the face on the side of the affected muscle is reduced (hemihypoplasia of the face, Fig. 16.7) and the ipsilateral trapezius muscle is wasted.

The aetiology is unknown, but prenatal or perinatal trauma is suspected in some cases. On histology, there is endomysial fibrosis around individual muscle fibres, which undergo atrophy.

Clinical features

The 'tumour' is so characteristic that it is diagnostic; a hard, painless spindle-shaped swelling 2–3 cm long in the substance of the sternomastoid muscle. Sometimes the fibrosis may affect the whole length of the muscle.

Angulation of the head is not always present, and the infant can turn the head towards the opposite side without angulation. Plagiocephaly [Chapters 12 and 15] is evident in the first 3 months of life as a result of this preferred position, and can be limited by putting the infant down to sleep on each side in turn.

Hemihypoplasia of the face [Fig. 16.7] describes the decreased growth of one side which may occur as a non-specific result of any type of immobilisation and is not directly attributable to fibrosis in the sternomastoid.

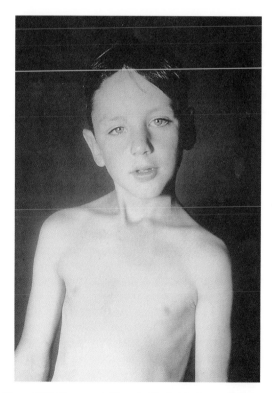

Figure 16.7 Sternomastoid torticollis. A tight (scarred) right sternomastoid muscle is apparent with secondary hypoplasia of the right side of the face.

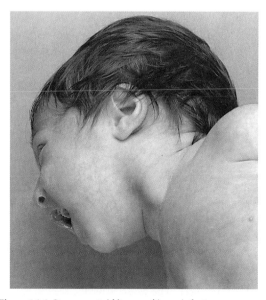

Figure 16.6 Sternomastoid 'tumour' in an infant.

Treatment

Babies with a sternomastoid 'tumour' should be managed non-operatively, because in 90% it will subside completely in 9–12 months.

In the remaining cases, the fibrosis causes permanent muscle shortening and persistent torticollis. Division of the sternomastoid muscle is indicated if there is persistent torticollis after the age of 12 months or hemihypoplasia of the face. The symmetry of the face improves after operation, but may take several years, and probably never recovers completely.

Developmental anomalies of the face

External angular dermoid

This is a common anomaly of fusion between the fronto-nasal and maxillary processes during formation of the head and face (Chapter 12). The cyst is noticed in infancy as it enlarges gradually and progressively [Fig. 16.8].

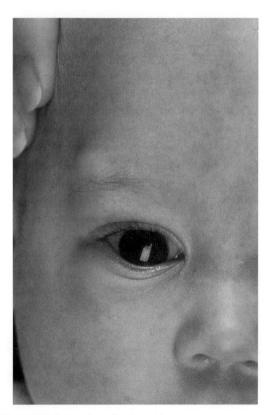

Figure 16.8 External angular dermoid.

Often it is beneath the pericranium, which gives it a firmer consistency than may be expected. Occasionally, it is misdiagnosed as a bony lump. Excision through a small eyebrow incision is curative.

Many varieties of facial clefts have been described and classified, but most of them are rare. Cleft lip and palate, by contrast, are very common. Clefts are described in Chapter 15.

Microsomia

Malformations of the structures derived from the first pharyngeal arch may cause microstomia, a misshapen ear, absence of the external auditory canal, a rudimentary middle ear, hypoplasia of the mandible and its teeth, hypoplasia of the malar-maxillary complex and, sometimes, facial paralysis. The condition may be bilateral.

Children with Treacher–Collins syndrome have bilateral absence of the malar bone, microtia, colobomata of the eyelids and hypoplasia of the masseter and temporalis muscles. Complex defects of the facial skeleton such as this are managed by craniofacial surgery (Chapter 15).

Deformities of the ear

Accessory auricles

Small tags of skin and cartilage may be present, usually close to the tragus, but sometimes along a line extending to the angle of the mouth. They are removed for cosmetic reasons.

Pre-auricular sinus

This is a common condition (1/50 in children of Asian origin), often bilateral and asymptomatic. There is a tiny hole just in front of the upper crus of the helix, from which an epithelial track extends deeply forwards. The track is often short, but sometimes extends deeply towards the pharynx and is extremely difficult to trace among the important structures in this area.

Where there are no symptoms or only an occasional bead of watery discharge, it is best left alone. If it becomes infected with purulent discharge and the opening becomes sealed, a large abscess may develop. In such cases, the abscess should be deroofed and the sinus excised, which is curative.

Microtia

A rudimentary ear of irregular skin and cartilage is associated with absence of the external auditory canal, a rudimentary middle ear and a small mandible on the same side [Fig. 16.9]. When the site of the ear is acceptable, it can be used as the basis for reconstruction, which is preferable to an artificial prosthetic ear.

Only when the condition is bilateral is it necessary to create an external auditory canal and it is important to provide a hearing aid within the first few months of life to enable the infant to hear and develop speech. Further operations are required in later years.

Bat ears

Bat ears, both unilateral and bilateral, are common and often familial [Fig. 16.10]. The concavity of the concha

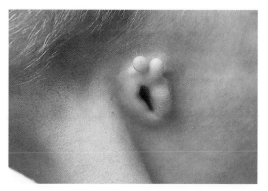

Figure 16.9 Microtia, associated with a maldevelopment of the dorsal ends of the first and second branchial arches. The external auditory canal is a shallow pit.

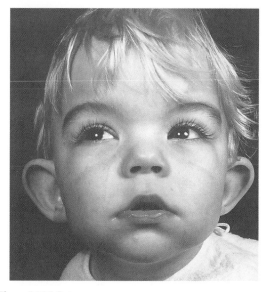

Figure 16.10 Bat ears.

extends to the rim which stands out farther than normal. The ear is often bigger than normal, as well as more protruberant.

Corrective surgery is advisable when there is gross protrusion, particularly when there are adverse comments from other children. Strapping in the neonatal period achieves nothing, and removal of skin from the post-auricular groove is inadequate. The fold of the antihelix must be fashioned, shaping and fixing the cartilages in a new relationship, and holding them in position for the approximately 3 weeks required for union of the cartilages. Surgery can be done any time after infancy.

'Shell' ears

Shell ears are similar to bat ears in protruding from the scalp, but they are small, and the rim of the helix is so short that the ear cannot be readily folded back into the normal position. Surgical repair usually has to be done in stages and is much more difficult than in bat ears.

Key Points

- Thyroglossal cyst presents as a midline neck lump fluctuating in size with inflammation.
- Cystic hygroma is a congenital anomaly of the jugular lymph sacs that frequently become infected. Early referral to a 'Vascular Anomalies Clinic' is recommended.
- Acquired neck lumps need excision biopsy if >3 cm in diameter and present for more than 4–6 weeks.
- Sternomastoid fibrosis with torticollis may need surgery to prevent facial asymmetry.
- External angular dermoids require excision.

Further reading

Beasley SW (2006) Torticollis. In: Grosfeld JL, O'Neill JA Jnr., Fonkalsrud EW, Coran AG (eds) *Pediatric Surgery*, 6th Edn. Mosby Elsevier, Philadelphia, pp. 875–882.

Smith CD (2006) Cysts and sinuses of the neck. In: Grosfeld JL, O'Neill JA Jr., Fonkalsrud EW, Coran AG (eds) *Pediatric Surgery*, 6th Edn. Mosby Elsevier, Philadelphia, pp. 861–874.

Abdomen

17 The Umbilicus

Case 1

The baby appeared quite normal at birth. The umbilical cord became desiccated and detached at 1 week, and a few weeks later the mother noticed an intermittent swelling at the umbilicus, covered with skin. It became quite large on crying, making the parents concerned about rupture. The lump often gurgled if compressed, but did not seem to upset the infant.

Q 1.1 Is this lesion dangerous, and what is its natural history?

Q 1.2 Is surgery needed?

Q 1.3 Why is there a hole in the abdominal wall?

Case 2

A week or two after separation of the cord stump, the umbilicus is still slightly red and damp. Despite careful drying the dampness persists and, at 6 weeks, a cherry-red mass is seen protruding from the umbilical scar.

Q 2.1 Why is this occurring and how is it treated?

Case 3

A 6-year-old boy presents with a small, mildly tender lump 5 cm above the umbilicus. He has a long history of recurrent epigastric pains, particularly after meals. Mother first noticed the lump in infancy but did not seek attention, as it appeared to be harmless.

Q. 3.1 What are the contents of the lump?

Q 3.2 Is it dangerous?

Q 3.3 Does it need treatment?

Embryology

Prior to birth, two umbilical arteries (branches of the internal iliac arteries) and one umbilical vein (via the falciform ligament and ductus venosus) form the umbilical cord. Vestigial connections between the midgut and yolk sac (vitello-intestinal duct), and between the bladder and allantois (urachus) may persist. After birth, the cord desiccates and separates, and the umbilical ring closes. Delayed contraction of the fibromuscular ring of the umbilicus allows the peritoneum and abdominal contents to bulge through the defect. Residual necrotic tissue from the cord stump may be colonised by bacteria to produce a low-grade, subacute infection leading to granulation tissue formation. Gaps in the criss-crossing fibres of the linea alba superior to the umbilicus may allow extraperitoneal fat to protrude, causing an epigastric hernia. When the gap is immediately adjacent to the umbilical scar, it may contain a peritoneal sac.

Failure of normal folding of the embryo to produce the umbilical ring, or persistence of the physiological hernia, may produce the more serious but rare conditions of exomphalos and gastroschisis [see Chapter 8]. The variety of umbilical abnormalities that can occur is summarised in Table 17.1.

Umbilical hernia

Some degree of umbilical herniation is present in almost 20% of newborn babies: still more in premature infants, or when there is any increase in intra-abdominal pressure, as in ascites, Down syndrome or cretinism. Because the anomaly occurs after involution of the umbilical cord, associated anomalies are rare, and the hernia is covered by skin.

While the infant lies quietly, the umbilical skin merely looks redundant, but on crying or straining, bowel fills

Jones' Clinical Paediatric Surgery, 6th edition. By Hutson, O'Brien, Woodward and Beasley. Published 2008 by Blackwell Publishing, ISBN: 978-1-4051-6267-8.

Table 17.1 Abnormalities of the umbilicus

Skin covered swelling	Umbilical hernia
Large membrane covered swelling	Exomphalos (or omphalocele)
Uncovered bowel protruding at birth	Gastroschisis
Infection of cord stump	Omphalitis
Mucus discharge	Umbilical granuloma
	Ectopic bowel mucosa
Air and faecal discharge	Patent vitello-intestinal (omphalomesenteric) tract
Urine discharge	Patent urachus

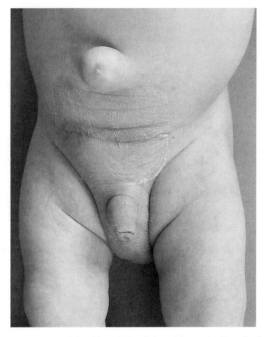

Figure 17.1 Umbilical hernia in a baby with repaired inguinal hernias.

the hernia and the lesion enlarges to become tense and bluish beneath the thin shiny skin [Fig. 17.1]. The bowel can be reduced easily, often with an audible gurgle.

Most umbilical hernias close spontaneously. However, there are several practical points that must be explained to the parents:

1 The time of natural closure. In the first 3–4 months of life, the bulge may actually increase a little before getting smaller. Resolution usually occurs in the first 12 months, but may take up to 3 years.

2 The skin never ruptures, and the thin skin of the first 4 weeks gradually becomes thicker.

3 Strangulation is virtually unknown and it is safe to wait. The size and tenseness of the hernia when the infant cries is often interpreted incorrectly as causing pain: umbilical hernias probably are symptomless.

Treatment

For the majority, no treatment is required. The use of strapping is contraindicated because it does not induce closure when this would not otherwise have occurred spontaneously, and because it may cause complications.

Surgery should be considered if the hernia is still present after the age of 3 years. If the neck of the sac is less than 1 cm in diameter at 12 months of age, eventual spontaneous closure is likely. Even if the neck is more than 1 cm in diameter at 12 months spontaneous closure may still occur and surgery is reserved for those that do not resolve, and deferred until after the third year.

Para-umbilical hernia

This is a defect in the linea alba separate from but adjacent to the umbilical cicatrix. Most are just above the umbilicus, rarely to one side or below it. The defect is a transverse elliptical slit with sharp edges, in contrast to the rounded shape and blunt edges of a central umbilical hernia. Spontaneous closure is unlikely and surgery is required in nearly all cases, as an elective procedure after the first year of life.

Epigastric hernia

Extraperitoneal fat from within the falciform ligament may protrude through a tiny defect in the decussating fibres of the linea alba. It produces a lump in the epigastrium that may be noticed incidentally. It may cause recurrent, vague epigastric tenderness or abdominal pain after eating, but often is asymptomatic. A firm fatty swelling is palpable in the midline of the epigastrium usually midway between the xiphisternum and umbilicus. Treatment is by excision or reduction of the protruding fat, and closure of the defect in the linea alba.

Umbilical sepsis

Umbilical sepsis (omphalitis) is a dangerous infection which occurs in the neonatal period in the exposed stump of the cord. The commonest causative organisms are *Staphylococci, Escherichia coli* and *Streptococci*. Consequently, an important aspect of preventive medicine is to keep the stump dry and dressed with antiseptics. In minor infections, the navel is red and swollen with a seropurulent discharge, but responds well to local and systemic antibiotics.

There may be little superficial evidence that infection has spread further through the lymphatics or the umbilical vessels. Septicaemia results when organisms enter the bloodstream through the superficial vessels, or through the recently patent vessels in the umbilicus: the two umbilical arteries retain a lumen for some time after birth and provide a route of infection to the internal iliac arteries. An abscess along this pathway is more common than entry of microorganisms into the circulation or into the peritoneal cavity.

Infection can also travel along the lumen of the umbilical vein to the portal vein and through the ductus venosus to the vena cava. Clinically overt infections in these structures are rare but serious, and latent infection can lead to thrombophlebitis and thrombosis of a segment of portal vein. Portal hypertension ensues with recanalisation and opening collaterals, leading to a cavernomatous malformation of the portal vein (Chapter 26).

The infant with a discharge from the umbilicus

A discharge from the umbilicus may be pus, urine or faeces.

Umbilical granuloma
An umbilical granuloma is a common lesion that presents as a small mass of heaped granulations, accompanied by a seropurulent discharge. It is assumed to be granulation tissue produced in response to subacute bacterial colonization of the cord stump. If there is a definite stalk, it can be ligated without anaesthesia, but if it is soft, deep or too broad, topical application of silver nitrate will enable epithelium to cover the surface and is curative. Sometimes, a small area of ectopic bowel mucosa at the base of the umbilicus has a similar clinical appearance, although tends to be a deeper cherry-red colour.

Ectopic mucosa
Discharge of mucus from the umbilicus may be caused by a small-sequestrated nodule of ectopic alimentary mucosa, which appears shiny, spherical, bright red and situated in the depths of the umbilical cicatrix. Crusts form on the cicatrix and surrounding skin. If it has a small opening on its surface a persistent vitello-intestinal (omphalomesenteric) duct may be suspected and a sinugram is indicated (see below).

Topical application of silver nitrate on one or two occasions is usually all that is needed to remove the alimentary epithelium, which is replaced rapidly by normal skin. Very occasionally, surgical excision is required.

Persistent vitello-intestinal duct
Persistence of the vitello-intestinal (omphalomesenteric) duct is a rare condition where there is ongoing communication between the intestinal tract and the umbilicus, reflecting the embryonic communication between the yolk sac and the midgut that normally disappears at about the sixth week of fetal life. Persistence of part or all of this tract gives rise to a group of lesions that usually present in early infancy, but on occasions are not recognised until some years later [Fig. 17.2].

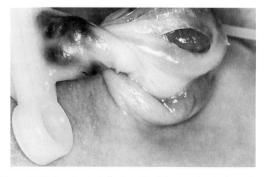

Figure 17.2 A patent vitello-intestinal duct and patent urachus may look similar: the diagnosis depends on whether the discharge is urinary or faecal.

A vitello-intestinal duct represents patency of the whole tract, and the contents of the ileum may discharge intermittently. A small mucosal opening is seen at the umbilicus. Very rarely, when the channel is short and broad, the ileum may intussuscept through it onto the surface of the umbilicus revealing the mucosal surface of the bowel. The Y-shaped segment of bowel, inside out, with two orifices is diagnostic.

A sinus or cyst is the result of partial obliteration of the duct; these may become infected, form an abscess, and discharge pus at the umbilicus.

A vitello-intestinal band is the remnant of the duct and runs from the deep surface of the umbilicus to the ileum. It may cause no symptoms throughout life or it may at any age cause intestinal obstruction when a loop of bowel becomes entangled beneath it.

Meckel's diverticulum is the patent inner segment of the duct, and sometimes it can be attached by a band to the underside of the umbilicus. The presenting features and complications are described in Chapter 23.

All remnants of the vitello-intestinal duct are excised, which may necessitate a laparoscopy or laparotomy to search for discontinuous segments of the tract.

Urachal remnants

Urinary discharge from the umbilicus results from a rare persistent communication through the urachus to the bladder [Fig. 17.2]. In rare cases , a persistent urachus may occur in association with obstruction in the lower urinary tract or with imperforate anus.

The surgical treatment is excision of the urachal remnant after investigation and relief of any underlying anomalies.

More commonly, a urachal remnant presents as a tender mass or abscess in the midline, at or below the umbilicus. The diagnosis is confirmed on ultrasonography. This partly obliterated urachus requires drainage and excision.

Key Points

- Umbilical hernia only needs treatment beyond 2–3 years of age.
- Infection of exposed necrotic umbilical cord stump leads to umbilical granuloma.
- Epigastric hernia contains extraperitoneal fat.
- A discharging umbilicus may indicate a patent vitello-mesenteric duct or urachus.

Further reading

Campbell J, Beasley SW, McMullin ND, Hutson JM (1986) Umbilical swellings and discharges in children. *Med J Aust* **145**: 450–453.

Cilley RE (2006) Disorders of the umbilicus. In: Grosfeld JL, O'Neill JA Jr., Fonkalsrud EW, Coran AG (eds) *Pediatric Surgery*, 6th Edn. Mosby Elsevier, Philadelphia, pp. 1143–1156.

18 Vomiting in the First Months of Life

Case 1

A 4-week-old breast-fed boy was completely well until 2 days earlier, when he began vomiting all feeds. He was otherwise well, and keen to feed despite the non-bile-stained vomiting. He had lost weight and had few wet nappies.

Q 1.1 What physical sign would you wish to elucidate to confirm the diagnosis you suspect?

Q 1.2 If you were unable to demonstrate this sign, what would you do if you still suspected the diagnosis?

Q 1.3 What initial investigation would you perform to assist you in resuscitation?

Case 2

A 9-day-old infant girl suddenly began severe bile-stained vomiting. There were no groin swellings. She would not feed. Earlier, she had been completely well.

Q 2.1 What diagnosis would you wish to exclude urgently?

Q 2.2 How would you do this?

Q 2.3 If this diagnosis was confirmed, what treatment is required, and how urgent would it be?

Case 3

A 3-month-old infant boy was always vomiting, irrespective of how frequently he fed. Initially, he had been breast-fed, but he was now on the bottle, and his grandmother assisted with night-feeds. He was vomiting small volumes of milk. He was not distressed by the vomiting, weighed 8 kg and was growing well.

Q 3.1 What is the most likely diagnosis?

Q 3.2 What measures could be suggested to reduce the vomiting?

Vomiting is common in the first months of life, when the evaluation of its significance is particularly important. The temptation to disregard it must be resisted: it is a symptom, not a diagnosis, and its cause must be established [Table 18.1].

Vomiting is significant when it is

1 bile-stained;
2 persistent;
3 projectile;
4 blood-stained; that is, 'coffee grounds', flecked with altered blood;
5 accompanied by loss of weight or failure to gain weight.

Most vomiting is due to non-surgical conditions or feeding difficulties. Neonatal infections (e.g. septicaemia,

meningitis or urinary tract infection) may present with a variety of clinical features, including vomiting, convulsions, diarrhoea, pallor, cyanosis and hypothermia. Gastroenteritis may be seen in bottle-fed babies, but is uncommon in fully breast-fed infants. In approximately 25% of those with the rare syndrome of congenital adrenal hyperplasia, there is a salt-losing metabolic disturbance with severe vomiting, and genital abnormalities in females (Chapter 10).

Malrotation with volvulus usually presents in the first week or so of life with bile-stained vomiting, but may occur at any age. The possibility of malrotation with volvulus must be entertained in any child with sudden onset of green vomiting. An urgent barium meal will diagnose malrotation if it shows that the duodenojejunal flexure is on the right and below the level of the pylorus. It can also be diagnosed on ultrasonography. If volvulus goes unrecognised, the entire midgut may be lost from ischaemia, because blood flow through the superior mesenteric

Jones' Clinical Paediatric Surgery, 6th edition. By Hutson, O'Brien, Woodward and Beasley. Published 2008 by Blackwell Publishing, ISBN: 978-1-4051-6267-8.

Table 18.1 Causes of vomiting at 1 month of age

Septic	Meningitis
	Urinary tract infection
	Septicaemia
Mechanical	Gastro-oesophageal reflux
	Pyloric stenosis
	Strangulated inguinal hernia
	Malrotation with volvulus
	(bile-stained vomitus)
Others	Congenital adrenal hyperplasia
	Overfeeding

artery is compromised, and the child will die. A child with volvulus needs urgent surgery.

Strangulated inguinal hernias are common in infants, and are easily diagnosed on examination. A hard, tender irreducible swelling at the external inguinal ring will confirm the diagnosis.

Pyloric stenosis

Congenital hypertrophic pyloric stenosis is the most common cause of vomiting that requires surgery in infants, and affects 1:450 children, of whom 85% are boys.

Pyloric stenosis is an important surgical condition in infancy because it is common, there is a risk to life and permanent relief is obtained by a relatively simple operation. The aetiology remains obscure and is partly genetic. Almost 20% of those affected have a family history of pyloric stenosis.

Symptoms
The usual presentation is with severe vomiting, which commences between 3 and 6 weeks of age in an otherwise well baby. Pyloric stenosis is exceptionally rare in infants younger than 10 days, or older than 11 weeks.

The vomiting occurs after all feeds and is copious. The vomitus contains milk with some added gastric mucus, and is practically never bile-stained. It may contain some brown coffee-ground flecks of altered blood, reflecting the gastritis secondary to the gastric outlet obstruction. Often the vomiting is projectile, and may occur well after the last feed. Initially, the child is active and hungry, and a key feature is his readiness and ability to feed again immediately after vomiting. Later, with increasing dehydration and electrolyte imbalance, he becomes weak, listless and lethargic, not unlike the clinical picture seen in a child with sepsis. He loses weight and looks scrawny. If untreated, he may ultimately die of dehydration and metabolic alkalosis.

Signs
Peristaltic waves of gastric contraction indicate hypertrophy of the gastric muscle secondary to slowly progressive obstruction: their observation makes pyloric stenosis likely. Palpation of the thickened pylorus in the epigastrium, however, confirms the diagnosis. The hypertrophic and thickened pylorus is traditionally called a 'pyloric tumour'. It feels like an olive or a small pebble and has been likened to the terminal segment of the little finger. It is relatively mobile. It is palpable most easily in the angle between the liver and the lateral margin of the right rectus abdominus muscle or in the gap between the two recti midway between the umbilicus and the xiphisternum [Fig. 18.1]. It is felt most easily when the baby is relaxed and not crying, and when the stomach is empty. When difficulty is experienced feeling the 'tumour', a nasogastric tube can be passed to empty the stomach.

Failure to palpate the pyloric tumour
If the initial palpation is not conclusive, further observation is necessary and a second examination is made a few hours later. Other manoeuvres which may assist in the palpation of an elusive pyloric tumour are summarised in Table 18.2. When the symptomatology is suggestive of pyloric stenosis but no tumour can be palpated, and

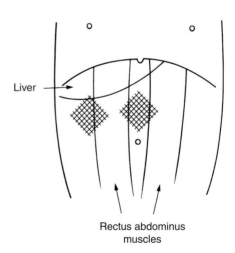

Figure 18.1 Schema showing the two places to palpate a pyloric tumour.

Table 18.2 Tips for palpating a pyloric tumour

1. Get baby relaxed	Be patient
	Palpate gently, avoid hurting infant
	Flex hips
	Wait until crying stops or infant is asleep
	Allow infant to feed or suck dummy
	Palpate at start of feed
	Repeat examination
2. Empty overfull stomach	Pass NG tube to empty stomach
3. Is the diagnosis wrong?	Check for sepsis/inguinal hernia if peristaltic waves are absent and pylorus is not palpable
4. Pyloric stenosis suspected but not proven	Ultrasonography Barium meal

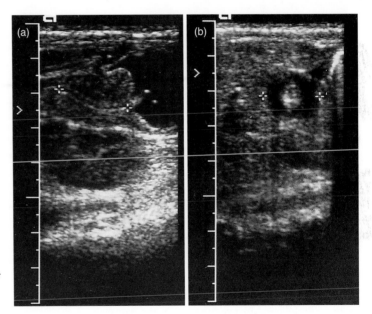

Figure 18.2 Ultrasonographic diagnosis of pyloric stenosis shows the thickened circular pyloric muscle in (a) longitudinal and (b) transverse planes.

septic causes of vomiting have been excluded, a paediatric surgeon should be consulted, and imaging of the pylorus may be required. Real-time ultrasonography may identify the hypertrophied pylorus [Fig. 18.2]. A barium contrast meal performed under fluoroscopic control will reveal gastric outlet obstruction [Fig. 18.3] and may show other pathologies, including gastro-oesophageal reflux, but is not often needed. These investigations are required in a minority of cases only.

The diagnosis may be delayed because vomiting has been attributed to pre-existing gastro-oesophageal reflux (which is present in many infants) or feeding problems. Often, there is a history of several changes in feeding patterns before the diagnosis is made. However, the palpation of a tumour is the *sine qua non* of diagnosis, and excludes all other causes. Other features, such as visible gastric peristalsis and the observation of projectile vomiting, are supporting evidence, but not in themselves diagnostic.

Investigation

The history and clinical findings reveal the degree of dehydration. The extent of the electrolyte and acid–base

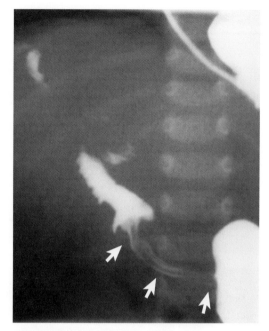

Figure 18.3 Pyloric stenosis demonstrated using a barium meal, showing the 'string sign'. The markedly narrowed pyloric canal (arrows) causes gastric outlet obstruction.

imbalance must be determined to guide appropriate resuscitation before operation. These infants often have a hypochloraemic, hyponatraemic, hypokalaemic metabolic alkalosis. Further estimations of the serum electrolytes and acid–base parameters after resuscitation should confirm complete correction of the electrolyte disturbance before surgery is undertaken.

Treatment

Treatment involves correction of the fluid and electrolyte abnormality followed by pyloromyotomy, the Ramstedt operation. There are numerous resuscitation protocols available, such as intravenous administration of 0.45% sodium chloride in 5% dextrose and supplementary potassium chloride. The rate of infusion is determined after estimation of the percentage dehydration, weight of the infant and maintenance requirements.

The Ramstedt operation can be done through a variety of approaches including a laparoscopic approach, an umbilical incision or a right transverse incision. In each, the hypertrophied pyloric muscle is split longitudinally allowing the pyloric mucosa to bulge through the gap, thus providing a wider channel into the duodenum. The best results are obtained when the muscle split includes

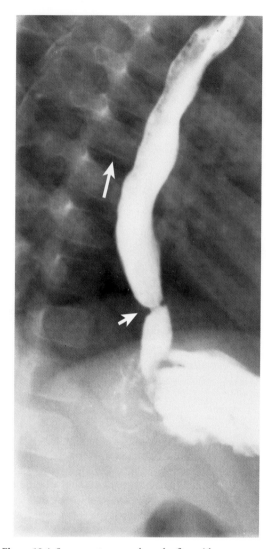

Figure 18.4 Severe gastro-oesophageal reflux with an oesophageal stricture secondary to reflux oesophagitis (arrow-head). The contrast can be seen to flow freely up the oesophagus (arrow).

the distal 1 cm of antrum. Normal oral feeds can be commenced 24 h after operation. The babies rapidly regain their lost weight.

Gastro-oesophageal reflux

Incompetence of the sphincteric mechanism at the oesophago-gastric junction causes vomiting in the neonatal period and tends to become less severe as the infant gets older. Vomiting occurs at any time during or between feeds, and usually is neither projectile nor bile-stained. If oesophagitis is present, bleeding may occur as bright blood in the vomitus, or more commonly, as 'coffee-ground' flecks of altered blood, or be revealed as anaemia. In some infants, severe gastro-oesophageal reflux is associated with repeated episodes of aspiration and pneumonia, or failure to thrive. Occasionally, an oesophageal stricture may develop.

Gastro-oesophageal reflux affects many infants and the diagnosis is made on clinical grounds.

Management

There is a natural tendency towards spontaneous improvement with age. For this reason, the initial treatment should be conservative, with the head of the cot elevated on blocks. Thickening of feeds and the use of mild antacids, such as Gaviscon, and anti-emetics, such as Maxolon, may also be helpful.

In severe cases, where there is evidence of oesophagitis, oesophageal stricture, anaemia, respiratory symptoms or failure to thrive, a barium swallow is advisable to confirm the presence of gastro-oesophageal reflux and to demonstrate any hiatus hernia or oesophageal stricture [Fig. 18.4].

Oesophagoscopy and oesophageal biopsy should be performed if haematemesis has occurred, when anaemia is present or when a barium swallow shows evidence of oesophageal obstruction, to assess the extent and severity of the peptic oesophagitis. Further information may be gained from 24-h pH monitoring and oesophageal manometry.

Surgery to control the reflux is indicated if the conservative regime fails, or if there is an oesophageal stricture or if a large 'sliding' hernia is present. This involves plication of the fundus of the stomach around the lower oesophagus [Nissen fundoplication], a procedure which is usually performed laparoscopically. The oesophageal hiatus is repaired at the same time. Oesophageal strictures secondary to reflux normally resolve spontaneously once the reflux has been eliminated.

Key Points
- Vomiting in babies is significant when it is blood- or bile-stained, persistent, projectile or accompanied by weight loss.
- Bile-stained vomiting in babies without sepsis should be treated as possible malrotation with volvulus, and referred urgently to a surgeon.
- If pyloric stenosis is suspected, the epigastrium should be observed for gastric peristalis.

Further reading

Hutson JM, Beasley SW (1988) Non bile-stained vomiting in infancy. In: *The Surgical Examination of Children*, Heinemann Medical, Oxford, pp. 71–76.
Schwartz MZ (2006) Hypertrophic pyloric stenosis. In: Grosfeld JL, O'Neill JA Jr., Fonkalsrud EW, Coran AG (eds) *Pediatric Surgery*, 6th Edn. Mosby Elsevier, Philadelphia, pp. 1215–1224.

19 Intussusception

Case 1

A 5-month-old boy is brought to you with a 48-h history of being unwell and vomiting. At times, he appears to have been in severe pain. He looks pale and lethargic. There is a vague impression of a mass on the right side of his abdomen.

Q 1.1 What is the likely diagnosis?
Q 1.2 How can the diagnosis be confirmed?
Q 1.3 Once treated, is it likely to happen again?

Case 2

Annabel, a 7-month-old infant, has been unwell for 5 days: she initially seemed irritable, and vomited her feeds, refused further feeds and soon became listless and dry. Her mother measured her temperature at 37.8°C. She has had few dirty nappies and has developed a distended and tender abdomen. There are no hernias.

Q 2.1 What conditions would be there in your differential diagnosis?
Q 2.2 What would be the initial management of this child?
Q 2.3 What is the likely definitive treatment that will be required?

In intussusception, one segment of the bowel (the 'intussusceptum') passes onwards inside the adjacent distal bowel (the 'intussuscipiens'). Once this telescoping phenomenon becomes established, intestinal obstruction follows. Intussusception represents one of the more common surgical emergencies in the first 2 years of life.

Aetiology

In 90% of the episodes, there is no obvious cause (so-called 'idiopathic intussusception'), although in older children, there is more likely to be a pathological lesion at the lead point of the intussusceptum, for example, a Meckel's diverticulum, a polyp or a duplication cyst.

In idiopathic intussusception, which usually affects infants in the first 2 years of life, it is possible that enlarged submucosal lymphoid tissue in the distal ileum (Peyer's patches) has undergone reactive hyperplasia and become the apex of the intussusception. This may be the result of a viral infection. The apex moves through the ileocaecal valve into the colon and occasionally may even reach the anus.

Incidence

The peak incidence is in infants 5–7 months old, and 70% of patients are between 3 and 12 months of age. Boys are affected more frequently than girls.

Clinical features

Table 19.1 presents features of intussusception.

Symptoms

Pain is the most important symptom (85%). It typically commences as a colicky pain lasting 2–3 min during which time the infant screams and draws up his knees. Spasms occur at intervals of 15–20 min. The infant becomes intermittently pale and clammy (similar to a syncopal episode in older children), exhausted and lethargic between spasms. After 12 h or so, the pain becomes more continuous.

Jones' Clinical Paediatric Surgery, 6th edition. By Hutson, O'Brien, Woodward and Beasley. Published 2008 by Blackwell Publishing, ISBN: 978-1-4051-6267-8.

Table 19.1 Presenting features of intussusception

1. Vomiting
2. Abdominal colic
3. Pallor
4. Lethargy
5. Abdominal mass
6. Rectal bleeding

(a)

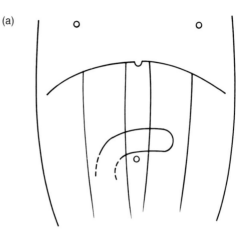

Vomiting almost always occurs as well, usually once or twice in the first hours and then again once the intestinal obstruction is fully established.

Signs

Children with intussusception look pale and lethargic except when they are aroused by a spasm of severe pain. A mass (sometimes described as being 'sausage-shaped') is palpable in more than half the infants and is usually found in the right hypochondrium, although it may be anywhere between the line of the colon and the umbilicus [Fig. 19.1]. The intussusception mass is most likely to be felt early in the course of the disease, before abdominal distension and increasing abdominal tenderness conceal it.

Normal or loose stools are often passed at or soon after the onset of symptoms, and any diarrhoea tends to be of small volume and short duration. About half the patients pass a stool containing blood and mucus ('red currant jelly'), formed by the diapedesis of red cells through the congested mucosa of the intussusceptum. Blood may be identified on the glove following rectal examination in many patients. Rectal examination may disclose the apex of the intussusceptum within the rectum.

The infant is pale, limp and tired, and has a tachycardia. If there is delay in diagnosis, the infant will become dehydrated, listless, and febrile, have abdominal distension and look ill. These are late signs and ideally, the diagnosis should be made before they appear.

Differential diagnosis

Wind colic is common in the first 3 months of life but rarely lasts more than an hour and usually is not accompanied by vomiting. Persisting severe colic for more than 1–2 h should arouse suspicion of an intussusception, particularly if accompanied by vomiting.

Gastroenteritis

Colic and the passage of blood and mucus in severe cases of gastroenteritis may mimic intussusception, except that the volume of diarrhoea is greater. In intussusception, the

(b)

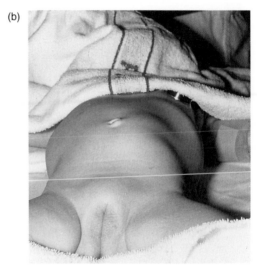

Figure 19.1 The site of the sausage-shaped intussusception in the abdomen, shown schematically in (a) and in a patient (b).

small loose stools passed early in the course of the disease simply represent evacuation of the colon distal to the obstruction. Persistent vomiting and pain without diarrhoea is unlikely to be gastroenteritis.

A strangulated inguinal hernia may present with abdominal pain, vomiting and distension, but is recognised easily when an irreducible lump is seen on examination of the groin.

Investigations

A plain x-ray of the abdomen may be normal, show nonspecific abnormalities, or reveal a small bowel obstruction with air-fluid levels in dilated small bowel. Occasionally, the apex of the intussusceptum can be seen.

The diagnosis is confirmed on ultrasonography and is usually the first investigation when intussusception is suspected [Fig. 19.2]. An air or barium contrast study will also confirm the diagnosis, and can be therapeutic (see below).

Treatment

Enema reduction of intussusception should be attempted in most cases, unless there is clinical evidence of dead bowel as demonstrated by peritonitis or septicaemia. Gas (air or oxygen) is more effective and probably safer than barium, and is the medium of choice if available [Fig. 19.3]. Enema reduction is slightly less likely to be successful if there is a long duration of symptoms (>24 h), outside the usual age range (<3 months or >24 months), or when there is an established small bowel obstruction with air-fluid levels on x-ray. Providing there is no peritonitis it is still worth attempting enema reduction in these children. If the child remains stable clinically after incomplete reduction on a first attempt, a delayed repeat enema 30 min to 2 h later is performed. Possibly, between 80% and 90% of intussusceptions should be reducible using a gas enema.

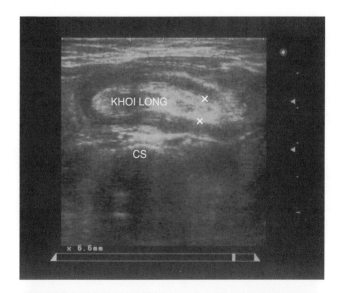

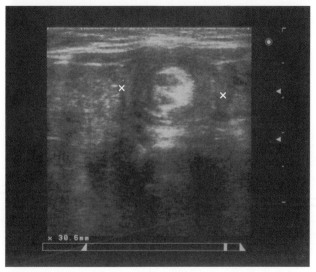

Figure 19.2 Ultrasonography is the first investigation in infants and children who are suspected of having intussusception. Upper panel shows longitudinal view of intussusceptum, while lower panel is a transverse section.

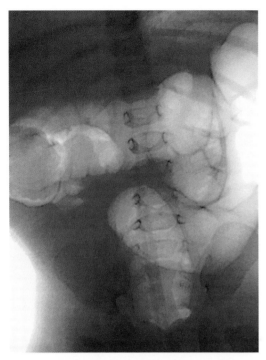

Figure 19.3 Gas enema showing end of intussusceptum, which confirms the diagnosis of intussusception. (Reproduced with permission from Phelan *et al.* [1988] *Amer J Radio*, **150**: 1349–1352.)

Technique of gas enema reduction

The infants should be resuscitated with intravenous fluids and kept warm. A Foley catheter is inserted into the rectum and the balloon inflated. The buttocks are strapped tightly together. Gas (usually oxygen from the wall supply) is introduced into the colon through the catheter, the pressure being controlled by a manometer [Fig. 19.3]. Under continuous fluoroscopic control, progress of the reduction is monitored. Sudden filling of the small bowel with gas suggests reduction is complete. The infant can be fed within hours of the procedure.

Surgery

Surgery is indicated when the delayed repeat enema fails to reduce the intussusception, where there is peritonitis clinically or where there is strong evidence of a pathological lesion at the lead point, for example, circumoral

pigmentation of Peutz-Jegher syndrome. Either laparotomy is performed through a transverse right supra-umbilical incision or a laparoscopic approach can be used. The intussusception is reduced by manipulation, although segmental resection may be required if there is gangrene, or where there is a pathological lesion at the lead point, for example, Meckel's diverticulum or polyp.

Recurrent intussusception

Recurrence of intussusception occurs in about 7% of patients. It is more likely after enema reduction than surgery. It usually occurs within 2 or 3 days of the first reduction. Recurrent intussusception usually presents early and is treated the same way as a first episode. The possibility of a lesion at the lead point should be considered.

> **Key Points**
> - Intussusception should be suspected when infants between 3 months and 3 years present with colicky abdominal pain, vomiting and intermittent pallor.
> - Diagnosis of intussusception is made by palpating a central/right-sided mass, and confirming with x-ray, ultrasound or gas enema.
> - Hydrostatic enema reduction corrects intussusception in about 85%, with 7% risk of recurrence.

References and further reading

Beasley SW, Hutson JM, Auldist AW (1996) Intussusception. In: *Essential Pediatric Surgery*, Arnold, London, pp. 45–51.

British Society of Paediatric Radiology: www.bsps.org.uk/intuss.htm

Doody DP (1997) Intussusception. In: Oldham KT, Colombani PM, Foglia RP (eds) *Surgery of Infants and Children: Scientific Principles and Practice*, Lippincott-Raven, Philadelphia, pp. 1241–1248.

Ein SH, Daneman A (2006) Intussusception. In: Grosfeld JL, O'Neill JA Jnr., Fonkalsrud EW, Coran AG (eds) *Pediatric Surgery*, 6th Edn. Mosby Elsevier, Philadelphia, pp. 1313–1341.

Ong N-T, Beasley SW (1990) The leadpoint in intussusception. *J Pediatr Surg* **25**: 640–643.

Phelan E, de Campo JL, Malecky G (1988) Comparison of oxygen and barium reduction of ileocolic intussusception. *Amer J Radio* **150**: 1349–1352.

20 Abdominal Pain: Appendicitis?

Case 1

Jeremy, a 6-year old, developed central abdominal pain and high fever yesterday. Today he presents with pain in the right iliac fossa. He looks flushed and has tenderness in both iliac fossae (*R>L*), but no peritonism. There is a 'gurgle' on deep palpation.

Q 1.1 What is the likely diagnosis?

Q 1.2 What tests are required?

Case 2

Alex is a 5-year old who has been vaguely unwell with abdominal pain for 2 days. Today he has pain in the right iliac fossa. He limps into the consulting room but does not look flushed, and his temperature is normal (37.2°C). There is tenderness and guarding that is lateral in the right flank.

Q 2.1 What is the likely diagnosis?

Q 2.2 Is a rectal examination necessary?

The knowledge that delay in diagnosis of appendicitis is potentially dangerous has probably been a major factor in reducing its morbidity in children. As a rule, abdominal pain in childhood lasting more than 4 h, should be regarded as evidence of a potential abdominal emergency until proven otherwise. Similarly, diarrhoea lasting more than 24 h, particularly if it is associated with lower abdominal pain, should suggest the possibility of a pelvic, retrocaecal or retro-ileal appendicitis. An illness may start with gastroenteritis and diarrhoea but later appendicitis may supervene. Only a minority of children presenting with acute abdominal pain are found to have a genuine surgical cause. Where there is a high index of suspicion of appendicitis the child must be re-assessed frequently with early referral to a paediatric surgeon.

The interpretation of abdominal pain in children

The interpretation of abdominal pain in small children can be difficult. Significant pain is often recognised late by parents and professionals alike, in large part because of

Jones' Clinical Paediatric Surgery, 6th edition. By Hutson, O'Brien, Woodward and Beasley. Published 2008 by Blackwell Publishing, ISBN: 978-1-4051-6267-8.

children's inability to voice their symptoms adequately, but also because the pain of appendicitis may not be as dramatic in this age group.

An infant, who prefers to lie still, refuses to be cuddled, wants to be left untouched and is reluctant to be examined, should raise concerns, because those factors suggest that movement exacerbates the pain, as in peritonitis.

If abdominal pain is persistent, observation must be continued and re-examination repeated until there are definite signs that indicate the need of surgery, or until the pain has subsided. In most children, whose pain is subsiding, operation should be deferred if the physical signs are not completely diagnostic.

Assessment of physical findings

Examination of the older co-operative child is relatively straightforward, whereas in a young, sick and frightened child, physical examination requires great skill. The examination must be unhurried, gentle, and performed with warm hands. The examiner should be seated beside the child. The child should be supine, straight, and with arms resting alongside. Useful assessment can sometimes be made if the child is asleep when first seen or, in the toddler, if the abdomen is palpated from behind with both hands while the mother cuddles the child's front against her.

However, with a continually crying child, adequate assessment is difficult and re-examination must be undertaken a short time later. Failure to acknowledge inadequate examination may result in serious diagnostic error.

Abdominal tenderness

Localised tenderness is found in conditions ranging from excess flatus, an overloaded colon or inflamed mesenteric lymph nodes, to acute appendicitis and strangulated gut; so that tenderness alone is an insufficient reason for operation. Localised tenderness can be elicited by direct palpation over any distended or inflamed loop of gut. This is a particular feature of the solitary distended loop in intestinal obstruction, but can also be observed in gastroenteritis. Irritated or inflamed visceral peritoneum will produce tenderness by direct, rather than by reflex, pathways.

Localised tenderness in the right iliac fossa, without guarding or a strongly suggestive clinical history, may be due to causes other than appendicitis. Although localised tenderness is often the earliest sign of appendicitis, children requiring operation soon develop guarding to support the diagnosis, whereas tenderness due to non-surgical conditions subsides in 1–2 days.

Guarding

Children with local or general peritonitis rarely display the board-like rigidity so often found in adults. More often, there is a variable degree of involuntary increased muscle resistance referred to as 'guarding'. Small differences in resistance in the lower and upper abdomen, or between right and left sides, may be significant when the findings are consistent.

Assessment of percussion tenderness is a sensitive test of peritoneal irritation in children. Similarly, pain in the abdomen during micturition is common in pelvic appendicitis, where the appendix lies close to the bladder.

There are no pathognomonic symptoms or signs of appendicitis itself, but when signs of peritonitis are localised to the right iliac fossa, appendicitis is likely.

Acute appendicitis may be missed when it presents with signs of local peritonitis other than in the right iliac fossa; the interposition of other tissues between the appendix and the anterior abdominal wall in pelvic, retrocaecal and retro-ileal appendicitis delays the appearance of abdominal signs until relatively late, and even then, they may be atypical.

In retrocaecal appendicitis, tenderness is maximal high and lateral on the right side, whereas in pelvic appendicitis or in retro-ileal appendicitis, the signs are more central and lower and may even be predominantly left-sided.

A palpable mass

Apart from faecal masses and symptomless masses in the loin (Chapter 25), the most common mass in the abdomen in childhood is an appendiceal abscess, particularly in children under 5 years of age, in the mentally handicapped child, or when the appendix is in an unusual position.

Scrotal examination

Torsion of the testis occasionally presents with referred pain in the iliac fossa, and can be mistaken for appendicitis. The scrotum should always be examined to exclude this.

Rectal examination

When appendicitis has been diagnosed on the basis of the history and anterior abdominal signs, a rectal examination is not indicated.

Rectal examination may be helpful in the diagnosis of a pelvis mass with a perforated pelvic appendicitis. However, informed consent must be obtained from the parents and a chaperone must be present. A pelvic mass also may be diagnosed with an ultrasound examination.

Signs arising in other systems

Infections in the ear, the tonsils or the respiratory passages may be accompanied by abdominal pain and vomiting and simulate an abdominal emergency. Measles or chicken-pox may produce abdominal signs, as can a wide range of other viral infections, by causing mesenteric lymphadenitis. Acute appendicitis can coexist with other conditions, so that the finding of pneumonia, tonsillitis or generalised lymphadenopathy, should not divert attention from any other abdominal signs which also may be present. Similarly, gastroenteritis may progress to appendicitis, so that even a well-established and undoubted diagnosis of gastroenteritis should be subject to review. Special diagnostic difficulties can be presented by the abdominal crisis of diabetic acidosis, Henoch-Schönlein purpura and various haematological disorders, including haemophilia – in all of which surgical intervention generally is contra-indicated.

Repeated observation and re-examination for signs of peritoneal irritation is essential.

Acute appendicitis

The mortality of acute appendicitis in children is less than 0.2% due to early diagnosis and the management of fluids and electrolytes before and after operation.

The abdominal findings are the crucial factors on which the diagnosis and the decision to operate is made. The value of history lies in arousing suspicion that an abdominal emergency is present, and in determining its most likely cause.

The clinical diagnosis is determined by the presence of localised tenderness and objective signs of local or general peritonitis. However, acute appendicitis is not only a common abdominal emergency, but also a great imitator, and it may appear in a variety of guises [Table 20.1].

Differential diagnosis

A perforated appendix is the only common cause of general peritonitis in childhood. In most children with an appendiceal abscess, there are signs of local or generalised peritonitis. Occasionally, however, an appendiceal mass may be present with little or no constitutional upset or localised signs of peritoneal irritation.

In acute appendicitis, mild pyuria (20–50 white blood cells/mm^3) may be seen and is due to an inflamed appendix adjacent to the ureter or bladder. Conversely, acute pyelonephritis may be present without pus cells or bacteria in the bladder and this must be distinguished from high retrocaecal appendicitis, in which tenderness often extends into the loin.

Infections in the lower urinary tract, particularly those associated with vesico-ureteric reflux, can mimic appendicitis in the right iliac fossa, but do not exhibit the guarding typical of peritoneal irritation. In pelvic appendicitis, the child may complain of low, abdominal pain during micturition.

Referred pain to the right abdomen may occur with right lower lobe pneumonia or right testicular torsion.

Peritonitis in the young child

Peritonitis is a frequent complication of appendicitis that may be difficult to recognise in infants and young children. Tenderness may be diffuse rather than localised and marked guarding may be absent, even when there is advanced general peritonitis. More often, a lesser degree of involuntary muscular rigidity or 'guarding' is encountered. Differences in muscle tone and the degree of guarding between the right and left sides or between the lower and upper abdomen, are highly significant.

As localised peritonitis progresses, the signs become more definite in the right iliac fossa. Paradoxically, as the

Table 20.1 The variety of presentations of acute appendicitis: presentation and differential diagnosis

Local tenderness in the right iliac fossa	**Local peritonitis [most often in right iliac fossa]**
• Simple colic	• Severe mesenteric adenitis
• 'Bilious attack'	• Primary peritonitis
• Gastroenteritis	• Meckel's diverticulitis
• Acute constipation	• Ruptured luteal cyst, ('apopletic ovary')
• Mild mesenteric adenitis	• Torsion of an ovarian cyst or ovary
• Urolithiasis	• Torsion of the omentum
• Deep iliac lymphadenitis	• Suppurating deep iliac lymph nodes
Generalised peritonitis	**'Urinary tract infection'**
• Primary peritonitis	• Urinary tract infection
• Perforated Meckel's diverticulum	• Acute pyelonephritis
An inflammatory mass	**Intestinal obstruction**
• Intussusception	• Adhesive bowel obstruction
• Duplication of the gut	• Internal hernia
• Ectopic kidney	• Meckel's band
• Retroperitoneal masses (Chapter 25)	
Acutely painful scrotum	**'Gastroenteritis' (from retro-ileal or pelvic appendix)**
• Torsion of testis	• Gastroenteritis
• Torsion of appendix testis	

peritonitis becomes more generalised and the abdomen more distended, the right iliac fossa signs may appear to diminish in some children. In this situation, abdominal distension and reluctance on the child's part to allow palpation of the abdomen are signs of great significance.

Even without distension, however, the persistence of pain, with or without accompanying diarrhoea, demands careful assessment, re-examination of the abdomen and, if required, rectal examination.

Treatment

The management of acute appendicitis involves
1 Adequate preoperative intravenous correction of fluid and electrolyte deficits.
2 Surgical removal of the appendix.
3 Irrigation of the peritoneal cavity to remove pus and contaminated free peritoneal fluid.
4 Effective antibiotic treatment to cover aerobic and anaerobic organisms commencing before surgery.

Fluid and electrolyte deficits are replaced by intravenous infusion, and if there is marked abdominal distension and vomiting, the bowel is decompressed by nasogastric suction. A dehydrated, toxic child with severely depleted fluid and electrolytes is a poor candidate for anaesthesia and operation. Obstruction of the airways by inhaled vomitus, unexpected cardiac arrest and prolonged 'surgical shock' with peripheral circulatory collapse, are less likely if surgery follows fluid resuscitation.

The aim of surgery is to remove the appendix and perform intraperitoneal toilet. The surgery may be performed by either a laparoscopic or an open approach.

Antibiotics are given to reduce the incidence of septic complications of appendicitis and peritonitis. Peritonitis is a polymicrobial infection caused by bowel organisms, so a wide spectrum of antibacterial activity is necessary. A combination of an anti-aerobic agent (cephaloridine derivative) and an anti-anaerobic agent (Metronidazole) is more effective than either alone. Wound infection results from intra-operative inoculation by peritoneal contaminants, and can be prevented by administering the antibiotics before the commencement of surgery.

Abdominal pain of uncertain origin

There remains a substantial group of children [Table 20.1] in whom the final diagnosis of abdominal pain remains in doubt. 'Indigestion', wind pains, acute constipation and other minor disturbances of bowel function, are impossible to establish as objective diagnoses, but are labels that tend to be attached to a number of children.

Perhaps the most troublesome condition is mesenteric adenitis ('non-specific viral infection'), because of the difficulty in distinguishing some cases from acute appendicitis. The combination of high fever, mild abdominal tenderness that varies in location, the absence of guarding and failure of the signs to progress, suggest mesenteric adenitis. A succussion splash in the right iliac fossa (consistent with an ileus) but no peritonism, is typical.

Abdominal emergencies in mentally handicapped children

Acute appendicitis is the commonest abdominal emergency in mentally handicapped children. Impaction, ulceration or perforation of the alimentary canal by an ingested foreign body, is more frequent than in children of normal intelligence.

The degree of difficulty in diagnosis is dependent on the severity of the mental handicap. In the most severely affected children, with hyperkinesia, hypertonia, inability to speak and a high threshold of pain, there may be few symptoms, and abdominal signs – for example tenderness or rigidity – may be difficult to detect or evaluate. Distension and the absence of bowel sounds although late developments, are usually present when attention is first drawn to the abdomen. Vomiting, fever and tachycardia may also be present.

As in normal children less than 5 years of age, appendicitis in mentally retarded children has frequently progressed to a local abscess or to spreading peritonitis by the time the diagnosis is made. A pelvic mass or, signs of intestinal obstruction from small bowel adhesions to the wall of an appendiceal abscess are common.

The delay in diagnosis leads to an increase in the incidence of complications and consequently, an increase in mortality.

Intestinal obstruction

A common cause of intestinal obstruction is strangulation of an inguinal hernia [Table 20.2] which, if recognised, presents few problems in diagnosis or management.

In children who have not had a previous abdominal operation, the cause of the obstruction may be a volvulus (Chapter 7), Meckel's band or diverticulum (Chapter 23),

Table 20.2 Causes of bowel obstruction in children beyond the neonatal period

Common	• Strangulated inguinal hernia
	• Intussusception
	• Appendicitis
Uncommon	• Adhesive bowel obstruction
	• Malrotation with volvulus
	• Meckel's band (closed-loop obstruction or localised volvulus)
	• Duplication cyst
	• Internal hernia

a duplication (Chapter 7) or very rarely, an internal hernia [see Table 20.2].

Most cases of obstruction in older children are due to bands or adhesions following a previous abdominal operation. Recurrent pain, accompanied by bilious vomiting, generally causes these patients to present early. Clinical evidence of distended loops of gut, either visible and palpable, or as air-fluid levels in an x-ray of the abdomen, will confirm the diagnosis.

Bowel obstruction is less obvious and more likely to be overlooked in the following cases:

1 In the early postoperative period after abdominal surgery, when pain is difficult to interpret and delay in recovery from paralytic ileus may mask the presence of an early fibrinous obstruction from adhesions.

2 In children in whom vomiting alone is the presenting feature of a high small bowel obstruction in which pain and abdominal distension may be absent.

Treatment

Oral fluids are withheld, the stomach is aspirated by a nasogastric tube, and intravenous fluid and electrolytes are commenced. Some children respond promptly to this regimen and the symptoms and signs subside within a few hours.

Continuing or increasing volumes of aspirate or persistent localised abdominal tenderness are sufficient grounds for laparotomy, preferably before a rising pulse rate, severe pain and increasing abdominal tenderness suggest impending strangulation of a loop of bowel.

Meckel's diverticulum

The tip of a Meckel's diverticulum may be joined to the umbilicus by a long thin band that can entrap and

obstruct the bowel: the child may develop a closed loop obstruction or a localised volvulus. Finally, a Meckel's diverticulum may become inflamed.

A Meckel's diverticulum is the commonest cause of major gastrointestinal bleeding in childhood (Chapter 23) and is evident when the child passes red brick stools, usually in association with dull abdominal pain and tenderness. Often the child looks pale and anaemic. A Meckel's diverticulum may also be suspected before operation in intestinal obstruction in a child who has not undergone a previous abdominal operation. The clinical manifestations are indistinguishable clinically from appendicitis, and the true diagnosis only becomes apparent at operation.

Primary peritonitis

Primary peritonitis presents with a sudden onset of high fever >39°C with diffuse abdominal distension and tenderness with guarding. This is a primary infection of the peritoneum and the abdominal contents are 'normal'.

The condition is more common in girls but often it is not related to tubal infection. Laparotomy/laparoscopy is performed as the presumed clinical diagnosis is appendicitis with secondary peritonitis. At laparotomy/laparoscopy odourless peritoneal fluid with a 'soapy' feel is found and a normal appendix is usually removed. Sometimes the infecting organism is *Streptococcus pyogenes*, but in most cases nothing is grown on culture. The prognosis is good and the peritonitis resolves rapidly.

Paediatric gynaecologic emergencies

In menarchal or pubertal girls, a gynaecologic disorder may present with acute abdominal pain. This group of conditions includes the exaggerated intraperitoneal bleeding at the normal time of ovulation (mittelschmerz bleeding) or rupture of a small luteal cyst. Tubal menstruation, torsion of the ovary and acute salpingitis are all uncommon. Physical examination of girls with any of these conditions will reveal lower abdominal tenderness and guarding.

Pelvic inflammatory disease may also present with fever and vaginal discharge.

Rectal examination of the pelvis is rarely performed and would require informed consent and a nurse chaperone. A pelvic/abdominal ultrasound examination will diagnose most conditions. Torsion of the ovary demands urgent surgery and the ovary can often be preserved after untwisting the torsion.

Key Points

- Abdominal pain requires careful physical assessment to determine the cause.
- Peritonitis is hard to diagnose in preschool children: beware the toddler who refuses examination.
- Local peritonitis in right iliac fossa is likely to be appendicitis.
- Pelvic appendicitis (by rectal exam or ultrasonography) and testicular torsion (by scrotal exam) need exclusion in children with vague RIF pains

Further reading

Beasley SW, Hutson JM, Auldist AW (1996) Appendicitis. In: *Essential Paediatric Surgery*, Arnold, London, pp. 52–57.

Dunn JCD (2006) Appendicitis. In: Grosfeld JL, O'Neill JA Jr., Fonkalsrud EW, Coran AG (eds) *Pediatric Surgery*, 6th Edn. Vol. 2, Mosby Elsevier, Philadelphia, pp. 1501–1513.

Puri P, Martell A (2006) Appendicitis. In: Stringer MD, Oldham KT, Mouriquand PDE (eds) *Pediatric Surgery and Urology: Long Term Outcomes*, 2nd Edn. Cambridge University Press, Cambridge, pp. 374–384.

21 Recurrent Abdominal Pain

Case 1

A 10-year-old girl presents with recurrent symptoms of abdominal pain.

Q 1.1 What underlying fears may the parents have about the nature of the pain?

Q 1.2 How can recurrent abdominal pain syndrome be distinguished from more serious causes of pain on the basis of history and examination?

Q 1.3 What is the role of the surgeon in this situation?

Recurrent abdominal pain syndrome is one of the most common problems seen in paediatric practice. The child usually has frequent short-lived episodes of abdominal colic, which are felt in the periumbilical area. The attacks are unpredictable in onset and last only a few minutes. Sometimes they may be brought on by or be more frequent when there is stress at school or home. Despite these psychological triggers, the pain itself is very real and although its exact nature remains uncertain, it may be due to gut colic. It can be compared to the psychosomatic stress headaches or gastric problems seen in adults. Constipation and gut upset brought on by 'food allergy' may also cause recurrent abdominal pain. The reason some families come to a surgeon with these symptoms is because of an underlying parental fear of a serious cause for the pain, such as cancer, appendicitis or a 'twisted bowel'. In fact, it is quite unusual to find a serious underlying cause for recurrent abdominal pain. Despite this, it is important to exclude these uncommon but more serious causes for abdominal pain, so that the family can then recognise the true nature of the problem which sometimes is stress-induced. The diagnosis depends on a careful history and physical examination.

History

The nature, severity and periodicity of the pain is the key to the diagnosis. Recurrent abdominal pain is mild to moderate in severity. The pain comes on suddenly in short-lived episodes lasting only a few minutes, and is usually situated in the periumbilical region. The episodes of pain are unpredictable and frequent, and scarcely a day goes by without pain. On the other hand, pain due to surgical causes such as obstructive hydronephrosis, appendicitis or malrotation with volvulus, is severe and persistent.

A child finds it difficult to quantify the severity of pain; this is best established by other factors. Severe pain will stop the child from normal activities such as play, or the child may be sent home from school with pain. Severe pain will wake the child from sleep, and may induce vomiting. Bile-stained vomitus is of particular significance in relation to the possibility of malrotation with volvulus. Surgical pain is prolonged, lasting for some hours, and may be localised in relation to the underlying cause: the pain of an obstructed kidney will be localised to one loin in the older child or in appendicitis to the right iliac fossa. Young children find it difficult to localise pain. The periodicity of surgical pain is different from that of recurrent abdominal pain. A child with obstructive hydronephrosis may be well for many months and develop severe prolonged episodes of pain lasting for a week, followed by many pain-free months.

The family and social histories are important. If a relative has recently developed cancer, the parents may have an underlying fear of a tumour in the child. On the other hand, a strong family history of renal anomalies may direct attention to the possibility of hydronephrosis in the child. As stress can be a key factor in recurrent abdominal pain, the social history is of great importance. Family breakdown, financial distress and moving house are common problems. Occasionally, abdominal pain may be a

Jones' Clinical Paediatric Surgery, 6th edition. By Hutson, O'Brien, Woodward and Beasley. Published 2008 by Blackwell Publishing, ISBN: 978-1-4051-6267-8.

presentation of child abuse. Stress at school may be due to many factors, such as poor student–teacher relations, bullying or unrealistic parental expectations. Sometimes when one asks the question, 'How does your child get on at school?' the parents answer that there is no problem because the child is always a 'straight A' student. The stress of trying to meet these high parental expectations is often the trigger for recurrent abdominal pain. Many parents spend considerable amounts of time away from home owing to work. The stress of separation may manifest itself in the child as recurrent abdominal pain.

Physical examination

In most patients with recurrent abdominal pain, the physical examination is normal. The child appears to be perfectly well, and a careful and complete physical examination, including measurement of the child's height and weight on a growth chart, offers a powerful reassurance to the parents. The most common abnormal physical finding is the presence of faecal masses in the left iliac fossa. Although this may not be the complete explanation of the pain, correction of the constipation may be very helpful.

A loin mass due to an enlarged hydronephrotic kidney is an uncommon finding. Weight loss associated with malaise and lethargy may indicate a serious underlying cause for the pain.

Special investigation

In the majority of children, special investigation is not helpful, although it may be useful to allay specific parental anxieties. Of all investigations, abdominal ultrasonography is the most useful and the least invasive: the kidneys, bladder, ovaries, gall bladder, liver, spleen and pancreas, can all be examined. Investigation should be reserved for patients with a possible surgical cause of the pain. The return on the investigation of recurrent abdominal pain is not particularly good, but occasionally a child is treated as recurrent abdominal pain for many years before a hydronephrosis is diagnosed on ultrasonography.

Gastroscopy or colonoscopy may be indicated in a select group of children who have upper or lower gastrointestinal symptoms. Children with Crohn disease may have weight-loss, growth failure and perianal disease. Oesophagitis, gastritis and duodenitis will usually have symptoms that distinguish these children from other children with recurrent abdominal pain.

Treatment

Following exclusion of significant pathology, recurrent abdominal pain is treated by reassurance, identification of the stress factors (if any) and by helping the family to understand the possible link between the stress and the child's symptoms. It is hard to 'cure' the pain, but if the family understands the pathology, they can live with the symptoms.

It is important to uncover any possible hidden fears the family may have, such as the risk of cancer. These underlying fears must be dispelled by demonstrating to the parents' satisfaction that the child is free of these problems. Tranquilisers have been used for children with recurrent abdominal pain, but they do not treat the underlying cause.

Constipation may be a factor aggravating recurrent abdominal pain. It is a simple matter to use laxatives to clear the faecal load, and in some children, this may be helpful in reducing the colic.

Some parents worry that their child has a 'grumbling appendix' or 'chronic appendicitis'. Although laparotomy or laparoscopy and appendicectomy are performed sometimes in a small, highly selected group of the more severely affected children, the results are variable and if the selection is poor, the symptoms can be made worse. The best results are obtained in those children who were well earlier, and who undergo frequent hospitalisation for pain, which is typical of acute appendicitis, but settles quickly. This diagnosis of 'chronic appendicitis' (repeated short-lived episodes of acute appendicitis) is uncommon, and surgical exploration should be a rare event.

The management of children with recurrent abdominal pain is a test of clinical acumen and counselling skills. The cases presenting for surgical opinion are usually more severe and it is important to exclude any underlying 'surgical' cause. A thorough clinical history and physical examination is the basis of diagnosis; extensive, traumatic or invasive investigations are rarely indicated, and if imaging is required, ultrasonography probably gives the best return.

> **Key Points**
> - Recurrent abdominal pains may be psychogenic, but occult organic causes need exclusion.
> - Detailed history and examination is usually sufficient.
> - Abdominal ultrasonography may reassure families with fears of cancer.

Further reading

Becmeur F, Varlet F (2005) Appendicectomy. In: Najmalden A, Rothenberg S, Crabbe DCG, Beasley SW (eds) *Operative Endoscopy and Endoscopic Surgery in Infants and Children.* Hodder Arnold, London, pp. 279–284.

Lee ACH, Stewart RJ (2005) Diagnostic laparoscopy. In: Najmalden A, Rothenberg S, Crabbe DCG, Beasley SW (eds) *Operative Endoscopy and Endoscopic Surgery in Infants and Children.* Hodder Arnold, London, pp. 197–204.

McCallion WA, Baillie AG, Ardill JES, Bamford KB, Potts SR, Boston VE (1995) *Helicobacter pylori,* hypergastrinaemia, and recurrent abdominal pain in children. *J Pediatr Surg* **30**: 427–429.

Zitsman JL (2006) Pediatric minimal-access surgery: update 2006. *Pediatrics* **118**(1): 304–308.

22 Constipation

Case 1

A 6-month-old baby presents with pain and rectal bleeding with defecation.
Q 1.1 What are the likely diagnoses and the management of this common problem?

Case 2

A 6-year-old boy presents with a long history of faecal impaction and soiling.
Q 2.1 Discuss the diagnosis and treatment of this condition?

Constipation is a common problem in infancy and childhood. Severe acute constipation presents to the surgeon with abdominal pain or rectal prolapse. Chronic constipation may present with soiling or an abdominal mass.

Acute constipation

This is mainly seen in babies at the age of 6 months. Dietary problems lead to the passage of a hard stool that tears the sensitive anal lining to cause an acute anal fissure with pain and bleeding. The pain on defecation makes the baby hold on to stool and a cycle of constipation is established. This problem is easily treated with dietary advice and the reduction of the volume of cow's milk. An excess of cow's milk satisfies the baby's thirst at the expense of other fluids, such as water or juice. Too much cow's milk also suppresses the baby's appetite for other foods. Dietary change is the long-term solution, but relief of the acute problem is obtained by laxatives, such as senna or paraffin, to soften the stool. Disposable enemas or suppositories are useful to clear the initial hard stool from the rectum. Parents also may have an underlying fear that the rectal bleeding is due to cancer, so this subject should be explored and the parents reassured. Acute constipation is sometimes seen in older children following an intercurrent viral illness, or time in bed after surgery. The results of treatment for acute constipation are excellent. In a child with earlier normal bowel habits the rectum maintains its muscle tone, and recovers rapidly with treatment, though laxatives should be continued until the precipitating factors are corrected.

Chronic constipation

This is a common debilitating problem in children and the treatment is difficult and prolonged. In most cases the anorectal mechanism and bowel is normal, but in rare cases, there can be an underlying cause, such as Hirschsprung disease [Table 22.1].

Chronic constipation presents with a history of many months or years with soiling, abdominal pain and abdominal distension. Generally, the diagnosis of constipation is made by the presence of hard faecal masses in the abdomen. These are felt along the line of the colon and especially in the sigmoid colon. These masses can be indented with digital pressure. This is a characteristic feature that differentiates faeces from other abdominal masses. Inspection of the anus may reveal faecal soiling with a lax, open anal canal.

In rare cases, other features on physical examination may indicate a serious underlying disease [Table 22.2]. Hirschsprung disease usually presents with neonatal bowel obstruction (Chapter 7) but occasional cases present at a later age with chronic constipation. These children are usually sick with poor nutrition and marked abdominal distension. The anal canal in Hirschsprung disease is tight, as against the lax anus seen in other causes of chronic constipation. Slow transit constipation with intestinal neuronal dysplasia describes a group of conditions with (presumed) congenital defects in bowel motility due to

Jones' Clinical Paediatric Surgery, 6th edition. By Hutson, O'Brien, Woodward and Beasley. Published 2008 by Blackwell Publishing, ISBN: 978-1-4051-6267-8.

Table 22.1 Predisposing factors in chronic constipation

1 Holding back – behavioural problems with toilet-training
2 Dietary factors – low fibre and fluid intake
3 Postoperative cause due to bed-rest, inactivity and narcotics
4 Intercurrent illness, for example, chicken-pox
5 Emotional upset at home or school
6 Uncommon organic causes: Hirschsprung disease, slow transit constipation with intestinal neuronal dysplasia, spina bifida, congenital anorectal anomalies

Table 22.2 Organic causes of constipation

Neurological anomaly
  Slow transit constipation
  Hirschsprung disease
  Spina bifida
  Spinal cord anomaly
  Sacral agenesis
Anatomical anomaly
  Anal stenosis
  Pelvic tumour
  Anorectal anomaly (postop)

functional anomalies of the neural plexuses of the bowel wall. These children present with chronic unremitting constipation that fails to resolve with normal treatment.

An early clue in both Hirschsprung disease and slow transit constipation is delayed passage of the first meconium stool beyond 24 h after birth. Another useful clinical feature is that, despite infrequent bowel actions, the retained stool in patients with intestinal neuronal dysplasia is usually soft. Many patients with intestinal neuronal dysplasia have a deficiency of substance P-immunoreactive staining of the myenteric nerves supplying the colonic muscle, or abnormalities of the interstitial cells of Cajal, although a small number have hyperplastic or hypoplastic ganglia.

Congenital anorectal anomalies usually present at birth with imperforate anus. However, some minor anomalies may present later with anal stenosis. The anus in this situation will be tight and anteriorly placed. Spina bifida anomalies are usually apparent at birth, but some cases of spinal dysraphism are not so obvious, and may present later with constipation. Diastematomyelia, sacral agenesis and spinal cord lipoma may all be diagnosed by careful clinical examination of the spine. Digital examination of the rectum is useful in assessing constipation, but should

only be undertaken after discussion with the parents and in their presence.

Special investigations

In most cases of constipation, special investigation is unnecessary. A plain x-ray is sometimes performed to assess the extent of faecal loading. Barium enema studies usually are not indicated.

If, on clinical history and examination, a rare underlying cause is suspected, further tests may be indicated, particularly if standard diet and laxative therapy has failed. Hirschsprung disease may be diagnosed with suction rectal biopsy showing aganglionosis. Diagnosis of slow transit constipation with intestinal neuronal dysplasia is a more complex procedure, entailing nuclear transit study to confirm delayed proximal colonic transit and multiple laparoscopic biopsies taken along the length of the large bowel to assess the level of neuropeptide staining.

Spinal dysraphism is diagnosed on a plain x-ray of the lower spine and anorectal anomalies are best assessed with an examination under anaesthetic.

Treatment
Although chronic constipation is easy to diagnose it is difficult to treat as this is often more prolonged than the parents expect. The essence of treatment is to empty the rectum and to keep it empty as often as possible for weeks or months until colonic and anorectal tone returns [Table. 22.1]. The normal rectum is empty most of the time except when a mass reflex of the colon conveys faeces into the rectum once or twice a day to stimulate rectal receptors to give the urge to defecate. This urge is suppressed until socially convenient. If the stool is left too long in the rectum, water resorption makes it hard and more difficult to pass. As more faeces accumulate in the rectum, distension of the smooth muscle reduces its contractility and sensation. Eventually, this process causes faeces to bank up in the colon and stools are only passed by overflow incontinence past a lax anal sphincter that dilates in response to a chronically distended rectum.

Treatment follows four lines:
1 Dietary advice with reduction of cow's milk and increase of fibre with a normal mix of the main food groups.
2 Behavioural training is required to establish normal toileting. This is initially difficult, as the child has diminished rectal sensation and motility due to chronic distension.
3 Laxatives both soften the stool and stimulate the bowel. The child may be quite dependent on continuous laxatives

for many weeks. New oral formulations containing polyethelene glycol have proved useful in severe, chronic constipation.

4 Enemas are the most invasive form of treatment but are only necessary in severe cases. Initially full bowel washouts in hospital may be required to clear gross faecal impaction. Less severe degrees of constipation respond well to small disposable enemas. In very severe cases, enemas can be given antegradely through an appendicostomy.

Treatment must be carefully supervised until a normal bowel habit is established. Constipation is often underestimated and undertreated. Soiling and abdominal pain in primary school children, are all too common as both parents and medical practitioners have an inadequate understanding of the problem. If the symptoms persist after 6 months of adequate therapy, the child should be referred to a tertiary centre for assessment and further investigation.

Rectal prolapse

Rectal prolapse is a particularly distressing consequence of constipation. Straining to pass a hard stool leads to prolapse of the poorly supported rectum in the young child. The rectum may reduce spontaneously leaving blood and mucus around the anus or the parents may reduce the prolapse. In children, this problem resolves quickly by treating the underlying constipation with laxatives and enemas. In rare cases, rectal prolapse may indicate an underlying anomaly such as malabsorption because of coeliac disease or cystic fibrosis. Rectal prolapse is also seen in spina bifida because of paralysis of *levator ani*.

Key Points

- Acute constipation is common and easily treated.
- Chronic constipation (+ soiling) is very distressing for families and often difficult to treat.
- Most children respond to good laxative and behaviour treatments.
- Persisting symptoms despite 6 months of adequate therapy needs referral for investigation for possible organic disorder.
- Delayed meconium stool beyond 24 h of birth is suggestive of an organic bowel disorder.

Further reading

Hutson JM, Catto-Smith T, Gibb S et al. (2004) Stephen L Gans Lecture. Chronic constipation: no longer stuck! Characterisation of colonic dysmotility as a new disorder in children. *J Pediatr Surg* **39**(6): 795–799.

Southwell, BR, King, SK, Hutson, JM (2005) Review article. Chronic constipation in children: organic disorders are a major cause. *J Pediatr Child Health* **41**: 1–15.

23 Bleeding from the Alimentary Canal

Case 1

A 2-year-old girl is being toilet-trained by her mother when a small amount of bright blood is seen at the anus.

Q 1.1 List the causes of minor rectal bleeding in childhood?

Q 1.2 What is the likely problem in this case?

Q.1.3 Describe the management of a fissure?

Case 2

James is a previously well toddler aged 8 months who presents with hypovolaemia after passage of two very large bowel motions containing dark red blood.

Q 2.1 What causes major rectal bleeding in children?

Haemorrhage, large or small, can occur from any part of the alimentary canal and at any age. Sometimes the haemorrhage threatens the life of the child; on other occasions, it is an important sign of other medical or surgical pathology.

Alimentary tract bleeding may present with a variety of symptoms, according to the level and rate of haemorrhage. It may be 'occult' and present as iron-deficiency anaemia, or it may be seen as blood passed per rectum; in this instance, there may be melaena (dark changed blood) or bright red bleeding [Table 23.1].

If bleeding occurs into the oesophagus, stomach or duodenum, it may present as either 'coffee grounds' or frank blood in the vomitus.

'Coffee grounds' vomiting

A small amount of blood mixes with the gastric contents, is denatured and changes to a brown colour. When vomited, these flecks of blood may have the appearance of coffee grounds. It is seen in a variety of conditions.

Jones' Clinical Paediatric Surgery, 6th edition. By Hutson, O'Brien, Woodward and Beasley. Published 2008 by Blackwell Publishing, ISBN: 978-1-4051-6267-8.

Pyloric stenosis

Obstruction of the pylorus results in gastritis and small amounts of blood mix with the gastric contents and may be vomited. Hypertrophic pyloric stenosis, which occurs in approximately 1:600 infants, causes vomiting at about 1 month of age. Cardinal clinical features are projectile vomiting, visible gastric peristalsis and a pyloric 'tumour' palpable in the epigastrium (Chapter 18).

Reflux oesophagitis

Acid reflux into the lower oesophagus sometimes causes ulceration of its mucosal surface. Small vomits occur after meals and when lying flat, often with epigastric discomfort. Initial treatment of this common condition includes general measures such as thickening of the feeds, and posturing the baby prone with the head elevated. More specific medical measures to reduce gastric acid include antacids, H_2 receptor antagonists (cimetidine) and proton-pump inhibitors (omeprazole, lansoprazole). Surgical treatment (fundoplication) is sometimes necessary for complications (especially oesophageal stricture; Chapter 18).

Non-specific gastritis

This condition may be due to a viral infection, and usually responds to measures which reduce gastric acidity.

Table 23.1 The causes of blood in vomitus

'Coffee grounds'	Pyloric stenosis
	Reflux oesophagitis
Frank blood	Oesophageal varices
	Peptic ulcer
Others	Nose bleeds with swallowed blood
	Nasogastric tube ulceration
Rare causes	Aneurysm in bed of tonsil
	Foreign body perforation of aorta

Mallory–Weiss syndrome

This may cause alarming haematemesis with bright blood and can occur in any child who vomits or retches continually, and is thought to be due to the formation of small longitudinal splits in the upper gastric mucosa. Fortunately, it responds to medical treatment if the vomiting can be stopped.

Haematemesis

The vomiting of large amounts of frank blood means that there has been significant loss of blood into the stomach.

Oesophageal varices

Oesophageal varices are the result of portal hypertension and, in children, this occurs in two main groups:
1 Extrahepatic portal hypertension, where thrombosis of the portal vein in the neonate results in 'cavernous malformation' of the portal system;
2 Intrahepatic portal hypertension due to (a) cirrhosis of the liver, caused by biliary atresia; (b) inborn errors of metabolism, such as alpha$_1$-antitrypsin deficiency; (c) chronic viral hepatitis; or (d) cystic fibrosis.

Oesophageal varices are best treated by prophylactic endoscopic sclerosant injections to prevent rupture and haemorrhage. However, they may bleed torrentially, and many require tamponade with a Sengstaken–Blakemore tube followed, if necessary, by emergency surgical treatment. Surgery consists of oversewing the varices or creating a shunt to join the portal system to the systemic venous system, aiming to lower the pressure in the portal system.

Peptic ulcer

Peptic ulcer disease is rare in children, but a 'stress ulcer' may occur in a child of any age with severe burns, cerebral tumour, head injury or other forms of severe stress. In all these conditions, there tends to be an increased production of gastric acid with resultant diffuse ulceration of the gastric lining or more localised ulceration in the duodenum. Peptic ulceration also may occur as a complication of drug treatment; for example, after administration of steroids. In adolescents who develop peptic ulceration, the aetiology is the same as in adults (i.e. *Helicobacter pylori* infection). There may be a strong family history of ulcer disease.

Management

For a bleeding peptic ulcer, the management is
1 Adequately resuscitate the patient with blood replacement.
2 Endoscopic upper G.I.T. examination.
3 Treatment of the cause, for example, H$_2$ antagonists and triple antibiotic therapy.
4 Surgery to the bleeding point is rarely required.

Iron-deficiency anaemia

Iron-deficiency anaemia in children is caused by poor dietary intake, but can be due to reflux oesophagitis or one of the other causes mentioned in Table 23.2.

Rectal bleeding

Rectal bleeding in children can be considered under various distinct clinical groups [Table 23.3].

Neonatal bleeding

There are two important surgical conditions and several important medical conditions that lead to rectal bleeding in children.

Necrotising enterocolitis [Chapter 7]

This is an important condition that has become more common with the advent of the modern neonatal nursery that cares for extremely premature babies. Most babies with necrotising enterocolitis respond to supportive treatment consisting of adequate ventilatory care, support of their circulation, resting the gastrointestinal tract and the administration of antibiotics. Some patients require surgery for full-thickness necrosis of the intestine, as revealed by free intraperitoneal gas on x-ray or by continued clinical deterioration despite intensive supportive care.

Volvulus neonatorum with ischaemia [Chapter 7]

Volvulus of the midgut occurs at any age, but is more likely in the neonatal period. In the presence of malrotation, the attachment of the midgut to the posterior abdominal wall is via a narrow mesentery that allows easy twisting of the entire midgut. The first sign results from obstruction of the lumen of the bowel with bile-stained

Table 23.2 Occult bleeding causing iron-deficiency anaemia

Reflux oesophagitis
Haemangioma of bowel
Polyps of the bowel
Inflammatory bowel disease

Table 23.3 Rectal bleeding in children

Neonatal
   Necrotising enterocolitis
   Volvulus with ischaemia
   Haemorrhagic disease of the newborn
   Gastroenteritis
   Anal fissure
   Maternal blood
Sick child with an acute abdominal condition
   Intussusception
   Gastroenteritis
   Henoch-Schönlein purpura
Major haemorrhage from the gastrointestinal tract
   Oesophageal varices
   Acute peptic ulcer
     gastric erosions
     duodenal ulcer
   Meckel's diverticulum
   Tubular duplications
Small amount of bright blood in well child
   Anal fissure
   Polyps
   Unrecognised prolapse
   Haemorrhoids
   Idiopathic
Chronic illness with diarrhoea
   Crohn disease
   Ulcerative colitis
   Non-specific colitis

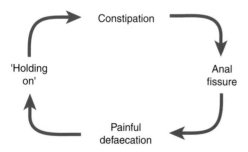

Figure 23.1 The cycle of anal fissure. The treatment aims to break the cycle.

vomiting; but the most serious event that may occur is ischaemia of the midgut, due to obstruction of the vessels in the twisted mesentery. Bleeding from the bowel is a late sign, and very urgent surgical treatment is necessary at this stage if there is to be any hope for the baby to become normal.

Non-surgical causes

Haemorrhagic disease of the newborn is due to Vitamin K deficiency and is prevented by routine administration of Vitamin K_1. Gastroenteritis may occur in the neonatal period, resulting in blood mixed with diarrhoea. An anal fissure may occur at any age, and is common in the neonate after a rectal examination. The baby may swallow maternal blood, either during delivery or from a cracked nipple.

A small amount of blood in a well child

A small amount of fresh blood may be passed in a well child. This is by far the most common clinical group, and the cause of the bleeding often may be distinguished on the history alone.

Anal fissure

Anal fissure occurs at any age and usually is due to constipation (Chapters 22 and 27). The child passes a large, hard stool which splits the anus, usually in the midline, either posteriorly or anteriorly. The child complains of pain on defecation and there is bright blood on the surface of the stool or immediately following it [Fig. 23.1]. The fissure can be seen by gently parting the anus. Rectal examination causes severe pain and is ill advised. The fissure heals quickly, and even when a fissure is not seen, the history may be quite diagnostic. Sometimes, a 'sentinel pile', a mound of oedematous skin just external to the fissure is visible. Anal fissures in children almost always respond to adequate treatment of the constipation. Local applications of anaesthetic agents achieve little, and surgical operations on the anal sphincter are rarely indicated in children.

Polyps

Juvenile polyps are relatively common in children and should be suspected when there is no constipation or no pain on passage of a stool (Chapter 27).

Rectal prolapse

Prolapse of the rectum is easily diagnosed on the history or by direct observation (Chapter 27). Sometimes, the rectal prolapse may become congested or traumatised, bleed and then reduce spontaneously; the parents observe the bleeding without knowing its cause. Rectal prolapse may occur with malabsorption or chronic diarrhoea, straining with constipation, and occasionally, as the presenting symptom of cystic fibrosis.

Haemorrhoids

Symptoms from haemorrhoids are rare in children but do occur. The presence of a venous malformation of the rectum should be considered. In older children, haemorrhoids may cause bleeding and can be treated conservatively. In some children, no cause for rectal bleeding can be found.

An ill child with an acute abdominal condition

In these children, the symptom of bleeding is not important in its own right, but points to another significant condition.

Intussusception

Intussusception presents with vomiting, colic, pallor and lethargy. In 50% of patients, the stools are blood-stained, the typical 'red-currant jelly stool' due to a mixture of blood and mucus (see Chapter 19).

Gastroenteritis

Patients with severe gastroenteritis often have vomiting, colic, and specks of blood mixed with the stool. The separation of these patients from those with intussusception can be difficult in the child under 2 years (see Chapter 19).

Henoch-Schönlein purpura

This condition causes arthralgia and a typical rash over the extremities and buttocks. Submucosal haemorrhages in the bowel with abdominal pain and passage of blood rectally also occur. Henoch–Schönlein purpura needs to be distinguished from intussusception.

Chronic illness with diarrhoea

Crohn disease may occur anywhere in the bowel and should be suspected in a patient with a chronic illness, unexplained fever, weight loss, bowel symptoms and chronic blood loss in the stools (Chapter 24). In patients with ulcerative colitis the diarrhoea is more prominent, and again it may contain blood. In non-specific colitis there is usually involvement of only the lower part of the large bowel with less general symptomatology.

Major haemorrhage per rectum

In these patients the haemorrhage is enough to cause anaemia or to require acute transfusion. The causes range

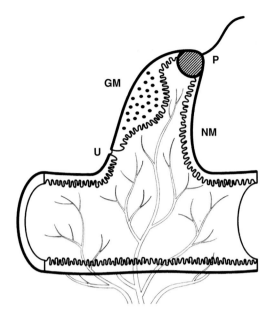

Figure 23.2 Meckel's diverticulum. A composite diagram showing ectopic pancreas (P) and gastric mucosa (GM). An ulcer (U) lies in the adjacent normal ileal mucosa (NM). The site of attachment of a vitello-intestinal or Meckel's band is shown at the tip.

from oesophageal varices and peptic ulcer (as discussed under the heading of vomiting) to Meckel's diverticulum and tubular duplications (both latter anomalies can contain ectopic gastric mucosa).

Meckel's diverticulum

Meckel's diverticulum occurs in 2% of the population, and in a small proportion of these patients, ectopic gastric mucosa forms part of the lining of the diverticulum [Fig. 23.2]. Acid produced by the gastric mucosa causes ulceration of the adjacent ileal mucosa. The bleeding usually presents as painless 'brick-red' stools with associated anaemia. The patient may require transfusion, but the bleeding usually stops spontaneously without the need for emergency surgery. The definitive investigation is surgery, but a technetium scan may show the ectopic gastric mucosa [Fig. 23.3]. A Meckel's diverticulum may result in a variety of other complications [Table 23.4].

Tubular duplications

These are much less common than a Meckel's diverticulum. Tubular duplications of the small bowel occur in the

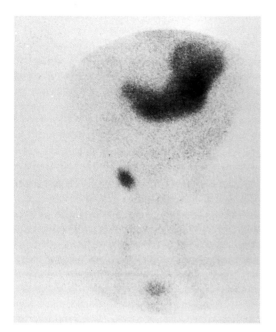

Figure 23.3 A technetium scan showing ectopic gastric mucosa in a Meckel's diverticulum.

Table 23.4 Complications of Meckel's diverticulum

1 Bleeding
2 Intussusception from an inverted diverticulum
3 An associated fibrous band causing a small bowel obstruction
4 Diverticulitis (rare in children)
5 Peptic ulceration with ileal perforation
6 Strangulation of diverticulum by its own band
7 Strangulation of diverticulum in an inguinal hernia

mesenteric side of the bowel and communicate proximally or distally with the bowel. They may be lined by gastric mucosa and cause bleeding when adjacent small bowel mucosa becomes ulcerated. Similar to a Meckel's diverticulum, they can be demonstrated by a technetium nuclear scan.

Key Points

- The cause of bleeding can often be determined from the site, colour and volume of blood passed.
- 'Coffee grounds' in vomitus suggests gastritis.
- Small volume, bright blood PR is characteristic with anal fissure.

Further reading

Arensman RM, Browne M, Madonna MB (2006) Gastrointestinal bleeding. In: Grosfeld JL, O'Neill JA Jr., Fonkalsrud EW, Coran AG (eds) *Pediatric Surgery*, 6th Edn. Mosby Elsevier, Philadelphia, pp. 1383–1388.

Cull DL, Rosario V, Lally KP, Ratner I, Mahour GH (1990) Surgical implications of Henoch-Schönlein purpura. *J Pediatr Surg* **25**: 741–743.

Previtera C, Guglielmi M (1990) Limitations and dangers of the Sengstaken-Blakemore tube in the treatment of haemorrhage from gastric varices. *Pediatr Surg Int* **5**: 422–424.

Tsang T-M, Saing H, Yeung CK (1990) Peptic ulcer in children. *J Pediatr Surg* **25**: 744–748.

24   Inflammatory Bowel Disease

Case 1

A 6-year-old girl presents with a 1-month history of weight loss and mild diarrhoea, containing blood and mucus.
Q.1.1 What is the likely diagnosis and how is it confirmed?

Case 2

A 12-year-old boy presents with vague pains in the abdomen, some weight loss and a perianal abscess.
Q.1.2 How is the diagnosis made?
Q.2.2 How are the different forms of inflammatory bowel disease distinguished?

Three categories of inflammatory bowel disease are encountered in childhood:
1 Crohn disease
2 Ulcerative colitis
3 Inflammatory bowel disease of indeterminate pathology.

Incidence

Crohn disease is by far the most common category of inflammatory bowel disease. During the past 25 years, there has been a dramatic increase in the incidence of Crohn disease in Australasia and in the Northern hemisphere. This disease was almost unknown in childhood before 1980. In contrast, the incidence of ulcerative colitis has remained relatively static.

Crohn disease

Crohn disease is a chronic inflammatory disorder of unknown aetiology, which can affect any part of the gastrointestinal tract from the mouth to the anus. It is a transmural inflammatory process that most commonly occurs in the terminal portion of the small intestine and colon.

Jones' Clinical Paediatric Surgery, 6th edition. By Hutson, O'Brien, Woodward and Beasley. Published 2008 by Blackwell Publishing, ISBN: 978-1-4051-6267-8.

There is a high incidence of involvement of the large bowel and rectum in paediatric patients.

Clinical features

Age of onset of symptoms
Most paediatric Crohn disease presents in adolescence but one third of the patients are aged 18 years or less at the commencement of symptoms.

Symptoms and signs
There is a broad spectrum of symptoms and signs associated with Crohn disease. Most common symptoms include recurrent abdominal pain and bowel disturbance, usually diarrhoea together with rectal bleeding. However, these symptoms may be relatively mild and the patient may present with the long-term effects of the disease such as weight loss, growth failure and delay of onset of puberty.

Delay in diagnosis often occurs because of lack of knowledge by medical practitioners concerning the relatively high incidence of Crohn disease in childhood and the variety of non-specific presenting symptoms.

Perineal inflammation
One of the commonest modes of presentation is perineal inflammation, occurring in one third of paediatric patients with Crohn disease, and this is invariably associated with rectal disease. Accordingly, paediatric patients particularly adolescents who present with a perianal

abscess and associated anal fistula should have a biopsy of the abscess wall at the time of drainage, to exclude underlying Crohn disease.

Extra-intestinal manifestations of Crohn disease

Examples of extra-intestinal manifestations include arthritis and erythema nodosum, which may be presenting symptoms.

Unusual modes of presentation of Crohn disease

Very occasionally, Crohn disease may present with acute right-sided abdominal pain and gastrointestinal disturbance, mimicking acute appendicitis. The diagnosis is then made at laparoscopy/laparotomy.

Cheilosis

Uncommonly, the patient may present with chronic inflammation of the oral cavity and lips, so-called cheilosis, manifested by oedema, erythema and fissuring of the lips. Biopsy reveals evidence of chronic inflammation including granulomas consistent with Crohn disease.

Investigations

Role of endoscopy

Endoscopy has a crucial role in diagnosis, initial evaluation and continuing assessment of Crohn disease.

Upper and lower ('top and tail') gastrointestinal endoscopy with biopsies is the key investigation for the diagnosis and initial assessment of the extent and severity of the disease. Colonoscopy together with biopsy provide a good chance of diagnosing Crohn disease because there is a high incidence of colonic involvement in paediatric patients with this disease. Gastroscopy is performed as well as colonoscopy because involvement of the upper intestinal tract is common.

Endoscopy has an important role in assessing the response to treatment and distribution of the disease, and is performed at periodic intervals.

In Crohn disease, the inflammation is typically segmental, and the characteristic appearance is single or multiple ulcers with the intervening mucosa appearing normal. In some instances, the diagnosis may be made by serial biopsies even when the macroscopic appearances are normal. Histological diagnosis depends on demonstration of granulomas, in association with other chronic inflammatory changes in the bowel wall.

Contrast imaging

CT scan with oral contrast

This imaging is performed to assess the small intestine that is not accessible to endoscopy [Fig. 24.1]. It also may provide valuable information concerning disease in the colon. Most commonly, abnormalities are demonstrated in the terminal ileum, and often in the colon. Abnormal findings include an irregular bowel contour, longitudinal ulcers and fissures, narrowing of the lumen by oedema and separation of loops by mural thickening. There may be evidence of stricture formation associated with dilatation of the proximal bowel. Bowel loops may be displaced by the presence of an inflammatory mass.

MRI

This imaging is used to assess pelvic Crohn disease. It provides information concerning ischio-rectal and peri-anal suppuration. It also demonstrates sphincter anatomy and distortion or damage related to the inflammatory process.

Other investigations

FBE is performed to detect evidence of anaemia, and liver function tests are performed to exclude associated liver disease.

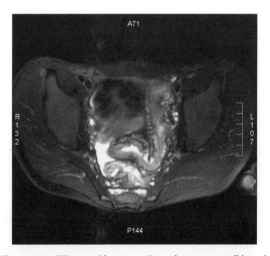

Figure 24.1 CT scan with contrast is used to assess small bowel affected by Crohn disease that is not accessible to endoscopy.

Stool cultures are performed to rule out chronic infection due to such enteric pathogens as Salmonella, Shigella, Campylobacter and Yersinia.

Treatment

The aetiology of Crohn disease is unknown, so treatment is directed at controlling the disease rather than curing it.

Medical treatment

High doses of oral steroids are used to induce a remission, for example, Prednisolone, 2 mg/kg (maximum 60–75 mg/day) for 4 weeks, with gradual reduction to nil after 8 weeks. Sulphasalazine, to prevent relapses, is introduced when the Prednisolone dose is down to 20 mg/day and is built up to a dose of 50 mg/kg/day twice daily. It may be necessary to continue low-dose Prednisolone (5 mg/day). Immuran can be used in resistant cases. Metronidazole may be helpful for perianal Crohn disease. Newer biological therapies such as Infliximab appear to be very effective.

Nutrition

Children with inflammatory bowel disease fail to grow because of the disease, not its treatment, and the reason the disease influences growth is its effect on appetite and caloric intake. High caloric dietary supplements, and occasionally enteral tube feeding or parenteral nutrition, all have their place in management.

Surgical treatment

The indications for surgical treatment of Crohn disease are as follows:
1 perianal disease;
2 intestinal complications;
3 acute abdomen – possible acute appendicitis.

Perianal disease

The most common indication for surgical intervention in Crohn disease is perianal disease [Fig. 24.2]. Perianal inflammation is invariably associated with rectal and colonic Crohn disease. There may be extensive involvement of the soft tissues of the perineum, scrotum, penis or vulval region.

Skin-tags and anal fissures are common and usually do not require surgical intervention. Perianal abscess is also common and requires incision and drainage. There

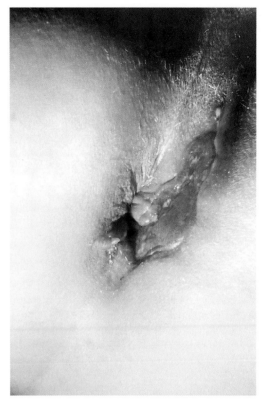

Figure 24.2 Perineal disease in a child with Crohn disease.

is usually an associated anal fistula that may need to be laid open, but healing will often subsequently be very slow. Occasionally, insertion of a seton suture along a chronic fistula tract may be appropriate to facilitate drainage of an infection associated with it and subsequent healing. More extensive suppuration may occur with development of an ischio-rectal abscess. Appropriate surgical management of this complication is drainage of the abscess and consideration given to faecal diversion in the form of a colostomy or ileostomy to help control the infection. Faecal diversion is usually effective in controlling the infection but it does not necessarily influence the activity of the Crohn disease. The potential end result of ischio-rectal sepsis is damage to the sphincters.

Perineal disease

Occasionally, there may be extensive involvement of the soft tissues of the perineum extending into the scrotum, penis or vulval region. This may be manifest by unsightly painful oedema and inflammation of the scrotal or vulval tissue.

The aim of surgical treatment for complicated perineal and perianal Crohn disease is to control infection and promote healing. In these regions, healing is often delayed and chronic inflammation may be protracted despite appropriate surgical and medical treatment.

Intestinal complications
These complications are due to transmural inflammation and include the following:
• localised stricture formation;
• localised disease unresponsive to medical treatment;
• localised disease associated with growth delay and often delay in pubertal development;
• inflammatory mass;
• intestinal fistulae;
• rectal stricture.

The aim of surgical treatment for these complications is to preserve as much intestine as possible.

Localised strictures may be treated by simple stricturoplasty (without loss of bowel) or resection. An important role for surgery is resection of localised disease associated with growth delay or delay in pubertal development, or both, despite maximal medical treatment. In the majority of these patients, a sustained remission can be expected, together with catch-up growth and resumption of normal schooling. The best results can be anticipated with resection of localised ileo-caecal disease before or at the onset of puberty.

Resection may be necessary for inflammatory masses and fistulae.

There is a high incidence of rectal strictures in paediatric Crohn disease. It is often associated with perineal inflammation.

The management of this complication includes steroid therapy, both systemic (as previously mentioned) and local steroid medication as administered in enema form. The surgery includes regular dilatations of the stricture under general anaesthetic (GA), usually conducted in association with endoscopic evaluation. The associated perineal inflammation tends to resolve with control of the rectal stricture.

Ulcerative colitis

Ulcerative colitis is a chronic inflammatory disease of the rectal and colonic mucosa, the aetiology of which is unknown.

Clinical features
The onset is usually insidious, but an acute onset similar to a Salmonella infection can occur. The onset of the disease is usually after 5 years of age, but can be as early as the first year of life.

The typical features are as follows:
1 unexplained bloody diarrhoea, with mucus, lasting more than 2 weeks;
2 anaemia;
3 fever;
4 weight loss.

All degrees of severity are encountered, and the predominating symptom varies from one patient to another.

Perianal complications occur in between 10% and 20% of patients, and include ulcers, abscesses and fistulae. As in Crohn disease, perianal complications may be the presenting problem, but more usually the development of perianal disease is preceded by a period of diarrhoea.

Investigations
Colonoscopy
Colonoscopy accurately assesses the extent of macroscopic disease and biopsies taken at colonoscopy achieve the diagnosis. In ulcerative colitis, inflammatory changes are seen in the rectum and extend for varying distances proximally in the colon. The changes range in severity from loss of the normal mucosal sheen and vascularity with associated mucosal friability to diffuse ulceration with blood and pus in the lumen. Numerous biopsies taken during colonoscopy will confirm the histological diagnosis and indicate the severity of inflammation at various levels. The histology can be reported, at best, as 'consistent with' ulcerative colitis, for there is no pathognomonic lesion.

In some instances, even when macroscopic appearances at endoscopy are normal, multiple biopsies will provide diagnostic histolological changes.

Contrast imaging
This investigation may show a 'saw-tooth' or marked irregularities in the mucosa, with deep ulceration. Later, the colon becomes narrow, rigid and devoid of visible peristalsis or haustration [Fig. 24.3]. Finally, there may be pseudopolyps or stenosis due to the development of a fibrous stricture.

Other tests
Other tests include an FBE, to demonstrate anaemia. Bacteriology tests should include a careful search for enteric pathogens, including Salmonella, Shigella, Campylobacter

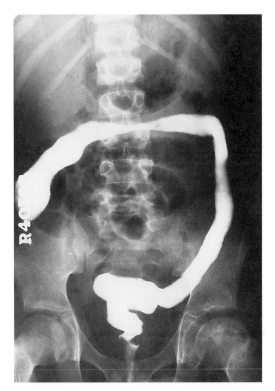

Figure 24.3 Ulcerative colitis. Featureless colon with 'saw-tooth' outline on barium enema.

and Yersinia. Blood for Yersinia antibodies should be collected.

Course of the disease

Improvements in medical treatment, with more aggressive use of steroids, have produced better control of the disease. Many children have remissions lasting several years, to the extent that the diagnosis is subsequently questioned. A small proportion continue to have recurrent lapses, and may require colectomy.

Risk of malignancy

The incidence of carcinoma is directly proportional to the duration of the disease. The risk in the first 10 years of disease is very low. After 10 years of disease, the rate increases by 10% for each decade.

Surveillance by regular colonoscopy and detection of dysplasia by biopsies as a predictor of potential malignancy is an important component of management of paediatric patients with ulcerative colitis. Colectomy is recommended after 10 years of proven disease.

Medical treatment of ulcerative colitis

The principles of medical treatment are similar to those for Crohn disease. These principles have been enumerated earlier. However, many of the drugs for ulcerative colitis can be given as enemas.

Surgical treatment of ulcerative colitis

Procto-colectomy is curative, but other surgical procedures have a place in the treatment of this disease.

The indications for surgical treatment are as follows:
1 Severe inflammation unresponsive to medical treatment;
2 Severe disease associated with growth delay and delay in pubertal development;
3 Long-term risk of malignancy (see above);
4 Acute haemorrhage;
5 Perforation;
6 Toxic megacolon.

It is most important to realise that absence of symptoms should not be taken as evidence of quiescent or inactive disease, or of healing. Surveillance by regular colonoscopy should continue in proven cases of ulcerative colitis.

Surgical options

Subtotal colectomy with ileo-rectal anastomosis: This procedure may be considered in a situation where there is minimal rectal inflammation, particularly in an adolescent entering young adulthood. This procedure may avoid the need for an ileostomy. However, this option requires continuing endoscopy surveillance, together with biopsies every 6 months. Removal of the rectum will be necessary after 10 years of disease.

Procto-colectomy: This procedure may be achieved with a number of techniques as follows:
• ileo-anal anastomosis with ileal reservoir;
• ileo-anal anastomosis without reservoir – Soave pull-through procedure.

Chronic inflammatory bowel disease of indeterminate pathology

In a small number of patients, the pathology is uncertain, and a diagnostic dilemma arises as to whether the patient has ulcerative colitis or Crohn disease. The principles of medical treatment are similar to those outlined earlier in this chapter. The principles of surgical treatment depend on what is considered to be the most likely condition as judged on clinical, endoscopic and histological evidence.

Key Points

- Crohn disease is now relatively common in children and adolescents.
- Recurrent abdominal pain with intermittent diarrhoea suggest IBD.
- Perianal sepsis in adolescents suggests Crohn disease.
- IBD diagnosis requires sophisticated imaging, endoscopy and biopsy.
- Surgical treatment is required if medical therapy fails, and for prevention of colonic cancer.

Further reading

Alexander F (2006) Crohn's disease. In: Grosfeld JL, O'Neill JA Jr., Fonkalsrud EW, Coran AG (eds) *Pediatric Surgery*, 6th Edn. Mosby Elsevier, Philadelphia, pp. 1453–1461.

Alexander F (2006) Inflammatory bowel disease in children. In: Stringer MD, Oldham KT, Mouriquand PDE (eds) *Pediatric Surgery and Urology. Long Term Outcomes*, 2nd Edn. Cambridge University Press, Cambridge, pp. 351–361.

Fonkalsrud EW (2006) Ulcerative colitis. In: Grosfeld JL, O'Neill JA Jr., Fonkalsrud EW, Coran AG (eds) *Pediatric Surgery*, 6th Edn. Mosby Elsevier, Philadelphia, pp. 1462–1474.

25 The Child with an Abdominal Mass

Case 1

A 9-year-old boy presents with a 2-week history of intermittent pain in the left loin and flank. Physical examination reveals a large smooth mass in the left side of the abdomen. The mass is firm, but not solid, and is 'ballottable'.

Q 1.1 What is the likely diagnosis?

Q 1.2 What investigations might be needed?

Case 2

A previously well 4-year-old girl presents with a large, smooth and solid mass in the right side of the abdomen, noted accidentally during examination. The blood pressure is 110/80.

Q 2.1 What is the differential diagnosis?

Q 2.2 What treatment might be needed?

Case 3

A 5-year-old girl has been 'unwell' and pale in recent weeks. The school nurse finds a large, hard and craggy mass in the upper abdomen.

Q 3.1 What investigations should be undertaken and what is the likely diagnosis?

Q 3.2 What would you tell the parents?

The following points need to be considered for a child with a mass in the abdomen:

1 The 'site' of the mass and its precise characteristics, to determine the probable organ of origin.

2 The age of the patient and the most likely pathological process arising in that organ at that age.

3 The length of history and the type of symptoms (e.g. fever and tenderness may suggest an infection).

Normal and abnormal masses

The most common abdominal masses in infancy and childhood are non-pathological. They are usually accounted for by the liver, which normally extends below the right costal margin until 3 or 4 years of age; faeces in the colon or a full bladder [Table 25.1]. In addition, there are three common pathological conditions that warrant special

Jones' Clinical Paediatric Surgery, 6th edition. By Hutson, O'Brien, Woodward and Beasley. Published 2008 by Blackwell Publishing, ISBN: 978-1-4051-6267-8.

consideration as a group presenting as an abdominal mass: hydronephrosis, Wilms' tumour of the kidney and abdominal neuroblastoma.

They have certain features in common:

1 They arise most frequently in infants and toddlers between 1 and 3 years of age.

2 At this age, the abdomen is normally protuberant and tends to conceal the mass, which is often quite large when first detected.

3 General or local symptoms are frequently minimal or absent. The mass itself is usually the presenting feature, and typically is discovered by the mother while drying the child's abdomen after a bath.

There may be a loin mass confined to one side of the abdomen extending below the rib margin towards the iliac fossa. Other masses are situated in the upper abdomen and may straddle the midline. Most masses are not tender unless there has been a complication such as infection or bleeding. When the mass is centred on the midline in the upper abdomen, a primary neuroblastoma is the most likely cause, particularly if the child is less than 4 years of age. Massive hepatic metastases (from a

Table 25.1 The more common normal and abnormal abdominal masses in children

Normal	Abnormal
Liver	Hydronephrosis
Faeces	Wilms' tumour
Bladder	Neuroblastoma
Lower pole of kidneys	

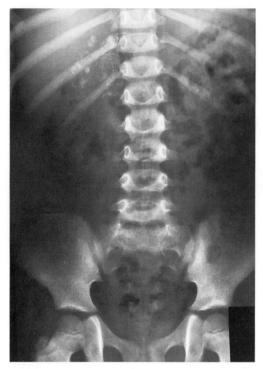

Figure 25.1 Neuroblastoma, showing calcification in the right paravertebral region.

neuroblastoma) and a primary hepatoblastoma are other possibilities. Loin masses may be due to hydronephrosis or Wilms' tumour of the kidney.

Investigations

The basic investigations are a plain abdominal x-ray and an abdominal ultrasound. The plain film of the abdomen may show calcification within the mass, more commonly in neuroblastoma [Fig. 25.1] than in Wilms' tumour, and not at all in hydronephrosis, unless there is a renal stone.

Abdominal ultrasound will determine whether a mass is 'cystic' or 'solid'. Cystic masses include hydronephrosis, polycystic kidneys, multilocular or simple renal cysts and a dilated kidney from severe vesico-ureteric reflux. Ultrasonography indicates the size, position and extent of a solid tumour, and gives an indication of blood vessel involvement (e.g. extension of a Wilms' tumour into the inferior vena cava). Lymph nodes, and even metastases, may be demonstrated. A nuclear scan of the kidneys will demonstrate function of a hydronephrotic kidney or one involved by tumour, as well as the degree of function of the contralateral kidney. A more extensive assessment may be necessary, including abdominal computerised tomography (CT) scan or magnetic resonance imaging and, rarely, angiography, to determine vascular supply. The management of hydronephrosis is described in Chapter 33.

Neuroblastoma

This is one of the common malignant tumours of early childhood. It arises from fetal neural crest cells, and the adrenal gland is the commonest site of origin [Fig. 25.1]; the tumour may also arise in the adjacent retroperitoneal sympathetic plexus, the mediastinum, the pelvis and less commonly in other sites.

Early metastases are found frequently and may be in the bone marrow, the cortex of long bones, the skull, the regional or distant lymph nodes, or in the liver. The numerous sites of origin and the occurrence of early distant metastases account for the variety of presenting features, including a rubbery lymph node in the neck or in the axilla (lymph node metastases); paraplegia of rapid onset (spinal involvement); a nodule in the skull or proptosis and periorbital-ecchymoses, or pain and tenderness in the long bones (bone metastases); fever, lethargy and loss of weight; fleeting pain in the limbs; failure to thrive with or without anaemia (bone marrow involvement); and diarrhoea caused by tumour metabolites.

In view of the highly malignant nature of neuroblastoma, it is a paradox that in a small number of cases, the tumour may regress completely with a spontaneous cure. This only occurs if there is a small primary tumour with bone marrow, liver, lymph node or skin metastases; and never if there is cortical bone disease. Almost all children in this group are under 1 year of age. In 65–75% of cases, disseminated disease is present already when the diagnosis is made.

Diagnostic criteria

When an abdominal mass is suspected to be a neuroblastoma, the diagnosis can be confirmed by the following:

1 a marrow biopsy for metastatic neuroblastoma, present at diagnosis in 65–75% of patients;

2 a 24-h collection of urine for biochemical analysis for tumour catecholamine metabolites (VMA, MHMA, [3-methoxyy-4-hydroxymandelic acid], dopamine, adrenaline, noradrenaline);

3 biopsy of either the abdominal tumour or other sites of suspected metastases, for example, lymph nodes.

The diagnosis is confirmed when neuroblastoma cells are identified within the bone marrow, or in a biopsy specimen. When tumour metabolites in the urine are elevated significantly and neuroblastoma cells are seen in bone marrow, a laparotomy can be avoided. A chest x-ray should be performed pre-operatively to look for paravertebral extension of the tumour and mediastinal involvement. The MIBG nuclear scan highlights active metastases when meta-iodobenzylguanidine is incorporated into functioning neuroblastoma tissue.

Treatment

Complete surgical excision of an abdominal neuroblastoma is not always possible and non-resectability is indicated by retroperitoneal extension of tumour encasing the aorta and inferior vena cava. If a small localised tumour is found, it should be removed. Treatment for large primary tumours and metastatic neuroblastoma involves intensive combination chemotherapy and reassessment after 3–6 months with surgical removal of the residual tumour, if feasible. Finally, high-dose chemotherapy is given with autologous bone marrow rescue. In rare cases, radiotherapy may be used.

The prognosis is poor, with less than 25% of children surviving when metastases are present at diagnosis. Survival is related to the tumour biology that is characterised by the *N-MYC* oncogene.

Wilms' tumour

Wilms' tumour, or nephroblastoma of the kidney, arises from primitive embryonic cells and produces a mixed histological picture of epithelial structures resembling tubules and a variety of mesenchymal tissues, including striated muscle fibres.

A bilateral Wilms' tumour is often seen in children. Where this is present there may be an underlying genetic defect, and chromosomal analysis should be performed, looking for an abnormality on chromosome 11 (eleven). There may be an increased risk of recurrent primary tumours.

Clinical features

A Wilms' tumour usually presents as a smooth mass in the loin that seldom crosses the midline, but extends downwards into the iliac fossa and upwards, under the costal margin. A right-sided Wilms' tumour may extend behind the liver, which if pushed downwards, can present as hepatomegaly. On the left side, a Wilms' tumour may be mistaken for an enlarged spleen.

Haematuria, often following minor trauma, is the presentation in some children, but does not indicate a poor prognosis. Clinical examination of the child should always include a blood pressure measurement, as this may be elevated due to unusual metabolites from the tumour tissue.

Investigation

Ultrasonography provides detailed information of the site, size and extent of the tumour [Fig. 25.2a, Table 25.2]. Ultrasonography also identifies renal vein and inferior vena cava involvement. The liver is examined for the presence of metastases and a chest x-ray excludes the presence of pulmonary metastases. A CT scan is employed on occasions [Fig. 25.2b] for large and complex tumours. CT is also used for needle biopsy guidance in large tumours.

Treatment

The kidney is removed, if possible. In Stage 1 tumours, adjuvant chemotherapy is given for a period of 3 months. In Stage 2 tumours, two-agent chemotherapy will be used for 12–15 months, and in Stage 3 tumours, three-agent chemotherapy is used for 12–15 months, with radiotherapy as an occasional adjunct. If the tumour is large, chemotherapy may be used to 'shrink' the tumour before surgical removal. In Stage 4 tumours, chemotherapy is the mainstay of treatment.

Table 25.2 Staging of Wilms' tumour

Stage	Tumour spread
I	Confined to kidney and removed completely
II	Microscopic local disease after resection
III	Macroscopic residual disease after resection
IV	Distant metastases

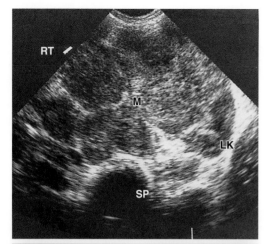

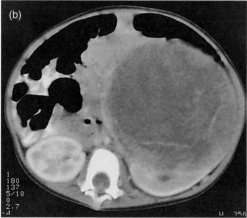

Figure 25.2 (a) Ultrasound showing a large Wilms' tumour (M) arising from the left kidney (LK); (b) CT scan showing the same tumour in cross section.

Two rare causes of a renal mass, mesenchymal hamartoma and multilocular cyst of the kidney cannot be completely excluded by investigations or on their macroscopic appearance at operation, and are removed with the kidney.

Prognosis

Wilms' tumour, in contrast to neuroblastoma, usually has a good outcome. In Stage 1, the cure rate is greater than 95%. Even in unfavourable circumstances, for example, with pulmonary metastases, the results are better than 50% 5-years' survival. Late recurrence locally, or as pulmonary metastasis, is very rare after 1 or 2 years, but careful follow-up with abdominal ultrasonography and chest x-ray, is required, particularly in the first 12 months of treatment.

Liver tumours

Hepatoblastoma is the most common malignant tumour presenting as a right upper quadrant mass in children less than 1 year of age. Alternative diagnoses include arteriovenous malformation (which may be accompanied by thrombocytopenia) and mesenchymal hamartoma, both of which are benign liver masses. Elevation of serum alpha-fetoprotein – a tumour marker – is highly suggestive of hepatoblastoma with a liver mass. Accurate preoperative assessment is necessary with imaging techniques including ultrasonography, CT scan, MRI and angiography. Surgical resection of the lesion, either locally or by lobectomy, remains the mainstay of treatment for all primary liver tumours. Preoperative chemotherapy has been shown to improve survival significantly. Liver transplantation occasionally is used if the tumour is unresectable after chemotherapy.

Key Points

- A child with an abdominal mass needs immediate clinical assessment and investigation to exclude malignancy.
- Abdominal masses in toddlers may be huge before diagnosis.
- Ultrasonography is an effective screening test for malignancy.
- A patient with a presumed abdominal tumour needs immediate referral to the regional surgical and oncology centre.

Further reading

Grosfeld JL (2006) Neuroblastoma. In: Grosfeld JL, O'Neill JA, Fonkalsrud EW, Coran AG (eds) *Pediatric Surgery*, 6th Edn. Mosby Elsevier, Philadelphia, pp. 467–494.

Ikeda H, Suzuki N, Takahashi A et al. (1998) Surgical treatment of neuroblastomas in infants under 12 months of age. *J Pediatr Surg* **33**: 1246–1250.

Tagge EP, Thomas PB, Otheson HB (2006) Wilms' tumour. In: Grosfeld JL, O'Neill JA Jr., Fonkalsrud EW, Coran AG (eds) *Pediatric Surgery*, 6th Edn. Mosby Elsevier, Philadelphia, pp. 445–466.

26 Spleen, Pancreas and Biliary Tract

Case 1

A 4-year-old girl presents with a distended epigastrium and paralytic ileus. On physical examination, there are several old fractures with callus formation.

Q 1.1 What causes pancreatitis?

Q 1.2 How is pancreatitis diagnosed?

Q 1.3 What is a pseudocyst?

Case 2

A 3-week-old infant develops gastroenteritis from her older siblings. After resolution of diarrhoea, she is noted to be jaundiced.

Q 2.1 How would you determine whether obstructive jaundice was present?

Q 2.2 What differences in management are there between a bile duct stone and biliary atresia?

The spleen

Splenectomy is indicated for a variety of conditions in childhood [Table 26.1]. Most splenectomies are performed using a laparoscopic technique.

Overwhelming post-splenectomy sepsis (OPSI)

The OPSI occurs in between 1% and 5% of children following splenectomy. Sepsis is caused by encapsulated organisms such as pneumococcus, meningococcus and haemophilus. The risk of OPSI is lifelong and has a mortality rate of 50%. The younger the age of the child at the time of splenectomy, the greater is the incidence of OPSI; or when the spleen is removed for haematological conditions, the incidence of OPSI increases. Preoperative immunisation against encapsulated organisms and lifelong penicillin is an essential part of splenectomy.

Hereditary spherocytosis

Hereditary spherocytosis is an autosomal dominant condition resulting in auto-immune haemolytic anaemia. In spherocytosis the red cells are abnormally spherical and are destroyed in the spleen. This tends to result in

1 chronic anaemia;

2 episodic haemolytic jaundice;

3 a tendency to form pigment gallstones.

These complications can be controlled by splenectomy, but unless they are severe, splenectomy is delayed until at least the age of 7 years of age because of the risk of post-splenectomy sepsis. Cholecystectomy may be required at the same time.

Idiopathic thrombocytopenic purpura

Idiopathic thrombocytopenic purpura is an auto-immune condition of unknown aetiology causing destruction of platelets. It presents most commonly in an acute form that usually resolves spontaneously. Administration of gamma globulin is sometimes required in severe episodes to control the platelet count. Splenectomy is rarely indicated. A small percentage of children will develop a chronic form of the condition. In selected children not responding to medical treatment, splenectomy may be required, to improve the platelet count.

Jones' Clinical Paediatric Surgery, 6th edition. By Hutson, O'Brien, Woodward and Beasley. Published 2008 by Blackwell Publishing, ISBN: 978-1-4051-6267-8.

Table 26.1   Indications for splenectomy in childhood
Hereditary spherocytosis
Idiopathic thrombocytopenic purpura
Thalassaemia
Sickle-cell anaemia
Storage diseases
Hypersplenism
Neoplasms
Congenital cysts
Trauma

Table 26.2   Common causes of pancreatitis in childhood
1. Trauma (handlebar injury, motor accident, child abuse)
2. Drugs – steroids, azathioprine
3. Viral
4. Biliary tract disorders – choledochal cyst, gallstones
5. Hereditary
6. Metabolic – hyperlipidaemia

Thalassaemia

In thalassaemia major, a homozygous condition, the production of abnormal haemoglobin results in chronic haemolytic anaemia. In the past, chronic anaemia, blood transfusions and subsequent increasing iron stores have resulted in the patient developing a very large spleen, producing the added problem of secondary hypersplenism. The enlarged spleen tends to destroy all cellular elements in the blood.

Transfusions keep the children healthy whereas regular parenteral desferrioxamine chelates excess iron liberated from haemolysed red cells and maintains normal serum iron levels. In thalassaemia splenectomy is indicated if the splenomegaly causes mechanical problems or if the secondary effects of hypersplenism are difficult to control.

Sickle-cell anaemia

The presence of abnormal haemoglobin S results in an abnormally shaped red cell during hypoxia. These 'sickle cells' tend to slow the blood flow through small vessels, causing ischaemia in the organ involved. Splenic infarcts can occur.

Splenectomy is usually contra-indicated as higher haemoglobin tends to be associated with increased 'sickling' of the red cells.

Trauma

Splenectomy for trauma is now exceptionally rare (see Chapter 38).

The pancreas

Acute pancreatitis

Acute pancreatitis in childhood is an uncommon clinical entity. The known aetiologies in the paediatric age group are extensive. A brief list of some of the more common causes of pancreatitis in childhood are listed below [Table 26.2].

Traumatic pancreatitis

The pancreas is the fourth most common abdominal organ injured in childhood trauma. Nearly all cases result from blunt abdominal trauma. Penetrating trauma is rare in childhood. The most common cause by far in most Western countries is a handlebar injury, but child abuse may present this way, secondary to a kick or punch in the abdomen. The morbidity associated with blunt trauma of the pancreas is determined by whether there is a disruption of the pancreatic duct. The initial investigation of choice is a CT scan. If the CT scan suggests disruption of the pancreatic duct, then further investigations to determine this may be indicated. In this situation a magnetic resonance cholangiopancreatogram (MRCP) or endoscopic retrograde cholangiopancreatogram (ERCP) can be of benefit. Most cases do not involve a duct injury and are managed conservatively. The management of duct disruption remains controversial. Some advocate conservative management, accepting the risk of a pseudocyst (see below), while others advocate an early distal pancreatectomy.

Pseudocyst

A pancreatic pseudocyst is a collection of pancreatic fluid within a non-epithelial-lined cavity. In theory, it can complicate pancreatitis from any cause, however, in children it is virtually only ever seen following trauma. Most pancreatic pseudocysts lie in the lesser sac. Treatment is initially non-operative. Many resolve spontaneously. The progress of the collection is followed by serial ultrasound scans. Intervention is indicated if the cyst is enlarging or causing symptoms. Internal drainage of the cyst into the stomach via an endoscopic cyst-gastrostomy or open cyst-gastrostomy is the preferred technique.

Hyperinsulinism (causing hypoglycaemia)

Excessive production of insulin may occur in several situations.
1 In babies of diabetic mothers as a temporary response to high sugar levels.

2 Beta-cell hyperplasia, a condition of unknown aetiology in which there is excessive production of insulin, which usually settles down with drug treatment (Diazoxide). Extensive pancreatectomy is only necessary occasionally.

3 Beckwith–Weidemann syndrome, a condition of newborn babies that is characterised by exomphalos; organomegaly (large tongue and abdominal organs); hemihypertrophy; and transient low blood sugar from excessive insulin and insulin-like growth factor production.

4 Islet cell tumours are a rare cause of hypoglycaemia; they can be cured if the tumour (usually benign) is localised and excised.

The biliary tract

Neonatal jaundice

Jaundice in the newborn most commonly results from a cause at the prehepatic or hepatic level. Posthepatic causes of jaundice result in conjugated hyperbilirubinaemia and may require surgical treatment. These causes include

1 biliary atresia;

2 choledochal cysts;

3 inspissated bile syndrome;

4 bile duct strictures;

5 spontaneous biliary perforation.

All cases of conjugated hyperbilirubinaemia in the neonatal period should be promptly investigated.

Biliary atresia

Biliary atresia is a condition of progressive obliteration of the extrahepatic ducts as a result of an inflammatory condition. This process may involve part or all of the extrahepatic biliary tree. The ducts may disappear or, more commonly, persist as a fibrous cord.

The incidence of biliary atresia is about 1 per 15,000 live births. The aetiology remains unknown although there is a wide range of hypotheses based on infective, embryological, metabolic and vascular studies. In up to 20% of cases, biliary atresia is associated with a distinct syndrome known as the biliary atresia-splenic malformation syndrome (BASM). Associated anomalies in this syndrome include splenic abnormalities (asplenia or polysplenia), situs inversus, malrotation, cardiac anomalies and preduodenal portal vein.

Biliary atresia presents as prolonged jaundice following the not infrequent period of neonatal physiological jaundice. Progressive obstructive jaundice occurs in the first 6 weeks of life with pale stools and dark urine. Typically, these infants are thriving at the time of presentation.

Diagnosis

Prompt diagnosis is essential in biliary atresia as the results of surgery are closely correlated with the timing of operation. Ultrasonography is the most important initial investigation. This will exclude other surgical causes of jaundice (see above). In biliary atresia a fasting ultrasound scan will usually show a small and contracted gallbladder. A presumptive diagnosis is best made by liver biopsy (open or percutaneous), which in experienced hands will yield a positive diagnosis in up to 95% of cases. The definitive diagnosis is made at laparotomy by confirming non-patency of the extrahepatic biliary tree. HIDA scans are of limited value as their interpretation in the newborn period is difficult.

Treatment

Biliary atresia is treated by porto-enterostomy (Kasai procedure). This operation involves dissecting out the obliterated extrahepatic ducts up to the portal plate and shaving off the inflammatory tissue at the portal plate flush with the liver surface. A Roux-en-Y loop of jejunum is then anastomosed to the edges of the portal plate. The operation relies on bile draining from microscopic bile ducts in the portal plate. Drainage rates of up to 60% can be achieved in good centres. There is a dramatic fall off in drainage rates if the operation is performed after 100 days of life. It is not possible to determine at the time of operation whether the operation has been successful. Liver transplantation is required if the operation fails.

Choledochal cysts

Choledochal cyst is a congenital dilatation of the extrahepatic biliary tree. There are various forms, but in the most common variant there is a dilatation of the gall-bladder, cystic duct, common hepatic duct and common bile duct. The dilatation is usually cystic, but fusiform variants are well described [Fig. 26.1].

The incidence in Western countries is between 1 in 100,000 and 1 in 150,000 live births with higher frequency in Asia. The cause remains unclear. The most popular theory relates to the so-called long common channel. Choledochal cysts are frequently associated with an anomalous junction between the terminal common bile duct and the pancreatic duct, whereby the ducts unite outside the duodenal wall and are therefore not surrounded by the normal sphincter mechanism. This situation encourages reflux of pancreatic juice into the common bile duct and it has been proposed that this may result in progressive damage of the biliary tree.

The most common presenting features of a choledochal cyst are obstructive jaundice and abdominal pain.

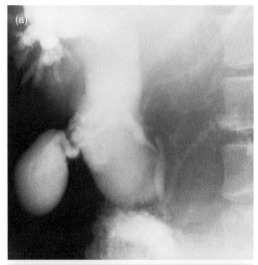

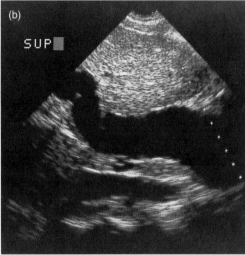

Figure 26.1 Contrast x-ray (a) and ultrasonography (b) of biliary tract showing the massive tubular dilatation of a choledochal cyst.

Pancreatitis is not uncommonly the presenting complaint. In rare cases, a choledochal cyst may present as an abdominal mass. The majority of choledochal cysts are present before the age of 10 years, and increasingly are being detected antenatally. Prenatal diagnosis may be made as early as 15-weeks' gestation. In some situations, differentiation from other congenital cysts in the upper abdomen such as duplication cysts, ovarian cyst and the rare cystic form of biliary atresia can be difficult.

Diagnosis

The diagnosis is easily made on ultrasonography. More detailed information of the nature of the dilatation is now obtained using an MRCP.

Treatment

Treatment is excision of the cyst and drainage of the proximal hepatic duct by a Roux-en-Y loop of jejunum. Choledochal cysts that have been diagnosed antenatally and remain asympomatic are electively treated at 6 months of age.

Inspissated bile syndrome

Inspissated bile syndrome is a condition causing obstructive jaundice in newborns resulting from inspissation of bile in the lower third of the common bile duct. This condition most commonly occurs in premature infants who have had prolonged total parenteral nutrition. It is also associated with extravascular haemolysis. It may occur in otherwise normal neonates.

The diagnosis is made on ultrasound which reveals a dilated proximal biliary tree in association with biliary sludge or stones.

Most cases resolve spontaneously. Resistant cases may be cleared by percutaneous transhepatic irrigation of the bile ducts or retrograde irrigation by ERCP. Surgery is only rarely required.

Bile duct strictures

Bile duct strictures are a rare but well-known cause of obstructive jaundice in newborns. Most strictures are idiopathic. A small proportion occur in association with a long common channel (see above), where the presumed aetiology is reflux of pancreatic juice into the common bile duct. The most common site of obstruction is the distal common bile duct. Diagnosis is made using percutaneous transhepatic cholangiography or ERCP. Relief of the obstruction may be achieved by balloon dilatation using the same modalities. If this is unsuccessful then biliary diversion is required by a formal operation.

Spontaneous biliary perforation

Spontaneous biliary perforation is a rare condition resulting in progressive obstructive jaundice and ascites in the newborn period. Most cases present between 1 week and 2 months of age. The site of the perforation is always at the junction of the cystic and common hepatic duct. The aetiology is unknown. The presentation is usually insidious. Ascites results from a localised biliary peritonitis and the jaundice occurs as a result of both proximal biliary obstruction secondary to oedema and reabsorption of bile through the peritoneum. The diagnosis is made on ultrasonography which demonstrates a loculated collection in the portal region. The treatment is surgical.

Cholelithiasis in children

In children, the cause of gallstones can be divided into the following groups:

1 *Haemolytic disorders.* Conditions such as sickle-cell anaemia, thalassaemia and hereditary spherocytosis are associated with the formation of pigment stones due to the increased red cell breakdown.

2 *Total parenteral nutrition (TPN).* The association of TPN and biliary sludge/cholelithiasis is well recognised. The exact cause is unknown, but biliary stasis due to impairment of the enterohepatic circulation of bile is probably important.

3 *Ileal resection.* Ileal resection is a well-known risk factor for cholelithiasis. In children, the most common cause of ileal resection is necrotising enterocolitis in premature infants. The traditional explanation for gallstones in this setting is that normal reabsorption of bile salts in the terminal ileum is impaired, leading to depletion of the bile salt pool in the enterohepatic circulation. This promotes lithogenic bile.

4 *Mechanical causes.* Any condition that leads to biliary stasis is associated with the formation of gallstones. These conditions include bile duct strictures, choledochal cysts and congenital gall bladder abnormalities.

5 *Specific conditions.* Certain conditions such as cystic fibrosis, Crohn disease and diabetes are associated with an increased incidence of cholelithiasis.

6 *Adult causes.* Adolescents with typical adult-type risk factors have the same tendency to develop gallstones. These risk factors include obesity, the oral contraceptive pill and genetic factors.

The ways in which a child with gallstones may present are summarised in Table 26.3.

Treatment

Treatment involves laparoscopic cholecystectomy (and removal of stones in the common bile duct if present).

Key Points

- Splenectomy is avoided in small children because of the risk of overwhelming post-splenectomy sepsis (1–5%).
- Ruptured spleen hardly ever needs splenectomy, as bleeding stops.
- Pancreatitis may occur with trauma.
- Prolonged jaundice in neonates needs investigation to exclude biliary atresia.
- Gallstones are now relatively common in children.

Further reading

Howard ER (2006) Biliary atresia. In: Stringer MD, Oldham KT, Mouriquand PDE, (eds) *Pediatric Surgery and Urology: Long-Term Outcomes*, Cambridge University Press, Cambridge, pp. 446–464.

Idowa O, Hayes-Jordan A (1998) Partial splenectomy in children under 4 years of age with hemoglobinopathy. *J Pediatr Surg* **33**: 1251–1253.

Miyano T (2006) The pancreas. In: Grosfeld, JL, O'Neill JA Jr., Fonkalsrud EW, Coran AG (eds) *Pediatric Surgery*, 6th Edn. Mosby Elsevier, Philadelphia, pp. 1671–1690.

Rescorla FJ (2006) Spleen. In: Grosfeld JL, O'Neill JA Jr., Fonkalsrud EW, Coran AG (eds) *Pediatric Surgery*, 6th Edn. Mosby Elsevier, Philadelphia, pp. 1691–1702.

Sawyer SM, Davidson PM, McMullin N, Stokes KB (1989) Pancreatic pseudocysts in children. *Pediatr Surg Int* **4**: 300–302.

Table 26.3   Presentation of the child with gallstones

1 Biliary colic: pain from a stone in the neck of the gall-bladder or in the common bile duct
2 Cholecystitis: chemical or bacterial inflammation of the gall-bladder usually associated with cystic duct obstruction
3 Obstructive jaundice: dark urine and pale stools due to a stone obstructing the common bile duct
4 Pancreatitis

27 Anus, Perineum and Female Genitalia

Case 1

A 3-month-old boy presents with a tender, red, indurated area (2×2 cm) adjacent to the anal verge. Twice in recent weeks antibiotics were prescribed for a similar problem that resolved. On palpation and compression of the mass a drop of pus appears at the anus.

Q 1.1 What is the diagnosis and its treatment?

Case 2

A worried mother rushes her 18-month-old daughter to the emergency department after noticing that no vaginal opening is visible. She is frightened something serious is wrong with the genitalia.

Q 2.1 What is the diagnosis?

Q 2.2 How is it treated and recurrence prevented?

Anorectal problems occur commonly in children with abscesses, fistulae and fissures affecting infants, pilonidal disease, haemorrhoids and polyps affecting older children.

Anal fissures

These are confined mostly to infants and toddlers in whom the passage of a hard stool splits the anal mucosa. There is a sharp pain and a few drops of bright blood on the surface of the stool.

When the area is examined the fissure often has already healed, an indication of its superficial nature and its rapid healing. When still present, it is visible usually anteriorly or posteriorly. A chronic fissure may be heralded by a sentinel skin tag. Multiple fissures and those that are not in the midline may be due to other pathology such as inflammatory bowel disease, infection or trauma.

Treatment

An acute anal fissure is of no consequence in itself and treatment is directed to the underlying constipation (see Chapter 22). A common association with anal fissure is spasm of the internal sphincter and many therapeutic

strategies have been directed for the relief of this spasm that is thought to cause a degree of ischaemia and be the source of the pain associated with anal fissures. Historically, multiple surgical strategies have been employed for chronic anal fissures (more so in adult patients) ranging from simple anal dilatation/stretch to open or closed internal sphincterotomy and even skin flap coverage of the fistula. Surgical treatment has been associated with a 90% cure rate but at the expense of continence (usually to flatus) in 10%. Interestingly, anal stretch has higher reported rates of incontinence than limited lateral sphincterotomy and as such should not be undertaken.

The risk of incontinence associated with surgical procedures stimulated a drive in the 1990s to find a topically active agent that could provide analgesia or sphincter relaxation. A wide variety of agents have been investigated including lignocaine, hydrocortisone, calcium channel blockers, such as nifedipine, nitroglycerin ointment (GTN) and more recently botulinum toxin (Botox). Overall, placebo has been associated with a 35% healing rate and GTN with approximately 55% healing rates. Unfortunately, GTN is associated with headaches in up to 40% of patients severe enough to stop treatment. Botox and Nifedepine have been shown to be as effective as GTN for the treatment of chronic anal fissure and all have been shown to be marginally better than placebo. The risk of late recurrence following medical therapy is approximately 50%.

Jones' Clinical Paediatric Surgery, 6th edition. By Hutson, O'Brien, Woodward and Beasley. Published 2008 by Blackwell Publishing, ISBN: 978-1-4051-6267-8.

After the relief of constipation the child may cry on defecation for several weeks because he or she may associate defecation with pain and react accordingly. The emotional tension built up around the act is more difficult to treat than the fissure itself and can be the forerunner of the whole vicious circle of constipation (Chapter 22).

Perianal abscess

This is fairly common in infants and arises from infection in the anal glands, which open into the crypts of the anal valves. Although the abscess almost always presents superficially, the fistulous tract passes through the lowest fibres of the internal sphincter to open at the level of the anal valves.

Treatment involves identification and laying open of the fistula and drainage of the abscess [Fig. 27.1]. Failure to deal with the fistula may result in recurrent infection.

Sometimes young children may develop a superficial subcutaneous abscess in the buttocks or near the anus, which is often secondary to a nappy rash and involves infection with skin organisms. Simple drainage and antibiotics are curative.

Rectal prolapse

Rectal prolapse is not uncommon in toddlers and it is an alarming experience for the parents [Fig. 27.2]. However, in most cases it disappears spontaneously after a few weeks or months without residual damage.

Aetiology
The two common predisposing factors are
1 Straining at stool by a child with constipation. Less frequently, diarrhoea as part of a malabsorption syndrome (e.g. cystic fibrosis or coeliac disease) may contribute.
2 Explosive or reluctant defecation. A healthy child occasionally develops a prolapse because the act is precipitate and little time is permitted for moulding of the stool by the muscles of the pelvic floor. Alternatively, the parents' ill-advised training may demand prolonged attempts to defecate, producing excessive straining in the absence of constipation.

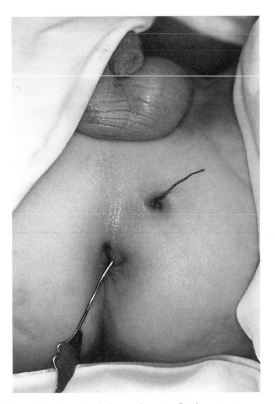

Figure 27.1 In perianal abscess there is a fistulous tract running from the abscess to the anus at the level of the anal valves. The tract is displayed by a lacrimal probe.

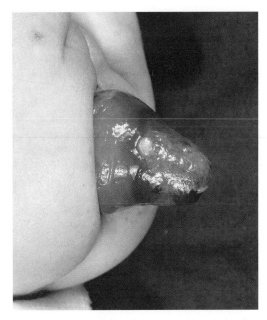

Figure 27.2 Rectal prolapse. The mucosa is congested and oedematous, and may bleed.

Rare, organic causes include
1 paralysis of anal sphincters (spina bifida);
2 hypotonia/starvation;
3 ectopia vesicae (abnormal pelvic girdle);
4 the after-effects of 'pull-through' surgery for an imperforate anus or Hirschsprung disease.

Clinical features

Most children with prolapse have normal anatomy. The prolapse rolls out painlessly only during defecation and usually returns spontaneously; manual replacement is required infrequently. The mucosa may become abraded while it is prolapsed and cause minor bleeding.

Differential diagnosis

A rectal polyp may prolapse (see below) and this can be identified by observation, digital palpation or proctoscopy. It is rare that the apex of an intussusception appears at the anus. This is accompanied by its own clinical features (Chapter 19).

External haemorrhoids do not occur in childhood, but congestion of the submucosal venous plexus during straining at stool sometimes produces a bluish sessile bulge.

Treatment

Constipation is the commonest cause and treatment for at least several weeks is required (Chapter 22). When there is no constipation the possibility of a malabsorption syndrome should be investigated.

A common error is to have the child squat over a potty on the floor to defaecate, which stretches the pelvic floor and the anal sphincters to the maximum disadvantage. A potty-chair or an insert for an adult seat enables the child to sit with support for the pelvic floor, and a reasonable time limit should be set.

It is rarely necessary to inject a sclerosant into the submucosal plane of the rectum to cause fibrosis and contraction of the rectal wall. This is reserved for the few stubborn cases that fail to respond to conservative measures; 0.5 mL of 5% phenol in almond oil is injected into the submucosa at three equally spaced points, 2 cm above the anal valves. It is even more rare that a suture needs be inserted into the subcutaneous tissues around the anus (Thiersch operation) and tied while a finger is held in the anus. This is applicable in certain neurogenic lesions and in severe hypotonia, but is contra-indicated in ordinary constipation. The extensive operations for rectal prolapse performed in adults are never justified in infants and children.

Rectal polyp

A rectal polyp is a benign hamartomatous lesion and a relatively common cause of rectal bleeding. Bright bleeding is produced painlessly at the end of defecation and is typically intermittent over long periods. Occasionally, the polyp prolapses through the anus [Fig. 27.3]. The polyp is almost always within reach of an examining finger. The diagnosis is discussed in the section on rectal bleeding (Chapter 23).

Treatment

On the rare occasions that the polyp presents through the anus, the base can be ligated without anaesthesia. Otherwise, under general anaesthesia the polyp can be located through the proctoscope and withdrawn to demonstrate its stalk, which is transected with diathermy or transfixed with a suture-ligature. Higher lesions can be similarly removed through a colonoscope. Recurrence is rare and malignancy unknown.

Multiple polyposis

This is a rare familial condition with malignant potential seen in adults, and even more rarely in children. It should

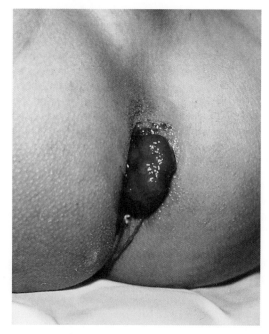

Figure 27.3 Prolapse of a benign rectal polyp through the anus.

be considered when more than three polyps are identi-fied, and when there is a family history of multiple polyposis. Colonoscopy and a double contrast barium enema are indicated. In children, major fluid and elec-trolyte losses may ensue and the colon should be removed.

Peutz–Jegher syndrome

This is an even rarer condition that has gained promi-nence because of the external evidence of its existence – the presence of pigmented freckles on the mucocutaneous margins of the lips and the anus. Polyps are found any-where in the gastrointestinal tract, especially in the jeju-num, and give rise to massive bleeding, intussusception or intestinal obstruction. The polyps may become malig-nant, but this is less common than in familial polyposis of the colon.

Postanal dimple (coccygeal dimple)

Many babies have a small shallow pit in the skin over the coccyx that is of no significance. Occasionally, it is narrow and deep and may become infected, in which case it should be excised.

A simple benign coccygeal dimple is not to be confused with a sacral sinus that, although rare, is potentially more dangerous. The sacral sinus lies over the sacrum, not the coccyx, and it is associated with an underlying spina bifida occulta (Chapter 9). The depths cannot be seen and there is likely to be a small track that communicates directly with the spinal theca or with an intraspinal der-moid cyst. This track is a source of recurrent meningitis and the child should be referred to a neurosurgeon for treatment.

Sacrococcygeal teratoma

A teratoma arising from and attached to the tip of the sacrum or the front of the coccyx occurs in 1:40,000 births, and slightly more frequently in females [Fig. 27.4]. It is usually obvious at birth and may be so large as to cause obstetric difficulties. Occasionally, the swell-ing is in the pelvis and does not protrude from the perineum.

The tumour is a mixture of solid and cystic areas aris-ing from all embryonic layers. The incidence of malig-nancy varies – from 5% to 35% – and it is a type known as an endodermal sinus or yolk-sac tumour. Malignant

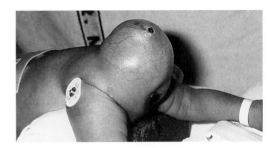

Figure 27.4 Sacrococcygeal teratoma of medium size; note distortion of the perineum and anal canal, and a small ulcer on the surface of the tumour. The prognosis for faecal continence after operation, however, is excellent.

degeneration is less likely when a teratoma is removed immediately after birth.

Management

Even very small lesions over the coccyx should be referred to a tertiary paediatric centre for excision soon after birth. Differential diagnosis includes other rare tumours (chor-doma or ganglioneuroma) or an anterior sacral menin-gocele. A magnetic resonance image may be required to determine the extent of the intrapelvic tumour. Excision is undertaken in the first few days of life if the infant has no other developmental anomalies that might take prior-ity. In spite of gross stretching of the pelvic floor, its nerve supply and the anal canal, the structures usually recover completely after careful surgery without any long-term neural deficit or lack of function.

Prognosis

Local malignant recurrence is uncommon, but more likely if

1 the tumour is uniformly solid and devoid of cysts;
2 the operation is not undertaken until after the age of 1 month.

The large benign teratoma presents at birth and could hardly be overlooked; it is removed in the neonatal period. However, a small malignant teratoma may escape diagno-sis until a rapid increase in size brings it to the notice later in the first year of life.

Pilonidal sinus

Pilonidal sinus derives from the Greek for 'nest of hairs' and commonly occurs in adults. In the paediatric population it is not seen until after puberty and then presents in a similar manner as in adult patients with either an uninfected sinus or an abscess. Though some people believe it is a congenital lesion most accept it is acquired. Treatment of the abscess requires incision, drainage and curettage of the hair mass. Treatment of the sinus is more controversial with many differing strategies from excision and healing by secondary intention to excision with primary wound closure and excision with either subcutaneous tissue flaps (Karydakis flap) or rotational skin flaps (Limberg flap) to provide both wound closure and minimise recurrence that is high. Recently, laser depilation has been added to the treatment algorithm in an attempt to reduce recurrence.

The female genitalia

Developmental anomalies are rare in girls: the commonest abnormality, adhesion of the labia minora, is caused by ulceration of the labia (nappy rash) with secondary adhesion during re-epithelialisation.

Labial adhesions

This is a common condition, which may cause discomfort during micturition, but is more often discovered on routine examination [Fig. 27.5a and b]. There is a delicate midline adhesion of the two labia minora that partially closes the posterior introitus, overlying the opening of the urethra, and may extend as far anteriorly as the clitoris.

Congenital absence of the vagina frequently is diagnosed in error, causing the parents much unnecessary anxiety. Labial adhesions never present at birth.

Treatment

In infants and young children the fused labia can be separated by exerting gentle lateral traction on the labia minora without anaesthesia or by sweeping them apart with the blunt end of a thermometer. In older children the labia may require separation under anaesthesia. Because of the tendency for the adhesions to recur, the mother should separate the labia daily for 2 weeks and apply petroleum jelly to the introitus to help prevent recurrent adhesion.

Imperforate hymen

This is a rare condition, which presents either at birth (the vagina secretes mucus that accumulates beneath the bulging imperforate hymen to form a mucocolpos; Fig. 27.6) or at puberty when apparent primary amenorrhoea, haematocolpos of even haematometrocolpos may be the presenting features, with cyclic attacks of abdominal pain. During childhood the condition is usually symptomless, except for possible urinary symptoms such as 'wetting', or dysuria when the cystic swelling distorts the urethra.

Treatment at birth sees the removal of a circular disc of membrane to provide drainage.

Vaginal discharge

The chief symptom is vulval irritation, but in some cases the discharge itself may be the only complaint. A profuse

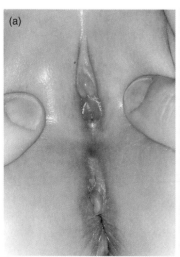
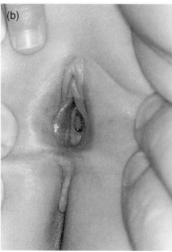

Figure 27.5 Adherent labia minora ('labial adhesions'). (a) The normal labia majora have been flattened by lateral traction to display the line of fusion. (b) Following the separation the introitus is fully visible.

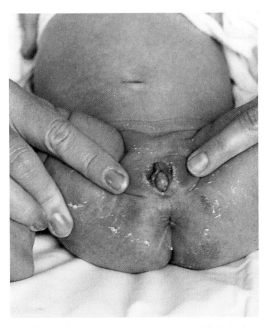

Figure 27.6 Imperforate hymen causing mucocolpos in a newborn infant.

offensive or blood-stained discharge suggests the presence of a foreign body. Small objects may be successfully removed by irrigation using a soft rubber catheter or instrumental removal under anaesthesia, through a miniature vaginoscope.

The possibility of sexual abuse must be considered, and where suspected, the discharge should be sent for microbiological examination (Chapter 36).

Key Points

- Pain of defecation associated with a few drops of bright blood suggests an anal fissure.
- Perianal abscess is common in the first year, and often leads to a fistula-in-ano.
- Both rectal prolapse and anal fissure resolve spontaneously with correction of constipation and good toileting behaviour.
- Any baby with an abnormal mass near the coccyx should be referred to a paediatric surgical centre at birth, as the diagnosis may be sacrococcygeal teratoma.
- Labial adhesion is acquired following ulceration with nappy rash, is easily distinguished from vaginal agenesis (imperforate hymen), and responds to simple separation and application of petroleum jelly to prevent re-adherence.

Further reading

Beasley SW, Hutson JM, Auldist AW (1996) The anorectum and perineum. In: *Essential Paediatric Surgery*, Arnold, London, pp. 58–66.

Beasley SW, Hutson JM, Auldist AW (1996) Labial adhesions. In: *Essential Paediatric Surgery*, Arnold, London, pp. 115–120.

Nelson R (2002) Outcome of operative procedures for fissure in ano. *Cochrane Database Syst Rev*, Issue 1. Art No.: CD002199.

Nelson R (2006) Nonsurgical therapy for anal fissure. *Cochrane Database Syst Rev*, Issue 4. Art No.: CD003431.

Rintala RJ, Pakarinen M (2006) Other disorders of the anus and rectum, anorectal function. In: Grosfeld JL, O'Neill JA Jr., Fonkalsrud EW, Coran AG (eds) *Pediatric Surgery*, 6th Edn. Mosby Elsevier, Philadelphia, pp. 1590–1602.

Stephens FD, Smith ED, Hutson JM (2002) *Congenital Anomalies of the Kidney, Urinary and Genital Tracts*, 2nd Edn. Martin Dunitz, London.

28 Undescended Testes and Varicocele

Case 1

At birth a baby boy was noted to have only one testis in the scrotum. Re-examination at 3 months showed that both testes were now in the scrotum.

Q 1.1 What is the likely natural history of the testis?

Q 1.2 Is treatment required later in childhood?

Case 2

No testes were palpable in the scrotum or groin in a baby at the 6-week postnatal check.

Q 2.1 What is the differential diagnosis?

Q 2.2 What is the management?

Case 3

Unilateral undescended testis is diagnosed at birth and confirmed at the 6-week check, in a baby with no other anomalies.

Q 3.1 What is the recommended age for surgery?

Q 3.2 What is the prognosis for fertility and cancer risk?

Definitions

Congenital undescended testis

A congenital undescended testis (UDT) is one that has failed to reach the bottom of the scrotum by 3 months of age. It represents the second most common problem in paediatric surgery after indirect inguinal hernia. At birth 4–5% of boys have undescended testes, but postnatal descent may continue for the first 3 months, when the incidence of cryptorchidism falls to 1–2%, which is about double the incidence 50 years ago. Further descent after 3 months is rare. Most undescended testes have no recognisable primary abnormality, but degenerative changes increase with the age of the patient at orchidopexy. These degenerative changes are likely to be secondary to the high temperature of the misplaced testis.

In the majority of patients, the cause of maldescent is unknown. Mechanical factors may be important as cryptorchidism is more common in boys with gastroschisis,

exomphalos and Prune Belly, all of which have a reduced intra-abdominal pressure *in utero*. A potential hormonal aetiology is suggested by association with IUGR, multiple pregnancies and previous stillbirth, all features suggestive of a degree of placental failure or insufficiency. It has been suggested that the increasing incidence of UDT, hypospadias, testicular cancer and low sperm counts in Northern Europe is caused by *in utero* exposure to environmental pollution with 'endocrine disruptors' (synthetic molecules that mimic oestrogen).

Acquired undescended testis

The concept of acquired undescended testes is controversial, but it explains the high frequency of children presenting later in childhood. The cause may be failure of the processus vaginalis to disappear completely after descent, thereby leaving a remnant in the spermatic cord which tethers the testis and prevents normal elongation with age (the length of the spermatic cord increases from about 5 cm in infants to 8–10 cm in adolescents).

Retractile testis

A normal retractile testis can be manipulated to the bottom of the scrotum, regardless of its initial position and

Jones' Clinical Paediatric Surgery, 6th edition. By Hutson, O'Brien, Woodward and Beasley. Published 2008 by Blackwell Publishing, ISBN: 978-1-4051-6267-8.

remains in the scrotum after manipulation. It is a normal size and is present in the scrotum on some occasions, such as during a warm bath. Testes may retract into an extension of the tunica vaginalis between the external oblique aponeurosis and the superficial abdominal fascia, known as the 'superficial inguinal pouch'. The position of the testis is controlled by the cremaster muscle which helps to regulate testicular temperature by retracting the testis out of the scrotum when cold; it also protects the testis from trauma. Cremasteric contraction is absent in the first few months after birth and is maximal between 2 and 8 years. Retractile testes may be normal, but in severe cases may represent acquired maldescent.

Ascending testis

An 'ascending' testis is one that is in the scrotum in infancy, but where the spermatic cord fails to elongate at the same rate as body growth, and the testicular position becomes progressively higher during childhood. There is often a history of the testis descending into the scrotum some weeks after birth. This anomaly is thought to be a form of acquired undescended testes.

Impalpable testis

Approximately 1 in 4 (25%) undescended testis will not be palpable. Of these 40% will be absent having undergone prenatal or perinatal atrophy; 20% will be intra-abdominal; 30% will be found within the inguinal canal and 10% in an ectopic location. The exact nature and location of an impalpable testis will only become apparent on exploration, either laparoscopic or open surgery.

Examination

The examination of the testis should take place in warm and relaxed surroundings, and is begun by placing one finger on each side of the neck of the scrotum to pull the scrotum up to the pubis and to prevent the testes from being retracted out of the scrotum by the other examining hand. Each side of the scrotum is then palpated for a testis; if it is not there, the fingertips are placed just medial to the anterior superior iliac spine and moved firmly towards the pubic tubercle [Fig. 28.1a], where the other hand waits to capture the testis if it appears [Fig. 28.1b]. Its range of movement is determined carefully, for the diagnosis depends on this. The precise classification of a palpable undescended testis is made by determining how far it can be manipulated into the scrotum.

More than two-thirds of undescended testes are located in the 'superficial inguinal pouch' (i.e. they are palpable in the groin) [Fig. 28.2]. The testes are normal in size and are within the tunica vaginalis, which makes them deceptively mobile. In rare cases, the testis may migrate to a truly ectopic position, such as the perineum, the base of the penis (prepubic), the thigh (femoral) or the opposite hemi-scrotum (crossed testicular ectopia).

Sequelae of non-descent

The higher temperature of the extra-scrotal testis is associated with failure of postnatal germ cell maturation and poor development of the seminiferous tubules. After

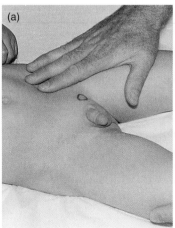
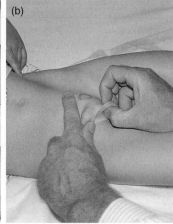

Figure 28.1 Examination to locate the position of the testis: (a) the fingers of one hand push the testis towards the neck of the scrotum, while (b) the other hand 'snares' the testis at the top of the scrotum to see whether it can be pulled right down to the bottom of the scrotum.

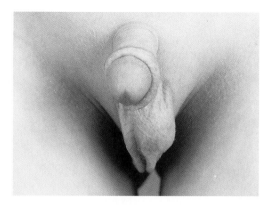

Figure 28.2 Undescended right testis. Once out of the scrotum, the testis is invisible, even though it is palpable in the groin.

puberty there may be oligospermia or azoospermia. The incidence of oligospermia, azoospermia and infertility is not significantly increased above that of the normal population in males with a history of unilateral UDT. However, the fertility rates for males with a past history of bilateral UDT is approximately half that of the normal population.

A testis in the inguinal region is more liable to direct trauma and torsion.

The risk of a seminoma arising in an undescended testis in later life is 5–10 times greater than in a normal testis after surgery at about 10 years of age. There is no proof that orchidopexy earlier in life, as is now routine clinical practice, significantly alters the incidence of malignant progression, though it is hoped it may. Orchidopexy does, however, place the testis in a location that is more amenable to self-examination making earlier detection of testicular malignancy easier.

Treatment of undescended testes

The object of treatment is to preserve normal spermatogenesis and increase comfort and achieve normal cosmesis. Hormone function at puberty (i.e. testosterone output) is normal regardless of treatment. The maturation of gonocytes to spermatozoa is adversely affected in undescended testes from the age of 4–12 months onwards, and to a degree proportional to the length of time the testis remains undescended beyond this age. Testes with acquired maldescent may descend fully at puberty, but they are poorly developed and spermatogenesis is deficient.

Orchidopexy for congenital cryptorchidism is recommended at 6–12 months of age. Orchidopexy usually is performed as a day surgery procedure. Acquired undescended testes should have orchidopexy once they can no longer reside spontaneously in the scrotum. There is no current role for hormone treatment.

Determination of hormone levels has no place in the investigation of unilateral UDT but should always be performed in boys with bilateral impalpable testes prior to surgical exploration. The diagnostic test, par excellence, for an impalpable UDT is laparoscopic exploration. Laparoscopy will detect the 40% of absent testes, enable removal of a useless and potentially neoplastic testicular nubbin and permit the initial surgical managment of the 20% that are truly intra-abdominal. A coexistent indirect inguinal hernia is almost universal but usually latent; when it becomes apparent clinically, herniotomy is necessary regardless of the boy's age, at which time orchidopexy is performed.

Absent testes

In rare cases, the testis is absent or excised because of torsion (and necrosis), tumours or dysgenesis. These boys may have psychological problems and may suffer significant embarrassment in the locker room. The use of prosthetic testes can be considered, but ideally insertion should be delayed until adolescence when adult-sized implants can be accommodated in the scrotum.

Varicocele

A varicocele is an enlargement of the veins of the pampiniform plexus in the spermatic cord and usually appears in boys over 12 years of age, at or before the onset of puberty. The mass of veins is best seen and felt when the patient is standing, and feels like 'a bag of worms'. Varicoceles are usually left-sided (80–90%), right-sided in 1–7% or bilateral in 2–20%. There is sometimes a small secondary hydrocele and the hemi-scrotum is redundant. The varicosites empty when the boy lies down (but the left hemi-scrotum remains more pendulous than the right), and clinical examination should always include getting the boy to stand up. It is usually on the left side and symptomless, though a dragging ache may develop when the varicocele is large.

The normal pampiniform plexus contributes to lowering the temperature of the testis, by cooling the arterial blood flowing to the testis through a counter-current heat exchange mechanism. The loss of this cooling mechanism affects both testes and the consequent rise of scrotal temperature to normal body temperature causes oligospermia. Varicoceles are found in 8–22% of the normal male population but a subclinical varicocele is found in 40–75% of infertile males.

Treatment

The optimal temperature for spermatogenesis (and the normal scrotal temperature) is 33°C, 4°C below body temperature. Relative infertility cannot be assessed until late adolescence, but secondary atrophy of the testis is well-recognised and if the affected testis is significantly smaller or softer in texture than the contralateral testis then early operation is indicated.

High ligation of the spermatic vessels or ligation of the cremasteric veins (dilated in 50% of varicoceles), which anastomose freely with the spermatic veins, should prevent recurrence in most patients.

Very rarely, a varicocele develops as the result of obstruction of the renal veins by a renal or perirenal tumour, for example, Wilms' tumour or a neuroblastoma, almost always on the left side, in a boy less than 5 years of age. The tumour can usually be palpated as an abdominal mass and usually has other associated symptoms, most notably haematuria.

Key Points

- UDT is common.
- Congenital UDT should be confirmed at 3 months of age after postnatal descent is complete.
- Congenital UDT should be referred for surgery at 6–12 months.
- Acquired UDT should be screened for in 4–10 year olds, and referred for surgery if testis does not reside in scrotum.
- Varicocele should be suspected in adolescents who have a pendulous left hemiscrotum.
- Varicocele diagnosis is confirmed on standing, and then referred for surgical assessment.

Further reading

Clarnette TD, Hutson JM (1997) Is the ascending testis actually "stationary"? Normal elongation of the spermatic cord is prevented by a fibrous remnant of the processus vaginalis. *Pediatr Surg Int* **12**: 155–157.

El-Saeity NS, Sidhu PS (2006) "Scrotal varicocele, exclude a renal tumour." Is this evidence based? *Clin Radiol* **61**: 593–599.

Hutson JM (2006) Undescended testis, torsion and varicocele. In: Grosfeld JL, O'Neill JA Jr., Fonkalsrud EW, Coran AG (eds) *Pediatric Surgery*, 6th Edn. Mosby Elsevier, Philadelphia, pp. 1192–1214.

Hutson JM (2006) Undescended testes. In: Stringer MD, Oldham KT, Mouriquand PDE (eds) *Pediatric Surgery and Urology. Long-term Outcomes*, 2nd Edn. Cambridge University Press, Cambridge, pp. 652–663.

Kirsch AJ, Escala J, Duckett JW *et al.* (1998) Surgical management of the nonpalpable testis: the Children's Hospital of Philadelphia experience. *J Urol* **159**(4): 1340–1343.

Thong MK, Lim CT, Fatimah H (1998) Undescended testes: Incidence in 1002 consecutive male infants and outcome at 1 year of age. *Pediatr Surg Int* **13**: 37–41.

29 Inguinal Region and Acute Scrotum

Case 1

A 6-month-old boy presents with an intermittent swelling in the left groin. Both testes are in the scrotum.
Q 1.1 What is the likely diagnosis?
Q 1.2 What is the treatment?

Case 2

A 7-year-old boy complains of pain and swelling in the right scrotum for 6 h. He had mumps recently.
Q 2.1 What is the differential diagnosis?
Q 2.2 Could he have mumps orchitis?
Q 2.3 What is the treatment?

The inguinoscrotal region is the commonest site for surgical conditions in childhood. Because the area is readily accessible to inspection and palpation, accurate diagnosis is easy, but depends on a knowledge of normal anatomy, and the many conditions which may occur in the area.

The inguinoscrotal region is not isolated from the rest of the body. Symptoms and signs can arise here in systemic diseases, and vice versa; for example, blood or meconium in the tunica vaginalis from intraperitoneal haemorrhage or meconium peritonitis; or torsion of the testis presenting with pain referred to the abdomen. A careful examination of the area, and of the whole patient, is necessary to avoid diagnostic errors.

The 'acute scrotum'

There are a number of conditions that cause a red, swollen and painful scrotum [Table 29.1]. There are wide variations in the speed of onset, the rate of progression and the local signs, and the severity of pain [Fig. 29.1].

Torsion of the testis

Testicular torsion is not the most common cause of an acute scrotum, but it is the most important. The spermatic cord undergoes torsion, obstructing the spermatic vessels, and is a surgical emergency because of the high incidence of necrosis of the testis if the cord is not untwisted promptly. The risk of torsion is highest just after the testis enlarges at puberty in 13–16-year olds. Also, the risk is increased in unoperated cryptorchid testes.

Two kinds of torsion occur

1 Intratunical (or 'intravaginal'), the most common, is made possible by an abnormally narrow base of the mesenteric attachment of the testis and epididymis within the tunica vaginalis. The predisposing abnormality is almost always present on the opposite side as well, and this testis should be fixed at the time of surgery to prevent torsion. In rare cases, torsion occurs between the testis and the epididymis, which are connected by a thin sheet of tissue. Unoperated cryptorchid testes are at risk as their fixation within the tunica is commonly tenuous.

2 Extratunical (or 'extravaginal') torsion is rare, and confined to the neonate in whom there is a plane of mobility in the areolar tissue outside the tunica to permit testicular migration to the scrotum. After testicular descent, the loose plane persists for a while before the tunica normally becomes fixed to the scrotum. The testis is almost always necrotic by the time the diagnosis is made.

Clinical signs

The onset is usually sudden, with pain in the testis and/or ipsilateral iliac fossa, nausea and vomiting. Sometimes the onset is more gradual, without severe pain, and the

Jones' Clinical Paediatric Surgery, 6th edition. By Hutson, O'Brien, Woodward and Beasley. Published 2008 by Blackwell Publishing, ISBN: 978-1-4051-6267-8.

Table 29.1 Causes of acute scrotum in children

1 Torsion of one of the testicular appendages (hydatid of Morgagni)	60%
2 Torsion of the testis	30%
3 Epididymo-orchitis	<5%
4 Idiopathic scrotal oedema	<5%

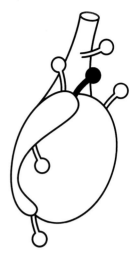

Figure 29.2 Torsion of a testicular appendage. The hydatid of Morgagni is the commonest (remnant of the cranial Mullerian duct), and is at the upper pole. In rare cases, there may be appendages on the spermatic cord and epididymis (upper or lower poles).

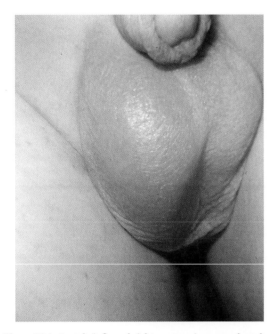

Figure 29.1 Acutely inflamed right scrotum in a prepubertal boy. The inflammation is confined by the right tunica vaginalis. Torsion of a testicular appendage or of the testis itself are likely causes.

diagnosis will be delayed if only the more acute form is accepted as typical.

An earlier history of similar but short-lived, even momentary pain, is suggestive of episodes of incomplete and spontaneously resolving torsion. A horizontal 'lie' of the testes when the child stands, often referred to as a 'bell-clapper testis', indicates the possibility of torsion, and should be taken as an indication for exploration and orchidopexy.

The swollen testis and epididymis are exquisitely tender (unless already necrotic) and may be partially obscured by overlying scrotal oedema and an effusion into the tunica (reactive hydrocele). The amount of swelling depends on the time that has elapsed and the rate of progression.

The hydrocele and the exquisite tenderness may make precise palpation of the testis difficult. As the pathology is within one tunica vaginalis, the inflammatory signs are confined to the ipsilateral hemiscrotum by the peritoneal membrane.

Treatment

Urgent exploration of the scrotum is arranged to untwist the testis and epididymis and to anchor ('pex') both it and the contralateral testis to prevent subsequent torsion. If the testis is completely necrotic, it should be removed.

Torsion of an appendage

Torsion of an appendage (e.g. 'hydatid of Morgagni') is the commonest cause of the acute scrotum in the prepubertal boy. The vestigial remnants are attached to the testis or the epididymis, and are present in about 90% of the male population [Fig. 29.2]. Recurrent attacks of pain also occur, sometimes very frequently, and the boy may present with a suggestive history, but few acute signs. A small tender lump at the upper pole of the testis is diagnostic.

Clinical signs

The boy complains of severe pain in his scrotum. A blue-black spot may be seen through the skin of the scrotum near the upper pole of the testis: palpation of it causes extreme pain, whereas palpation of the testis itself causes minimal discomfort. It may be impossible to distinguish torsion of a testicular appendage from testicular torsion once a secondary hydrocele has developed.

Treatment

Where torsion of the testis cannot be excluded on clinical examination, urgent exploration is mandatory, and at operation the appendix testis is removed. If the tender 'pea' of a twisted testicular appendage is palpable, surgical excision of it provides immediate relief of symptoms and prevents recurrence.

Epididymitis/epididymo-orchitis

Epididymo-orchitis is rare in childhood, and virtually never occurs between 6 months of age and puberty. It is common practice to refer to inflammatory conditions in the scrotum as 'epididymo-orchitis', even though the epididymis alone is usually affected.

Escherischia coli may be carried by retrograde flow along the vas deferens from the urinary tract. Predisposing factors include abnormalities of the urinary tract or urethral instrumentation.

Clinical signs

Babies with epididymitis due to urinary organisms should have a renal ultrasound and micturating cysto-urethrogram after the epididymitis has subsided; this is to identify anomalies of the lower urinary tract before irreversible damage to the kidneys has occurred.

Differential diagnosis

The clinical picture can mimic torsion of the testes so closely that in most if not all children, the diagnosis should be made only after exploration of the scrotum. True acute orchitis is very uncommon, but may occur in mumps or septicaemia. Mumps orchitis is extremely rare before puberty. The testis is larger and harder than in epididymo-orchitis. Infiltration of the testis is also rare, but does occur occasionally in leukaemia or with a primary neoplasm (embryonic adenocarcinoma, seminoma or a benign tumour of the interstitial cells of Leydig).

Treatment

Treatment of epididymitis consists of rest, antibiotics (e.g. Septrin, Furadantin), a high fluid intake and alkalinisation of the urine. Severe or repeated infections may lead to an abscess or progressive destruction of the testis, but sterility is rare when only one side is affected.

'Idiopathic' scrotal oedema

In this condition, there is rapidly developing oedema of the scrotum that may then spread to the inguinal region, penis and foreskin, or on to the perineum.

The scrotum is symmetrically swollen, pale pink or red, and there is slight discomfort rather than acute pain. The pathology is in the skin (and therefore spreads beyond the tunica vaginalis), and may represent allergic inflammation.

Careful palpation reveals non-tender testes that are normal in size and position. The oedema subsides in 1–2 days, but may occasionally recur some weeks later. There may be a history of allergy or of playing out of doors at the onset; a bite from an insect or a spider is a probable cause in some, but as a rule, the history is inconclusive.

Differential diagnosis

It can be distinguished from other causes of the 'acute scrotum' by the complete absence of tenderness in the epididymis and testis, and by the spread of oedema beyond the confines of the scrotum.

The spread of infection from a pustule in the perineum can produce an area of slightly reddened skin and subcutaneous oedema that extends beside or across one-half of the scrotum. A tender enlarged inguinal node at or near the external inguinal ring assists in the diagnosis of perineal lymphangitis.

A toddler who sustains a straddle injury or sits on a toy with a sharp projection may injure the urethra, causing extravasation of urine. Pain on voiding, blood at the urethral meatus, and progressive oedema of the perineum, scrotum and suprapubic region, are suggestive of urethral injury that is confirmed on urethrography (Chapter 38).

Fat necrosis of the scrotum

This extremely rare condition presents with tender, usually bilateral, comma-shaped lumps in the scrotal wall of stout boys. Trauma may be responsible, but often there is a history of swimming in very cold water, suggesting that cold injury is the cause. Treatment is supportive, as the necrotic fat gradually absorbs. If doubt exists, exploration is required.

Management of the acute scrotum

As a general rule, an urgent exploration is required in all cases of acute scrotum in which the possibility of testicular torsion cannot be completely excluded. The diagnosis of epididymitis or orchitis is unlikely, unless there is a history of urinary tract infection, a known developmental anomaly of the renal tract, or significant pyobacteriuria.

A midline scrotal incision has advantages: when torsion of the testis is found it can be untwisted and fixed, and exploration and fixation of the opposite testis is done through the same incision.

Inguinal lymphadenitis

The superficial inguinal lymph nodes drain the lower limbs, the perineum, the buttocks and the perianal region–all common sites of minor skin infections in the 'napkin area' in infants. Infections often reach the inguinal nodes, which become enlarged and may form an abscess after the initial focus has disappeared. Occasionally, atypical mycobacterial infection in pre-school children involves these nodes. The axilla, neck and spleen should be examined for evidence of a generalised lymphadenopathy. In small children, an inguinal abscess may be mistaken for a strangulated inguinal hernia. Treatment is incision and drainage when necessary.

Deep external iliac adenitis

The proximal drainage of the nodes of the femoral canal is a group of deep iliac nodes on the brim of the pelvis around the external iliac artery. For no apparent reason an infection may pass inconspicuously through the more superficial inguinal nodes to form an abscess in these iliac nodes on the front of the external iliac artery and the iliopsoas muscle.

Clinical features

These are vague; general signs of toxaemia and fever are variable, and the hip may be held in slight flexion. The abscess is at first too deep to palpate clearly, and the diagnosis may be delayed until the abscess is large enough to appear above the inguinal ligament.

On the right side it may resemble an appendiceal abscess, but a distinguishing point is that a deep iliac abscess is contiguous with the inguinal ligament, whereas in an appendiceal abscess, there is a gap between the two. The absence of vomiting and bowel disturbance is also helpful.

Treatment

Extraperitoneal drainage is required and pus is often present, even when fluctuation cannot be detected clinically because of the thickness of the intervening tissues.

Inguinal hernias

The testis descends into the scrotum during the seventh month *in utero* inside a diverticulum of peritoneum, the processus vaginalis. This begins to obliterate shortly before birth and closure is normally completed during the first year of life, leaving only the tunica vaginalis surrounding the testis [Fig. 29.3a].

Failure of obliteration of the processus vaginalis is associated with several clinical conditions in infancy and childhood: hernia, hydrocele and encysted hydrocele of the cord (and also possibly acquired undescended testes).

A hernial sac may extend from the internal inguinal ring to the tunica vaginalis – the so-called inguinoscrotal hernia [Fig. 29.3b]. More commonly, there is a so-called 'incomplete sac' proximal to an obliterated segment that intervenes between the sac and the tunica vaginalis [Fig. 29.3c]. This accounts for the vast majority of inguinal hernias in children.

A hydrocele in childhood is a collection of the fluid that lubricates the intestines, formed by the omentum within the peritoneal cavity; the fluid trickles down a narrow processus and collects inside the tunica vaginalis around the testis [Fig. 29.3d].

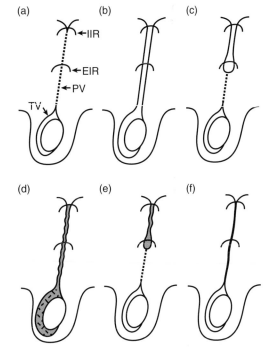

Figure 29.3 Hernias and hydroceles. (a) The normally obliterated processus vaginalis (PV) between the internal inguinal ring (IIR), external inguinal ring (EIR) and the tunica vaginalis (TV); (b) a completely patent hernia; (c) incomplete hernia; (d) hydrocele with narrow but patent PV; (e) Encysted hydrocele with fluid collecting as a 'cyst' in the spermatic cord; (f) residual fibrous remnant of PV that may cause 'ascending' testis. (Reproduced with permission from Clarnette & Hutson [1997] *Pediatr Surg Int* 12: 155–157.)

An encysted hydrocele of the cord develops in the same way; the peritoneal fluid collects in a loculus of the processus at some point along its course in the spermatic cord. This loculus usually retains its communication with the peritoneal cavity [Fig. 29.3e].

Combined abnormalities: multiple spaces or cysts developed along the processus, and it is not uncommon to find a proximal hernial sac communicating through a narrow tract with a distal hydrocele. Finally, a residual fibrous remnant of the processus may prevent elongation of the spermatic cord with age, leading to acquired UDT or 'ascending testis', later in childhood [Fig. 29.3f].

The higher incidence of abnormalities on the right side may be because the right testis descends later than the left and the processus on the right side is therefore more likely to remain patent. The higher incidence of hernias in premature babies is because the normally higher postpartum intra-abdominal pressure compared with the fetus makes it more difficult for the processus to close spontaneously.

In girls, the canal of Nuck undergoes the same obliteration as the processus vaginalis in boys. The obliteration is more likely to be complete, with a lower total incidence of hernias but a higher incidence of bilateral hernias.

Indirect inguinal hernia

Nearly all inguinal hernias in children are indirect, with an incidence of 1 in every 50 live male births. This is the commonest condition requiring surgery during childhood and there is a high familial incidence.

Some 12% of indirect inguinal hernias occur in girls, in whom they appear more evenly throughout childhood than in boys. In boys, the greatest incidence is in the first year of life, especially the first 3 months [Fig. 29.4]: 60% are on the right side, 25% on the left and 15% bilateral. The sac usually contains loops of small bowel, and sometimes omentum. In girls, the ovary is often palpable in the sac, and may be difficult to reduce.

Diagnosis

The child's mother reports that there is an intermittent swelling overlying the external inguinal ring. It is usually painless but on occasions may cause discomfort. It is often present when there is an episode of crying or straining, and in infants is seen during nappy changes. It may reach the bottom of the scrotum, as in the case of a 'complete' sac, and there is an impulse on crying or straining.

When the history is suggestive but the hernia is not seen during examination, the index finger can be rolled transversely across the spermatic cord at the point where it lies on the pubic crest; when there is a hernial sac, the

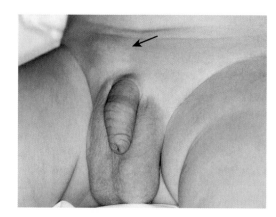

Figure 29.4 Right indirect inguinal hernia (arrowed) in an infant.

spermatic cord is thickened in comparison with the side on which no swelling has been seen, and the 'rustle' of contiguous layers of peritoneum represents the empty hernial sac – sometimes referred to as a 'silken sleeve'.

One source of confusion between the history and the clinical signs arises when the parents mistake a testis in the superficial inguinal pouch for a hernia, and the site of the reported swelling should be precisely indicated and the concurrent presence of a testis in the scrotum documented. If doubt still exists, a further examination is made a few days later.

The opposite side should always be examined, and both testes confirmed to be descended in the scrotum.

Differential diagnosis

The primary distinction to be made is between a hernia and a hydrocele; the latter is cystic, brilliantly transilluminable and irreducible, (even though there is a connection, it is too narrow to squeeze the water out quickly) with no impulse on crying or straining, and its proximal pole is identifiable distal to the external ring.

Femoral and direct inguinal hernias are rare but should be kept in mind; a retractile or undescended testis may mislead the unwary, and in young children, an inguinal lymph node may be situated close to the external inguinal ring.

Treatment

Surgery is necessary in all cases because of the danger of strangulation, which occurs most commonly in the first 6 months of life. Operation should be performed as soon as is practicable, unless there is an intercurrent condition that requires attention, for example, a skin infection or bronchitis.

A herniotomy is performed through an incision in the transverse inguinal skin crease, and is a relatively simple operation in experienced hands, even in the newborn.

Exploration on the opposite side is usually undertaken in boys under 6 months of age, in whom a significant contralateral sac is present in more than 50% of the cases. In 75% of girls of any age, a sac is found on the opposite side.

Incarcerated/strangulated inguinal hernia

Incarceration is the only significant complication of an indirect inguinal hernia; it is common in infancy but somewhat less common in older children. A loop of small bowel becomes trapped in the hernial sac, and although the blood supply is not compromised immediately in most cases, a hernia that is even temporarily irreducible should be considered as being potentially strangulated. The obstruction in the sac is at the external inguinal ring, unlike in adults where the obstruction is often at the internal ring.

Strangulated hernias are seen more often in infants less than 6 months of age, such that up to 30% of infants with an inguinal hernia initially present with a strangulated hernia.

Clinical features

The infant cries and cannot be pacified; when the mother changes the nappies and a swelling in the groin is noted – perhaps for the very first time. There is a tense, tender swelling at the external inguinal ring, and no impulse on crying. There may be generalised colicky abdominal pain, vomiting, abdominal distension and constipation when complete intestinal obstruction supervenes – but this may occur 12 h after the onset. With delay in diagnosis, there may be redness and induration overlying the lump, or signs of peritonitis, suggesting bowel ischaemia.

Differential diagnosis

The differential diagnosis includes an encysted hydrocele of the cord, which may appear suddenly – but the swelling is not tender, the cyst moves readily with traction on the cord, and abdominal signs and symptoms are lacking.

Absence of a testis in the scrotum on the affected side may point to torsion of an undescended testis or of a descended testis that has been elevated out of the scrotum with torsion.

Lymphadenitis or a local inguinal abscess may be as confusing in young children as to warrant exploration to clarify the diagnosis.

Secondary effects

The testicular vessels can be severely compressed by a tense, strangulated hernia. Some degree of testicular atrophy had been reported in 15% of boys after an episode of irreducibility and strangulation. For this reason, early reduction is as important for the testis as for the imprisoned bowel. Occasionally, in infant girls, the ovary can be strangulated inside the sac.

Treatment

An incarcerated hernia may reduce spontaneously *en route* to the hospital, but more often than not, persists. The strangulated hernia should be reduced by taxis. The tips of the fingers of one hand are applied to the fundus of the hernia while the fingertips of the other hand are cupped at the external ring. Gentle pressure is exerted initially to disimpact the hernia from the external ring, and then the contents of the hernia are reduced along the line of the inguinal canal. Nothing seems to be accomplished for a minute or two, and then the bowel suddenly gurgles and returns to the abdomen. Taxis is a manipulative trick, not a matter of force, and if necessary can be attempted several times. A distressed child can be sedated with chloral hydrate or midazolam. There is virtually no chance of producing reduction *en masse* and in over 90% of cases, taxis is successful. When it is successful, the patient should not return home until herniotomy has been performed, usually after 24 h, to give time for oedema of the sac and its investing tissue to subside.

When taxis is unsuccessful, the child should be transferred immediately to a tertiary paediatric surgical centre for operation. The friable sac is difficult to handle and the surgery should always be performed by a paediatric surgeon. In exceptional cases, the bowel is gangrenous and a segmental excision with anastomosis may be necessary. The need for resuscitation before operation will be obvious from the clinical findings.

Direct inguinal hernia

Direct inguinal hernias are rare in paediatric practice, forming less than 1% of inguinal hernias. They are occasionally seen in premature infants who develop bronchopulmonary dysplasia after prolonged ventilation, and in teenage children with cystic fibrosis. Repair of the posterior wall of the inguinal canal medial to the epigastric vessels is required.

Femoral hernia

Femoral hernias are equally rare. The diagnosis is made clinically when the swelling is below the inguinal ligament and lateral to the pubic tubercle.

As in adults, femoral hernias are more common in females, usually between 5 and 10 years of age. The hernia is usually small and irreducible, for most of it is composed of a fibro-fatty investment of the fundus. The hernia can be repaired easily from below the inguinal ligament.

Hydroceles

Almost all hydroceles in infancy and childhood communicate with the peritoneal cavity through a patent processus [Fig. 29.3]. Much less common is the development of an 'acute' hydrocele secondary to some affliction of the testis or epididymis, for example, torsion, infection, trauma or tumour.

Clinical signs

A hydrocele is a painless cyst containing peritoneal fluid that has tracked down a narrow but patent processus vaginalis [Fig. 29.3d]. It is situated around the testis, is brightly translucent and cannot be emptied by pressure because of a 'flap valve' at its junction with the processus. When the hydrocele is lax, the testis within it can usually be palpated with ease, or, when the hydrocele is tense, its shadow can be demonstrated by transillumination.

The upper limit of the hydrocele is clearly demonstrable; that is, the palpating finger 'can get above it', except in unusual varieties that extend up to the inguinal canal. There is no impulse on crying or straining.

Hydroceles in infants

Unilateral or bilateral hydroceles are common in the first few months of life. They are often large, lax and nearly always symptomless and have a strong tendency to close and absorb spontaneously. Most will have disappeared by the age of 1 year and surgery is only required if the hydrocele persists beyond about 2 years.

An encysted hydrocele of the cord is a loculus of fluid located above and separate from the tunica vaginalis [Fig. 29.3e]. It does not require surgery in infancy, and may be considered as a variety of the natural process of obliteration. After 2 years of age, or after observation for a year, operation to close the communication with the peritoneal cavity may be required.

Hydroceles in older children

In boys more than 2 years of age, there is often a diurnal variation in its size. It is small or absent in the mornings and at its biggest in the late afternoon, when it may cause a dragging ache. These changes reflect the narrow communication with the peritoneal cavity along which the fluid returns during recumbency, and reaccumulates by the effect of gravity during the day. Despite the patency of the processus, the fluid can almost never be expelled by pressure.

A hydrocele in this age group rarely disappears spontaneously and surgery is required. The processus is transfixed and divided at the internal inguinal ring (i.e. herniotomy). The whole sac need not be removed but the fluid in it can be released.

Key Points

- In acute scrotum, urgent exploration is mandatory unless testicular torsion can be excluded on clinical examination.
- The scrotum contains two peritoneal sacs (tunica vaginalis) that limit spread of inflammation arising from within one of them.
- The processus vaginalis normally closes shortly after testicular descent (i.e. perinatally).
- Inguinal hernia in a baby is dangerous as incarceration is very common.
- Hydrocele (with a narrow peritoneal connection) only needs surgery after 2 years of age if spontaneous closure does not occur.

References and further reading

Azmy AAF (1994) Acute penile and scrotal conditions. In: Raine PAM, Azmy AAF (eds) *Surgical Emergencies in Children: A Practical Guide.* Butterworth-Heinemann, Oxford, pp. 256–271.

Beasley SW, Hutson JM, Auldist AW (1996) *Essential Paediatric Surgery,* Arnold, London, pp. 67–76, 90–94.

Clarnette TD, Hutson JM (1997) Is the ascending testis actually 'stationary'? *Pediatric Surgery International* 12: 155–157.

Clift VL, Hutson JM (1989) The acute scrotum in childhood. *Pediatric Surgery International* 4: 185–188.

Glick PL, Boulanger SC (2006) Inguinal hernias and hydroceles. In: Grosfeld JL, O'Neill JA Jr., Fonkalsrud EW, Coran AG (eds) *Pediatric Surgery,* 6th Edn. Mosby Elsevier, Philadelphia, pp. 1172–1192.

Hutson JM (2006). Undescended testis, torsion and varicocele. In: Grosfeld JL, O'Neill JA Jr., Fonkalsrud EW, Coran AG (eds). *Pediatric Surgery,* 6th Edn. Mosby Elsevier, Philadelphia, pp. 1193–1214.

Hutson JM, Beasley SW (1988) Inguinoscrotal lesions. In: *The Surgical Examination of Children.* Heinemann Medical, Oxford, pp. 35–54.

30 The Penis

Case 1

A mother brings her 6-week-old son to her general practitioner for advice on the care of the foreskin.
Q 1.1 Should she retract and clean the foreskin?
Q 1.2 At what age does the foreskin become easily retractable?

Case 2

A 5-year-old boy presents with a non-retractable foreskin.
Q 2.1 How do you differentiate between normal preputial adhesions and phimosis?
Q 2.2 What types of treatment are available for phimosis?

Case 3

A mother of a newborn baby boy asks for advice on the pros and cons of circumcision.
Q 3.1 What advice would you give on neonatal circumcision?
Q 3.2 If circumcision has to be performed, discuss the standards of surgery involved.
Q 3.3 What are the complications of circumcision?

Case 4

A newborn baby presents with hypospadias.
Q 4.1 At what age is corrective surgery performed?
Q 4.2 What are the aims of surgery for hypospadias?
Q 4.3 What are the principles of hypospadias surgery?

The prepuce and glans penis

The prepuce (foreskin) is lightly adherent to the glans in the first few days of life, but becomes more densely adherent during the first year.

Forcible retraction of the prepuce should be avoided until spontaneous separation occurs. This is usually in infancy, but it may take 5 years or even longer. The normal process of separation of preputial adhesions is by a combination of pressure of urine and the build-up of shed skin cells from the inner aspect of the foreskin (smegma). This sebaceous deposit of white cheesy material builds up under the foreskin to lift it off the glans; the discharge of this material is often mistaken for infection.

Accumulations of smegma may produce yellowish bulges under the preputial skin [Fig. 30.1], often referred to as 'smegma pearls' and may be mistaken for a sebaceous cysts or even a tumour!

Jones' Clinical Paediatric Surgery, 6th edition. By Hutson, O'Brien, Woodward and Beasley. Published 2008 by Blackwell Publishing, ISBN: 978-1-4051-6267-8.

Care of the normal foreskin

The normal foreskin needs no special care in young children. If the foreskin is healthy, it need not be retracted and does not have to be more specially cleaned than any other part of the body. After puberty the foreskin should be retracted for cleaning. Young children do get problems with infection in the foreskin, but this is due to phimosis and the foreskin cannot be retracted in this pathological condition. Three abnormal conditions arise in the prepuce.

Phimosis

Phimosis is tightness of the preputial orifice that prevents retraction of the foreskin over the glans [Fig. 30.2]. It may be either physiological – the normal prepuce with residual adhesions or pathological. In the case of normal preputial adhesions, gentle retraction opens out the foreskin to reveal the tip of the glans, but the adhesions prevent further retraction. Pathological phimosis may be caused by ill-advised forceful retraction of physiological phimosis, recurrent balanitis, an incomplete circumcision or

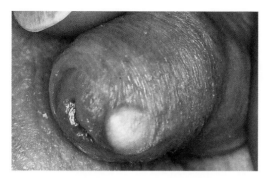

Figure 30.1 Accumulation of smegma beneath the foreskin appears as a yellowish bulge at the level of the coronal groove.

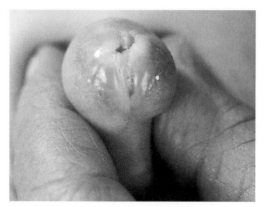

Figure 30.2 Phimosis. Scarring of the distal foreskin causes stenosis of the opening.

Balanitis Xerotica Obliterans (BXO). Phimosis may impair drainage of the space between the foreskin and the glans leading to accumulation of stagnant urine and smegma. The urea in the stagnant urine becomes converted to ammonia and may cause an ammoniacal dermatitis of the prepuce which may then become secondarily infected to cause balanitis.

Phimosis may be treated by the local application of steroid cream applied daily to the phimotic skin for 2 weeks. This steroid treatment is successful in many cases, but circumcision will be necessary if steroid treatment is not successful. It is important to treat phimosis actively as persisting phimosis in adults causes pain during intercourse due to the damaged foreskin. Chronic low-grade infection will occur under the foreskin and if this low-grade infection persists for many decades, it can lead to squamous cell carcinoma of the glans in later adult life. Originally described in chimney sweeps during the

industrial revolution, this is uncommon now due to marked improvements in personal hygiene.

Ballooning of the foreskin that persists after micturition is a sign of obstruction requiring circumcision.

Paraphimosis

This occurs when a tight foreskin has been forcibly retracted. The retracted foreskin forms a constriction ring around the coronal groove of the glans causing venous engorgement and painful swelling of the glans [Fig. 30.3]. Retention of urine occurs and the problem demands urgent resolution. Reduction of the paraphimosis can often be achieved by patient, gentle compression in a patient who is awake but occasionally this requires a general anaesthetic.

Balanitis

Balanitis is an infection of the glans penis, infection of the foreskin is called posthitis and the combination balanoposthitis. It usually starts as an inflammatory process due to ammonia in urine that is retained under the prepuce which becomes secondarily infected. This infection responds quickly to topical or systemic antibiotics. Recurrent infection can occur until the preputial adhesions have separated completely. Further episodes of infection may be prevented by simple hygiene measures, gentle retraction of the foreskin or the topical application of a steroid ointment to expedite preputial adhesiolysis. A topical barrier ointment at the first sign of inflammation may prevent bacterial infection.

Balanitis Xerotica Obliterans

Balanitis Xerotica Obliterans is a scarring condition of the foreskin causing a pathological phimosis that if left untreated may extend onto the glans penis and into the urethra causing urethral stricturing. It is a chronic dermatitis of unknown aetiology similar to lichen sclerosis et atrophicus. If detected early enough it may respond to topical steroids but usually warrants circumcision.

Circumcision

Phimosis and the complications of phimosis, paraphimosis and balanitis, are the medical indications for circumcision. However, the application of steroid cream may cause a rapid resolution of phimosis and this has reduced the need for circumcision [Table 30.1].

Circumcision also may offer some protection against urinary tract infection (UTI), with a reported 10-fold reduction in the incidence of UTI in circumcised males from 1% to 0.1%. This is not of great significance for the

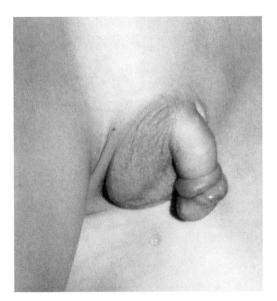

Figure 30.3 Paraphimosis. The penis is red, swollen and painful. The prepuce has been retracted behind the glans and is compressing the shaft, causing oedema and venous congestion.

Table 30.1 Indications for circumcision

Medical	Phimosis
	Paraphimosis
	Balanitis
	Serious urinary tract anomaly
Non-medical	Religious
	Social

Table 30.2 Complications of circumcision

Bleeding
Infection (local/septicaemia)
Ulceration of glans/meatus
Penile deformity

normal child but circumcision is often performed in a child with severe urinary tract abnormalities to prevent recurrent UTI.

Apart from these medical indications circumcision is also performed for religious and social reasons. The pendulum of opinion has swung back and forth, but circumcision for social reasons is now performed less frequently.

The most common reason given for circumcision is cleanliness and convenience, in that the foreskin does not have to be retracted. However, general standards of hygiene are now so high that prophylactic circumcision is not recommended. Carcinoma of the foreskin does occur as a rare tumour in adults with long-standing phimosis; but the lesson here is that phimosis should be treated, rather than the normal foreskin removed.

There can be complications after circumcision [Table 30.2]. The penis has a very good blood supply and postoperative bleeding may occur. In the neonatal period, any bleeding is of major concern as the blood volume of the average newborn is 80 mL/kg, which is 240 mL for a 3 kg baby. Any blood loss over 25 mL is life-threatening. By the age of 6 months, a baby has doubled its birth weight and the safety factor on blood loss is more acceptable. Infection with coliform organisms on the open wound in the napkin area may lead to septicaemia in the neonatal period as the baby's own immunity is poorly developed. By the age of 6 months, the baby is better able to cope with infection. The other common complication of circumcision is ulceration of the thin delicate epithelium of the glans. This can occur at any age, and sometimes leads to meatal stenosis from scar contraction around the meatus. The glans needs to be protected after circumcision with copious amounts of moisturising cream applied via nappy liner cloths for 2–3 weeks after the surgery.

Circumcision for religious reasons will be performed at the age and situation decreed by the religion. Circumcision for medical or social reasons needs to be performed at the optimal time for the best standards of medical practice. The standards of safety and skill expected of surgery and anaesthesia are very high, and the previous methods of circumcision performed in the neonatal period do not meet these standards. Circumcision should be performed after the age of 6 months in an operating theatre under general anaesthesia, with careful surgical technique. The parents should receive counselling and education, so they can give informed consent. In years gone by, the large numbers of babies presenting for social circumcision gave rise to the practice of circumcision in the neonatal period without anaesthesia, with a surgical technique in which speed, rather than meticulous tissue-handling, was the main consideration. The situation today is quite different, and circumcision should be judged by the same standards that apply to any important operation.

Meatal stenosis

This occurs as an acquired lesion caused by ulceration of the glans following circumcision. It leads to a thin urinary stream with dysuria and bleeding due to meatal ulcer-ation. The problem can be prevented by protection of the glans with moisturising cream for 2 weeks after circumcision. Scar contracture after meatal ulceration leads to meatal stenosis, and this requires surgical meatoplasty to correct the problem. It is more common if circumcision is carried out while the child is still in nappies.

Hypospadias

Hypospadias is caused by failure of the development of the tissues forming the urethra, on the shaft of the penis. The urethral orifice opens on the ventral surface of the penis and does not reach the end of the glans. In severe cases, the urinary meatus may open into the scrotum or perineum. There is deficiency of the ventral foreskin and the skin on the ventral penile shaft [Fig. 30.4]. The lack of tissue on the ventral surface of the penis leads to a tight 'bowstring' effect causing a ventral bending of the penis, known as chordee. This chordee deformity is more marked during erection and will cause difficulty with intercourse in later life, if it is not corrected.

The malposition of the urinary orifice and the chordee deformity are usually present together, but in some cases, severe chordee may be present with an orifice at the end of the penis. Hypospadias affects 1 in 350 boys.

Severe 'hypospadias' with a bifid scrotum and unde-scended testicles is actually a presentation of a disor-der of sexual development with ambiguous genitalia [Chapter 10].

The clinical findings in hypospadias are
1 Downward deflection of the urinary stream from the ventrally placed meatus.
2 The penis is bent ventrally with chordee, which causes difficulty with intercourse.
3 The foreskin forms a dorsal hood and is deficient ven-trally, which gives an abnormal cosmetic appearance to the penis.

These disabilities are primarily functional, as the boy may find it difficult to direct his urinary stream, and in later life, intercourse may be difficult if there is signifi-cant chordee. The disabilities are also psychological, as severe anomalies of the penis or a poor cosmetic result following surgery may interfere with the development of the normal male body image. Therefore the age for cor-rection of hypospadias has been made younger, and now the recommended age for commencement of surgery is 6–12 months.

Investigation
Hypospadias is associated with some increase in other anomalies of the genito-urinary system (9% incidence of cryptorchidism, 9% inguinal hernia, 3% renal anomalies) and investigation with renal ultrasonography is recom-mended. More severe penoscrotal hypospadias is associ-ated with a Utriculus Masculinus, a remnant of the vaginal anlagen that may predispose to recurrent urinary tract infections, epididymo-orchitis or stone formation. Severe hypospadias with bifid scrotum and/or unde-scended testes (ambiguous genitalia) requires full investi-gation for disorders of sexual development.

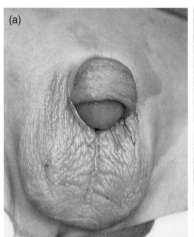
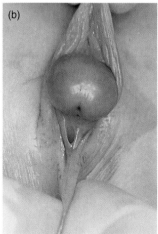

Figure 30.4 Hypospadias. Incomplete fusion of the inner genital folds leads to a proximal urethral meatus, a dorsal hooded prepuce and chordee. The penis may look fairly normal (a) until the foreskin (dorsal hood) is pulled upwards, revealing the proximal urethral meatus (b).

Treatment

The four aims of treatment are

1 to correct the chordee;

2 to bring the urinary meatus to the tip of the penis;

3 to provide a good cosmetic appearance;

4 to achieve the above aims with the minimum complications.

Hypospadias surgery is one of the most difficult areas of surgery in children. As the primary defect is failure of tissue development, there is tissue missing from the ventral surface of the penis and any simple attempt at closing the defect has a high failure rate. There are over 250 different operations described for hypospadias, most of which are no longer performed having been superseded by procedures with better cosmetic and functional outcomes. However, with modern surgical techniques the results of surgery are quite good and the success rate should be 95%. The principles of surgery are as follows:

1 Relocate the meatus to the tip of the penis using locally based skin flaps.

2 Correct the chordee by releasing the ventral skin that tethers the penis.

3 Achieve a cosmetic outcome with either a circumcised or uncircumcised appearance by reconstructing the prepuce.

4 Postoperative urinary drainage is usually aided by a urinary catheter or a urethral stent.

5 In most cases of hypospadias, the surgery is performed in a single stage; however, in severe cases, the surgeon may elect to correct the chordee first and go on to do the urethroplasty at a later operation to reduce the complication rate.

Complications

Failure of healing with complete breakdown or a partial breakdown with urinary fistula formation, is a distressing problem. Strictures may occur in the neourethra, and poorly corrected chordee will lead to troubles in adult life. These complications used to be common, but the standards of surgery for hypospadias are now quite high, and one could expect good results.

Epispadias

In this condition, the urethra opens at the base of the penis, on its dorsal aspect. It is part of the spectrum of lower abdominal wall defects in which ectopia vesicae is the most severe form (Chapter 8). Most boys with epispadias are incontinent of urine because the bladder neck is deficient; epispadias as an isolated abnormality in a continent child is exceptionally rare, even rarer than ectopia vesicae itself, which occurs in 1 in 30,000 live births.

Apart from the problem of the repair of the urethra, using the same type of urethroplasty as in hypospadias, there are many of the same major difficulties that arise in ectopia vesicae.

> **Key Points**
> - The normal foreskin needs no special care in young children.
> - Indications for circumcision include phimosis, recurrent balanitis and complex urinary tract anomalies.
> - Neonatal circumcision should be discouraged.
> - Hypospadias requires surgery at 6–12 months.
> - Severe 'hypospadias' needs investigation for disorders of sexual development.

Further reading

Beasley SW, Hutson JM, Auldist AW (1996) The penis. In: *Essential Paediatric Surgery*, Arnold, London, pp. 98–106.

Cuckow PM (2006) Circumcision. In: Stringer MD, Oldham KT, Mouriquand PDE (eds) *Pediatric Surgery and Urology: Long-term Outcomes*, 2nd Edn. Cambridge University Press, Cambridge, pp. 664–674.

Gargollo PC, Kozakewich HP, Bauer SB, Borer JG, Peters CA, Retik AB, Diamond DA. (2005) Balanitis xerotica obliterans in boys. *J Urol* **174**: 1409–1412.

Murphy JP, Gatti JM (2006) Abnormalities of the urethra, penis and scrotum. In: Grosfeld JL, O'Neill JA Jr., Fonkalsrud EW, Coran AG (eds) *Pediatric Surgery*, 6th Edn. Mosby Elsevier, Philadelphia, pp. 1899–1910.

Shankar KR, Rickwood AMK (1999) The incidence of phimosis in boys. *BJU International* **84**: 101–102.

Wiswell TE, Hachey WE (1993) Urinary tract infections and the uncircumcised state: an update. *Clin Pediatr (Phila)* **32**(3): 130–134.

Urinary Tract

31 Urinary Tract Infection

Case 1

Stacey is a 5-year-old girl who presents with dysuria, pyrexia and haematuria. There is no relevant past history.

Q 1.1 What investigations should be done?

Q 1.2 What is the likelihood of an underlying urinary tract anomaly?

Q 1.3 If there is no urinary tract anomaly, why has the infection occurred?

Case 2

Thomas is 6 months old and presents with fever, lethargy and smelly, turbid urine. He is not gaining weight.

Q 2.1 How would a UTI be confirmed?

Q 2.2 What tests are needed to document a possible urinary tract anomaly?

A urinary tract infection (UTI) is best defined as the symptomatic occurrence of pathogenic microorganisms, usually bacteria, in the urinary tract. It is a common cause of illness in infants and children, may herald an underlying urinary tract anomaly, be associated with the occurrence of renal scarring and subsequently the development of hypertension. UTI are commonly misdiagnosed in children. Dysuria and the passage of cloudy urine are common symptoms in children with a febrile illness and do not necessarily reflect UTI. On the other hand, many children with a UTI have non-specific symptoms, or have unexplained fever, vomiting or even failure to thrive: in these patients, the diagnosis may be overlooked.

The diagnosis of UTI is based on the presence of a single type of bacteria growing in large numbers in an appropriately collected specimen of urine. The standard required for a significant culture is $>10^5$ colony forming units (cfu)/mL. This figure of 10^5 cfu/mL is based on samples of urine obtained from clean-catch voided specimens. Lesser counts are regarded as significant in specimens obtained in a more sterile manner, for example, 10^3 cfu/mL for specimens obtained by urethral catheterisation and 10^2 cfu/mL for specimens obtained by suprapubic aspiration. Asymptomatic bacteriuria has been reported in the urine of 8% of infants and 6.6% of children.

The diagnosis of a UTI is further supported by the detection of white blood cells (WBCs) in the urine, ($>5 \times 10^6$/L in boys and $>4 \times 10^6$/L in girls). However, this is not a prerequisite for the diagnosis. Children on immunosuppressant therapy may not be able to produce an immune response and some infants with overwhelming sepsis may have bone marrow suppression. WBCs can also be found in the urine of patients without a UTI such as those with intra-abdominal infection (appendicitis, etc.) and other pyrexial illnesses; however, there will not be a significant bacteriuria.

Incidence/prevalence

There is considerable variation in the reported incidence of UTI. By the age of 7 years, approximately 8% of girls and 3% of boys will have been treated for a UTI. UTI is more common in neonates and decreases steadily after the first month of life. A large Swedish population-based study of infants under the age of 2 years reported an incidence of UTI in 2.2% of boys and 2.1% of girls. After this age, UTI becomes more common in girls such that by the age of 16 years 3.6% of boys and 11.3% of girls will have been diagnosed with a UTI.

Jones' Clinical Paediatric Surgery, 6th edition. By Hutson, O'Brien, Woodward and Beasley. Published 2008 by Blackwell Publishing, ISBN: 978-1-4051-6267-8.

Table 31.1 Presentation of urinary tract infection

Infants	Older children
Pyuria of unknown origin	Abdominal pain
Septicaemia	Dysuria
Listlessness and lethargy	Pyrexia
Haematuria	Haematuria
Vomiting	Pyelonephritis
Failure to thrive	Dysfunctional voiding
Persistent neonatal jaundice	

UTIs are responsible for 1–5% of febrile illnesses in children under 2 years of age. A UTI is more common in children with higher temperatures, with UTI as the cause of pyrexia >38°C in 9% infants less than 2 months old. It was diagnosed in 7% of infants with a maximum temperature of <39°C and in 16% of those whose temperature was 39°C or higher.

Clinical presentation

The symptoms and signs of UTI vary in children of different age groups [Table 31.1]. In older children a UTI presents with typical symptoms of cystitis – such as frequency, dysuria, hesitancy, secondary enuresis and suprapubic pain, or upper UTI – pyelonephritis – such as fever, vomiting, malaise and loin pain. All children with unexplained pyrexia should have a UTI excluded.

History
A detailed history is important and should include antenatal and perinatal history, fluid intake and voiding patterns as well as bowel habits. A history of previous UTI or any previous episodes of unexplained fever is important. Bed-wetting or voiding disorders do not necessarily indicate a urinary tract abnormality, except in a child who has been previously continent, although bladder instability may often present with recurrent UTIs. On the other hand, a history of constant dribbling of urine is abnormal, and requires investigation to exclude an ectopic insertion of a ureter. The family history is pertinent, as vesico-ureteric reflux and duplex kidneys are known to be common among siblings.

Clinical examination
A general physical examination should include blood pressure measurement, because hypertension in a child with a UTI indicates significant renal pathology. The abdomen should be examined carefully for a renal mass or an overdistended or expressible bladder, which in a neonate is suggestive of a neurogenic bladder. The perineum should be inspected carefully to check perianal sensation and anal tone. Labial adhesions, phimosis, meatal stenosis (and even rarities such as prolapsing ureterocele in a female) can be diagnosed on inspection. 'A urological examination includes a neurological examination', as a neurogenic bladder is an important cause of UTI. The lower limbs are examined for signs of muscle-wasting, sensory loss and orthopaedic deformities (e.g. talipes), which suggest neurological abnormality. The bony spine is inspected and palpated for occult forms of spina bifida or sacral agenesis. An overlying patch of abnormal skin (e.g. pigmented naevus, hair, haemangioma, lipoma or sinus) may indicate the presence of a serious spinal lesion.

Many abnormalities can be diagnosed from the history and physical examination, prior to organ imaging. Radiological investigations often confirm clinical suspicions.

Diagnosis

In the presence of pyuria, a definite diagnosis of UTI can be made when there is a pure culture of a urinary pathogen in an appropriately collected specimen before antibiotics were started or changed. The choice of method for sample collection will depend on the age and condition of the patient.

Children
There are considerable difficulties in collecting a mid-stream specimen of urine (MSSU) in infants and toddlers, but it should be possible to collect a clean mid-stream specimen in the older child. In circumcised boys, the glans should be cleaned with soap and water, rather than antiseptic solutions, using a soft flannel. The urine is collected mid-stream in a universal container during continuous voiding. Boys who have not been circumcised probably do not need to retract the prepuce to clean the glans. Similarly, in the older female child, the labia should be parted, cleansed with a flannel, soap and water from the front to the back three times, and the child asked to void while holding the labia parted. A disposable funnel may facilitate sample collection in girls. The urine is collected mid-stream during continuous voiding. Alcoholic preparations should not be used, as these cause intense pain on delicate mucosa.

Younger children

Toddlers who have recently been toilet-trained are often reluctant to void on request into a container but a reliable sample can be obtained by having the child void into a pottie that has been cleaned with hot water and detergent, rather than an antiseptic, or that has a disposable insert.

Infants

Getting a usable sample from infants can be difficult, although a number of reliable methods can be used. A clean-catch specimen of urine, obtained by stripping the child from the waist down and waiting for him/her to void provides a sample that is as reliable as that obtained by suprapubic aspiration, and better than those obtained by pad or bag collection. Micturition in infants may be encouraged by tapping the suprapubic region or caught when the baby is first exposed to cold, as he/she is undressed. Parents generally consider this to be a time consuming and a messy method.

A sterile adhesive urine collection bag is one of the most commonly used collection systems. The bag is applied to the skin around the genitalia after cleaning. Some bags are designed with a secondary inner bag into which the urine drains to minimise skin contact and potential contamination. The bag should be removed as soon as the child has voided and the specimen decanted into a sterile container by cutting a hole in a corner of the bag. Bag specimens are particularly prone to skin contamination but clearly in an appropriately processed specimen should not yield a false negative and a false positive is unlikely in the presence of significant pyuria.

An absorbent pad can be placed inside the nappy, for those parents who do not like the erythema that adhesive bags produce, and have been shown to produce samples as reliable as bag specimens if properly monitored.

The most reliable technique of collecting urine is by suprapubic aspiration (or by 'in/out' catheterisation). In infants up to about 18 months of age, the bladder is an intra-abdominal organ, making suprapubic needle aspiration of urine simple, quick and reliable. A 'bladder tap' should be performed in any sick infant to exclude UTI, particularly if a urine specimen obtained by other means is inadequate. In a 'septic workup', it is important to do the suprapubic aspiration first, as infants will void during painful procedures, such as venepuncture or lumbar puncture.

A 10 mL syringe with a 23-gauge 4 cm needle is used for the procedure [Fig. 31.1]. The child is nursed supine and restrained by an assistant. The suprapubic area is swabbed with skin disinfectant, and the needle

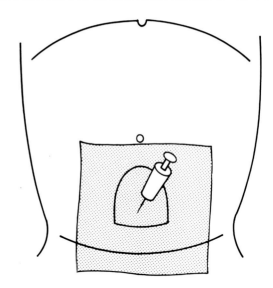

Figure 31.1 The method of suprapubic aspiration for urine culture. The shaded area is the area of aseptic skin preparation.

introduced in the midline, 1 cm above the upper margin of the symphysis pubis. The needle should be introduced by aiming it perpendicular to the floor: in the neonate insert the needle about 2 cm; insert further in older infants. The needle is then withdrawn while aspirating on the syringe, until urine is drawn into the syringe. If the child starts passing urine, the urethra should be gently occluded or a clean-catch specimen obtained, so be prepared. It is sent for culture in a sterile container.

Suprapubic aspirates are the 'gold standard', as any concentration of bacteria is considered significant, although false positive rates of between 10% and 30% have been reported. Furthermore, suprapubic aspiration does not always yield a sample with success rates from 25% to 90%, but this can be improved through the use of ultrasonography.

Once obtained the specimen has to be processed as promptly as possible to minimise overgrowth of contaminating bacteria. Samples should be refrigerated at 4°C if there is to be any delay in processing. At 4°C the sample will remain suitable for culture for up to 2 days.

Sample analysis

Dipstick analysis

Urine dipsticks are now the most commonly used test for UTI and used to screen samples for further processing. The most useful components are the nitrite and leucocyte esterase tests. Most pathogenic bacteria produce nitrite by reduction of nitrate. There may be insufficient quantities to be detectable, hence the sensitivity is only 50%, but the specificity approaches 100%. False positive tests may result from prolonged storage of urine. The urinary frequency in children with a UTI may lead to a false negative. Leucocyte esterase is a marker for WBCs and has similar false positives and negatives. Dipstick tests cannot be relied upon to confirm or exclude a UTI. They are most useful in children with vague symptoms, in whom the clinical suspicion of a UTI is low. A negative dipstick suggests that the probability of UTI is low and patients can await the result of microscopy or culture before starting therapy. Regardless of the dipstick result, all children with a suspected UTI should have urine cultured to yield a definitive diagnosis.

Urine microscopy

The absence of bacteria or WBCs on microscopy makes a UTI unlikely. Bacteria are rendered more readily visible by either Gram-staining or using phase-contrast microscopy, as now recommended in some renal units.

Urine culture is the definitive test for UTI and takes up to 24 h. A further 24 h sub-culture in the presence of antibiotic-impregnated discs is required to define antibiotic sensitivities.

Pitfalls in diagnosis

The urine specimen may be clear in a child with early pyelonephritis, and upper tract obstruction. In this instance, the child should be treated empirically and further specimens of urine should be taken during treatment, as it is common for bacteriuria to be detected on the second or third day.

The child with an infected urinary calculus may have more than one urinary pathogen cultured from the urine specimen.

Cloudy urine does not always signify UTI. In many instances, the cause of the cloudiness is simply precipitation of phosphate crystals when urine cools rapidly.

Organisms

Most UTIs are caused by a single organism originating from the bowel. *Escherichia coli* is the causative organism in approximately 75% of cases. More than 90% of *E. coli* upper tract UTIs are caused by *E. coli* possessing P fimbriae, which allow the bacteria to adhere to the urothelial lining and avoid elimination by micturition. Other causative agents include Klebsiella, *Streptococcus faecalis* and

Proteus mirabilis. Proteus, a preputial commensal found in 30% of uncircumcised boys but only 2% of circumcised boys, produces urease and therefore promotes stone formation. Urease splits urea, forming ammonia and increases urinary pH, which precipitates calcium and magnesium phosphate salts. Less common species such as Pseudomonas, *Staphylococcus aureus*, Enterobacter, Citrobacter, *Serratia marcescens* and Acinetobacter are more likely in children with urinary tract anomalies. *Candida albicans* rarely presents in the community at large but is now the second most common pathogen in hospital-acquired infections, especially those with indwelling catheters or on immunosuppressants.

There are a number of risk factors for UTI, such as incomplete bladder emptying from dysfunctional voiding or vesico-ureteric reflux. UTIs are more common in uncircumcised boys (see Chapter 30) and those with constipation (Chapter 22).

Recurrence

Approximately a third of patients will have a further UTI within 3–6 months, especially in younger infants and girls. In girls who develop a second UTI, roughly half will go on to develop a further UTI and so on. Recurrence is more common in children with high grades of vesico-ureteric reflux.

Management

Treating a UTI aims to eliminate the acute infection, providing symptomatic relief and reducing or preventing renal scarring. The American Academy of Pediatrics has made a number of recommendations in relation to the treatment of children with suspected or proven UTIs [Table 31.2].

Treatment

Choice of antibiotics

The choice of antibiotics is governed by the sensitivities of the urinary pathogen, usually *E. coli*. Trimethoprim, nitrofurantoin and cefalexin are first-line options for empirical treatment whilst awaiting the results of urine culture. If the patient has been taking antibiotics recently, then a change of antibiotic may be appropriate unless they are clinically responding. *E. coli* resistance to trimethoprim

Table 31.2 American Academy of Paediatrics Recommendations for UTI management

- Suspect UTI in infants with unexplained fever
- Await culture results before treatment if non-toxic
- In unwell child, start treatment before culture result in hospital with IV especially if <1-year old
- Reassess with repeat culture if no better in 48 h
- Antibiotics should be given for 7–14 days

Table 31.3 Urinary tract investigations

Renal ultrasonography
Good screening test for obstruction and anatomical variants

Radio isotope imaging
MAG3/DTPA
Excretory scans measuring function and degree of
   obstruction
DMSA
Static renogram showing state of parenchyma
   (scar/inflammation/dysplasia)
MCU
'Gold standard' test for V-U reflux

Plain radiograph
Useful for spinal anomalies + calculi

is increasing and 15–40% of studies report resistance. Co-trimoxazole (trimethoprim and sulphamethoxazole) is now seldom used in children because of the association of sulphamethoxazole with Stevens–Johnson syndrome.

Nitrofurantoin is effective but more likely to cause nausea and vomiting so is best taken with meals. Resistance to nitrofurantoin is also on the increase and it is ineffective against *P. mirabilis*. For patients with a history of previous antibiotic resistance or with breakthrough infections whilst on antibiotic prophylaxis second-line choices include co-amoxiclav, an oral cephalosporin or pivmecillinam. Amoxycillin alone is not suitable because 50% of urinary pathogens are resistant to it. Nitrofurantoin and nalidixic acid are poor antibiotics in the ill child, as they do not achieve adequate tissue levels. Similarly, the new quinalones, although highly effective for treating adult UTI, are not suitable for children, as they may cause erosion of articular cartilage. Aminoglycosides are useful in serious upper UTI, but need careful monitoring in the child with poor renal function, because of nephrotoxicity.

Investigations

Investigation of patients with UTI aims to prevent progressive renal scarring and its consequences – hypertension and renal insufficiency [Table 31.3]. Scarring is a recognised complication of upper UTI, therefore imaging is aimed at detecting scarring and to identify children at risk of further scarring. Therefore, the first investigation should be to determine the location of the infection, that is, upper or lower urinary tract. Lower UTIs are not associated with the development of renal scars and further investigations are less useful. Clinical suspicion based on symptoms and clinical findings may be suggestive of an upper UTI but not conclusive. The gold standard test for the detection of pyelonephritis is a nuclear medicine scan – technetium dimercaptosuccinic acid (DMSA). Power Doppler ultrasonography may be as effective as DMSA in detecting acute pyelonephritis and renal scars but this is not proven. Routine ultrasound scanning is not as effective as DMSA in the detection of upper UTIs.

The incidence of urinary tract abnormality in children with one proven UTI is at least 30%, and higher in the first year of life. The most common abnormality found is vesico-ureteric reflux (VUR). The incidence of VUR in children <1-year old with a UTI is >50%. A causal association between VUR and renal scarring was first proposed in the 1960s, secondary to reflux of infected urine. In recent years, there has been a paradigm shift in our understanding of the significance of VUR, following the detection of renal 'scars' in neonates without a documented UTI. These defects probably represent congenital renal dysplasia that has developed in association with an abnormal ureteric insertion into the bladder. Whilst VUR is a significant risk factor for recurrent UTIs, it is a weak predictor of renal damage in children hospitalised with a UTI. Added to the significance of detecting or excluding VUR is the uncertain clinical benefit of treating children with VUR. Whilst there is no doubt about the benefits of treating an acute UTI, there is no evidence of prevention of renal scarring by long-term prophylactic antibiotics. A large systematic review has failed to find evidence to support the clinical effectiveness of routine investigation of children with a confirmed UTI. This is not because the investigations do not yield positive results but rather because of a paucity of evidence of the significance of those findings or evidence of a change in disease progression in response to therapy.

This suggests investigation of children with UTI should be targeted on those children at higher risk of renal scarring such as the very young (<2 years old), those with recurrent UTIs and those with known anatomical abnormalities. It cannot be over-stated, that adequate documentation of UTI is important, and a clinical diagnosis of 'UTI' without urine culture is inadequate. Given the low-cost, low-risk nature of renal ultrasonography it seems reasonable to perform a renal ultrasound scan with pre- and post-micturition images on all patients with a proven UTI. In infants it is a useful screening tool for obstruction, duplication and other congenital anomalies and in older children may suggest a degree of voiding dysfunction with incomplete emptying of the bladder on micturition.

Renal ultrasonography

Ultrasonography is a good study for children as there is no ionising radiation involved and there is no need for painful injections. This is an accepted preliminary investigation to exclude urinary obstruction. If the scan shows severe hydronephrosis with obstruction and pus, an emergency percutaneous nephrostomy should be considered to drain the infected urine. This is minimally invasive, and similar to draining an abscess, provides immediate relief of symptoms, enables antegrade studies to detect level of obstruction and may save the kidney. Ultrasonography is also valuable in the diagnosis of double systems and ureteroceles.

Nuclear isotope imaging

Nuclear imaging of the renal tracts is useful for assessment of renal function, but does not give good anatomical information. The main renal isotope scans available are the technetium-mercaptoacetyltriglycine (MAG 3), the technetium-diethylenetriamine pentaacetic acid (DTPA) and the DMSA.

The MAG 3 and DTPA are excretory scans providing dynamic renography that measure differential renal function and an estimate of glomerular filtration rate. They suggest obstruction when the clearance after the administration of Lasix is delayed; however, they must be interpreted with caution as there is a high rate of false positive detection of obstruction. The DTPA scan is unreliable in the neonate up to about 6 weeks post-term, due to the immaturity of the kidney, and for this reason, the MAG 3 is used in these patients. Dehydration interferes with assessment of obstruction, as low urine flow causes delayed excretion. Increasingly the dynamic renogram is being extended to look for VUR but cannot accurately grade the degree of reflux.

The DMSA scan is a static renogram and a more useful test in the neonatal period. DMSA is taken up by functioning renal cortical tissue, but does not give any indication of the excreting or concentrating ability of the kidney. It is useful in determining renal damage in reflux-associated nephropathy, and whether there is any functioning renal tissue in the neonate with gross hydronephrosis.

Micturating cystourethrogram

A micturating cystourethrogram (MCU) is performed by the insertion of a small catheter into the bladder, filling the bladder with conventional radiological contrast and screening the patient during voiding to detect abnormalities. An MCU remains the 'gold standard' for the detection and grading of reflux (see Chapter 32). In the male child, it is mandatory to examine the urethra during voiding to exclude outlet urethral obstruction.

Plain abdominal radiographs

These may be useful for showing spinal abnormalities, renal or ureteric calculi or faecal loading.

Key Points

- UTI is common in infancy and needs confirmation by culture and screening for underlying anomalies.
- Recurrent pyelonephritis predisposes to hypertension and renal damage.

Further reading

Brindle MJ (1990) Children with urinary tract infection: a critical diagnostic pathway. *Clin Radiol* **41**: 95–97.

Hansson S, Hjalmas K, Jodal U, Sixt R (1990) Lower urinary tract dysfunction in girls with untreated asymptomatic or covert bacteriuria. *J Urol* **143**: 333–335.

Rickwood AMK, Carty HM, McKendrick T *et al.* (1992) Current imaging of childhood urinary infections: prospective study. *BMJ* **304**: 664–665.

Schroeder AR, Newman TB, Wasserman RC et al. (2005) Choice of urine collection methods for the diagnosis of urinary tract infections in young, febrile infants. *Arch Pediatr Adolesc Med* **159**(10): 915–922.

Westwood ME, Whiting PF, Cooper J, Watt IS, Kleijnen J (2005) Further investigation of confirmed urinary tract infection (UTI) in children under five years: a systematic review. *BMC Pediatr* **5**: 2.

32 Vesico-Ureteric Reflux

Case 1

Melanie is a 5-year-old girl who presents with a history of recurrent urinary tract infection.

Q 1.1 What further investigations should be performed?

Q 1.2 What are the pros and cons of the micturating cystourethrogram?

Q 1.3 Are there any alternatives to the micturating cystourethrogram?

Case 2

A 1-year-old child with severe right-sided vesico-ureteric reflux and recurrent urinary tract infection is found to have reflux nephropathy with defects in the upper and lower poles of the right kidney.

Q 2.1 Is reflux nephropathy congenital or acquired?

Q 2.2 If the recurrent urinary tract infections are kept under control, will further renal damage occur?

Q 2.3 What are the indications for corrective surgery?

Vesico-ureteric reflux (VUR) – the retrograde passage of urine from the bladder up the ureter is the most common abnormality detected in children with a urinary tract infection (UTI). It is found in up to a third of all children presenting with a UTI and in >50% of those less than 1-year old. Frequent and complete micturition protects against UTI by 'flushing' the urinary tract and removing any bacteria. Children with reflux do not empty completely and are therefore at risk of UTI. Furthermore, reflux allows transfer of bacteria from the bladder to the kidney with the risk of developing pyelonephritis and renal scarring.

Incidence

Micturating cystourethrogram (MCU or MCUG) demonstrates VUR in 1–2% of healthy children, although it is an active and intermittent phenomenon and may be missed in 15% of the studies [Table 32.1]. VUR is 5 times more common in girls than boys and is up to 50 times more common in siblings of children with reflux.

Jones' Clinical Paediatric Surgery, 6th edition. By Hutson, O'Brien, Woodward and Beasley. Published 2008 by Blackwell Publishing, ISBN: 978-1-4051-6267-8.

Pathogenesis

VUR may be a primary, congenital anomaly or secondary to abnormal bladder function that may itself be congenital or acquired.

Primary VUR is due to a failure of the one-way valve at the vesico-ureteric junction. The normal ureter runs inside the bladder muscle and under the epithelium for some distance before opening into the bladder cavity. This part of the ureter, known as the sub-mucosal tunnel or intra-mural ureter is compressed against the muscular bladder wall by the increased intra-vesical pressure associated with bladder filling or micturition. If the sub-mucosal tunnel length is too short then the ureter may not be adequately compressed to prevent reflux. It is the increasing length of this sub-mucosal ureter with growth that is responsible for spontaneous resolution of low grades of VUR with age.

Secondary VUR describes reflux due to impaired bladder outflow. This impairment to outflow with a subsequent increase in intra-vesical pressure may result from physical or functional impediments to bladder emptying. Congenital anatomical causes of secondary VUR include posterior urethral valve and neuropathic bladder in patients with spina bifida. VUR may develop secondary to voiding dysfunction seen in older girls or in patients with 'dysfunctional elimination syndrome' hence the association of VUR and constipation.

Table 32.1 International Reflux Study Committee definitions of grades of VUR, percentage incidence of each grade together with likelihood of spontaneous resolution

Grade	Definition	Percentage incidence	Spontaneous resolution (%)
I	Reflux into ureter only	7	83
II	Non-dilating reflux to level of renal calyces	53	60
III	Mild to moderate calyceal dilatation with minimal blunting of calyces	32	46
IV	Moderate dilatation with loss of forniceal angles but preservation of papillary impressions	6	9
V	Gross dilatation and tortuosity	2	0

Consequences

The detection of reflux per se is of little significance rather it is the consequences of its presence that matter. It used to be thought that there was a clear association between VUR, UTI and renal 'scarring' but in recent years the margins have become blurred (see Chapter 31 – UTI). We now know that renal dysplasia can exist prior to any infection, that sterile reflux does not produce scars and that pyelonephritis can cause scarring in the absence of reflux. In children found to have VUR after a UTI, static isotope renography, DMSA scan, reveals photopenic areas suggestive of inflammation or scarring in 25–40%. Some of these 'scars' will not be due to infection but rather represent congenital renal dysplasia. Fifteen to thirty per cent of infants born with antenatally suspected VUR (based on ultrasonographic findings) will have isotope evidence of renal dysplasia antenatally, usually in the form of a global reduction in renal size. Infective renal scarring on the other hand tends to result in focal areas of renal damage usually at the poles of the kidney where the renal papillae are most susceptible to reflux.

Some patients with renal scarring, regardless of the aetiology, will develop hypertension. Raised blood pressure has been found in about 15% of patients with VUR, UTI and dysmorphic kidneys. Reflux nephropathy is responsible for about 22% of patients with paediatric end-stage renal failure.

Presentation

Urinary tract infection
VUR is found in 30–50% of children presenting with a symptomatic UTI (see Chapter 31 – UTI).

Antenatal diagnosis

There is no accepted ultrasonographic definition of antenatal hydronephrosis (ANH) but we would investigate all infants where the anterior–posterior (AP) diameter of the renal pelvis is 5 mm or more. VUR is detected postnatally in 10% of all neonates with ANH, is more likely when the AP diameter is less than 15 mm; more severe ANH tends to be associated with anatomical obstruction. Postnatal confirmation of ANH is undertaken with an ultrasound scan within the first week of life and again at 6 weeks of age. If hydronephrosis is confirmed then an MCUG is done to look for VUR. Interestingly, 25% of babies with normal postnatal ultrasound scans have reflux on MCUG, but mostly this is of no consequence.

The diagnosis of reflux on an MCUG at this early stage, before the development of UTI, enables administration of prophylactic antibiotics which it is hoped, by preventing reflux of infected urine, will limit renal scarring. There is some evidence that long-term prophylactic antibiotics prevent recurrent UTIs but no evidence that renal scarring is reduced. So, whilst it is uncertain whether prophylactic antibiotics will reduce the long-term risks of scarring, hypertension and renal failure, the benefits of UTI reduction in infants are worthwhile, especially as these children are often hospitalised.

Family history

VUR has been found in a quarter to a half of siblings of children with VUR. Given the current debate regarding the significance of VUR, investigation of asymptomatic siblings is even more controversial. There is some evidence that a normal renal ultrasound scan obviates further testing. VUR, if present, is likely to be of low grade and in these patients, the benefit of prophylactic antibiotics has not been proven.

Diagnosis

There are no clinical symptoms or signs specific to VUR; it can be diagnosed only by special investigations.

Lower tract studies

The MCU is the gold-standard test for the diagnosis of VUR [Fig. 32.1]. The bladder is catheterised and filled with x-ray contrast and the child is then screened while voiding. Although invasive and uncomfortable, as well as documenting the presence of reflux, MCU allows the severity of VUR to be graded [Table 32.1] – which has implications for prognosis and potential spontaneous resolution – and provides detailed anatomical information about the bladder and urethra. Because of the discomfort associated with urethral catheterisation and the risk of causing a UTI, MCUs should not be requested in every patient. Some factors to consider when deciding on whom to order an MCU include

1 *Age:* Urethral catheterisation is easier and the diagnosis more important in infants less than 12-months old.

2 *Recurrent UTI:* A child with recurrent UTIs proven on urine culture should have an MCU to check for VUR or other associated anomalies. The zeal with which an MCU is sought will depend on the age of the child, as VUR is probably less significant in older children in terms of further management.

3 *First UTI:* A child who has one documented UTI should have an MCU if (a) under 15 months of age; (b) clinical or sonographic evidence of pyelonephritis; (c) abnormalities, for example, hydronephrosis, scarring, duplex on ultrasonography; (d) there is a strong family history of urinary tract abnormalities (controversial).

If the patient is due for an examination under anaesthetic (e.g. cystoscopy) anyway then a catheter can be inserted under GA and the MCU carried out later the same day.

If clinician or parental concerns relate to the use of radiation to the gonadal region then a Direct Isotope Cystogram can be performed. This test also involves urethral catheterisation and bladder instillation with a radioisotope. This test will allow for a longer period of assessment making the detection VUR more likely but does not enable accurate classification.

The Indirect Isotope Cystogram avoids the need for urethral catheterisation by extending the dynamic renogram using either DTPA or MAG-3 isotope, which having passed through the kidneys accumulates in the bladder, and may indicate the presence of VUR by showing a second increase in radioactivity within the renal region of interest.

Upper tract studies

The performance of investigations to examine the upper tracts is less controversial. Routine renal ultrasonography is a well-tolerated, non-toxic, inexpensive investigation that can be repeated periodically to assess renal growth and scar progression.

Isotope renography, though more invasive, provides a more accurate assessment of the presence of renal scars, differential renal function, and indirectly VUR.

Timing of investigations

Ultrasonography can be performed at any stage, potentially detecting pyelonephritis early or scars late in the clinical course of infection. The MCU, if undertaken, is usually delayed until the UTI has resolved, as VUR may be more likely to cause a UTI. The MCU is usually carried out prior to discharge. If the isotope study is carried out during the acute episodes, it may detect photopenic areas suggestive of either pyelonephritis or scars. Approximately

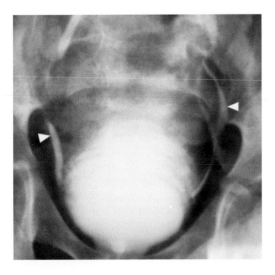

Figure 32.1 Bilateral Grade I VUR shown on MCU. The contrast in the lower ureters is arrowed. There is a high chance that reflux of this grade will resolve spontaneously.

50% of these photopenic areas will disappear within 2 months. For long-term prognosis, it is the presence of permanent scars that is significant and hence the isotope scan is best delayed for at least 2–6 months after UTI.

Natural history

There is a strong tendency for primary VUR to resolve spontaneously in the preschool years with the normal growth of the bladder muscle offering better support to the intra-vesical ureter. Nearly all cases of mild VUR without ureteric dilatation (Grades I and II; Table 32.1) resolve spontaneously. More severe cases of VUR with dilatation of the ureter (Grades III, IV and V; Fig. 32.2) have a lower rate of spontaneous resolution and may require surgical correction. As well as grade of reflux, the probability of spontaneous resolution is influenced by laterality and age of patient at diagnosis. As the spontaneous resolution of reflux is associated with bladder growth

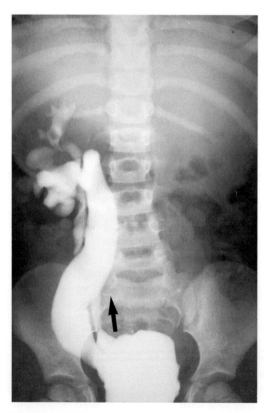

Figure 32.2 MCU showing gross right-sided VUR (arrow) up both ureters in a duplex system. There is no reflux on the left.

it seems self-evident that reflux presenting in older patients is less likely to resolve. Similarly, reflux is less likely to resolve in patients with bilateral as opposed to unilateral reflux.

Management

Medical management

The initial management of VUR is always medical, and aims to prevent symptomatic pyelonephritis and renal scarring whilst awaiting spontaneous resolution. Medical management is based on preventing or minimising UTIs on the premise that reflux of infected urine is harmful. This is achieved by ensuring a normal fluid intake and regular toileting, proper perineal hygiene – more important in girls, elimination of constipation, if present, and administration of low-dose prophylactic antibiotics. The optimum dose schedule and duration of treatment has not been established. Most clinicians will start newly diagnosed infants with VUR on low-dose continuous antibiotic (Trimethoprim or Nitrofurantoin) administered at night (as this is usually the longest time that urine dwells in the bladder), stopping either when the child is toilet-trained or has been without a proven UTI for 12 months. Some clinicians would question the need for prophylactic antibiotics at all.

The critical factor in medical management is vigilance and prompt, appropriate treatment of UTIs as they occur. This requires close medical supervision and well-informed, motivated parents with ready access to medical attention to prevent pyelonephritis leading to renal scarring and potential long-term damage.

Surgical management

Where medical management has been a failure, as evidenced by recurrent breakthrough UTIs, surgical intervention may be appropriate. Structural anomalies such as para-ureteric diverticulae, ureteric duplication, ureterocele may make spontaneous resolution of VUR less likely but do not negate the potential benefit of a trial of medical therapy. Secondary VUR such as that seen in association with a neuropathic bladder or posterior urethral valve is best managed by treating the underlying condition rather than surgical reimplantation of the ureters.

There are a number of surgical strategies that may be employed in patients with VUR. Circumcision may be appropriate in boys with VUR, especially if the UTI is due to *Proteus mirabilis*, a known preputial commensal.

A nephro-ureterectomy may be appropriate if the reflux is into a non-functioning dysplastic kidney. In the very young/small infant a temporary vesicostomy – permitting the bladder to drain at low pressure onto the abdominal wall, decompressing the upper tracts and minimising reflux may be appropriate. However, the primary aims of surgical therapy for VUR are to prevent reflux and this can be achieved either endoscopically or surgically with ureteric reimplantation.

Endoscopic treatment ('STING' or 'HIT')

Endoscopic injection with synthetic polysaccharide is gaining increasing acceptance worldwide with published success rates of 75% or more following a single injection, 85% with 2 injections and 95% following three injections. Endoscopic therapy offers a number of advantages over open surgery, namely, that it is a day-case procedure, can be easily repeated and does not make surgery, for those patients in whom it fails, more difficult. Disadvantages are lingering doubts about its long-term safety and efficacy and some concerns about over-treatment in patients who may have resolved spontaneously anyway (i.e. Grades I and II VUR).

Ureteric reimplantation

For many years, ureteric reimplantation has been the mainstay of surgical management of VUR. This is because the reported success rates for reflux resolution are in excess of 95%. There are a number of differing surgical approaches that traditionally have involved detaching the ureter from the bladder and creating a new sub-mucosal tunnel and neo-ureterovesicostomy largely from within the bladder. More recently, it has been shown that minimally invasive ureteric reimplantation can be done with pneumo-vesicum (bladder filled with CO_2) although the merits of this new approach have yet to be demonstrated.

Key Points
- VUR is associated with both primary abnormal development of the kidney (dysplasia) and secondary scars of pyelonephritis.
- VUR is common in fetuses and babies as the bladder (and ureteric valve) is small: resolution is common with growth.
- VUR may be diagnosed antenatally but postnatal MCU is needed for confirmation.

Further reading

Cass DT (1990) Surgical aspects of primary vesico-ureteric reflux. *J Pediatr Child Health* **26**: 180–183.

Elder JS, Peters CA, Arant BS Jr. *et al.* (1997) Pediatric vesicoureteral reflux guidelines panel summary report on the management of primary vesicoureteral reflux in children. *J Urol* **157**(5): 1846–1851.

Ewalt DH (1998) Renal infection, abscess, vesicoureteral reflux, urinary lithiasis and renal vein thrombosis. In O'Neill JA, Rowe MI, Grosfeld JL, Fonkalsrud EW, Coran AG (eds) *Pediatric Surgery*, 5th Edn. Mosby, St Louis, pp. 1609–1622.

Voort JH van der, Jones KV, Gough D (2006) Vesico-ureteric reflux a) Definition and Conservative Management b) Surgical Treatment. In: Stringer MD, Oldham KT, Mouriquand PDE (eds) *Pediatric Surgery and Urology Long Term Outcomes*, 2nd Edn. Cambridge University Press, Cambridge, pp. 555–582.

33 Urinary Tract Dilatation

Case 1

Antenatal ultrasonography at 18 weeks shows bilateral hydronephrosis in the fetus, which is still present in the third trimester, when oligohydramnios develops.

Q 1.1 What is the natural history of antenatal hydronephrosis?

Q 1.2 What conditions cause antenatal hydronephrosis?

Q 1.3 What treatment is required at birth?

Case 2

An 18-month-old male infant presents with fever and dysuria. Urine culture shows an infection and an ultrasound shows hydronephrosis and hydroureter (bilateral).

Q 2.1 What causes 'hydroureter'?

Q 2.2 What investigations are needed for urinary tract infection (UTI)?

Hydronephrosis is defined as an abnormal dilatation of the kidney, specifically the renal pelvis, and sometimes referred to as pelviectasis. More severe cases have an associated dilatation of the calyces (calyectasis) and possible also the ureter (hydroureter). The presence of hydronephrosis implies a degree of partial outflow obstruction (which may still be present or have resolved), but can also be found associated with retrograde flow of urine or vesico-ureteric reflux (VUR). Differentiating those patients with hydronephrosis secondary to a persisting and potentially harmful partial obstruction from those in whom the dilatation probably represents the sequelae of an obstruction that is now resolving or has resolved presents an interesting clinical challenge. Having determined the level of the likely obstruction, we must then ascertain the potential for renal injury or loss of function.

Hydronephrosis is diagnosed by ultrasonography. A normal kidney will not have any dilatation of its collecting system, and therefore any dilatation is defined as hydronephrosis. The Society of Fetal Urology has proposed a grading system for hydronephrosis, but most units adopt descriptive documentation of the maximum antero-posterior renal pelvis diameter in a transverse plane at the level of the renal hilum, often referred to as

the renal pelvis diameter (RPD) or renal antero-posterior diameter (APD). Consistently measuring the renal pelvis at this point standardises repeated observations to look for trends towards progression or regression and also to compare with the published literature for predicting outcome. A precise APD threshold above which investigation should be pursued cannot be found but most surgeons would investigate a patient with an APD >5 mm.

Clinical presentation

Prior to the advent of routine antenatal screening patients with urinary tract dilatation typically presented with pain or UTIs. Pain is the most common presenting feature in the older child, and may be accompanied by infection or haematuria, especially after minor trauma [Table 33.1]. A distinguishing clinical feature is lateralisation of the pain to the loin, and accompanying nausea or vomiting. Symptoms are exacerbated by a fluid load and sometimes by position. Intermittent loin pain precipitated by a fluid load (known as a Dietl's crisis) is caused by stretching the renal capsule with a sudden worsening of hydronephrosis.

Nowadays most neonates and infants with hydronephrosis are detected by antenatal ultrasonography. For that small proportion not detected antenatally, hydronephrosis in the neonate may manifest as a UTI or as a palpable abdominal mass. Presentation as a loin mass is unusual

Jones' Clinical Paediatric Surgery, 6th edition. By Hutson, O'Brien, Woodward and Beasley. Published 2008 by Blackwell Publishing, ISBN: 978-1-4051-6267-8.

Table 33.1 Clinical presentation of urinary tract obstruction

Child	Infant/neonate
Pain	Antenatal hydronephrosis on ultrasound
Infection	Incidental finding
Haematuria	Infection
Loin mass	Loin mass
Incidental finding	Haematuria
	Pain

except in a neonate, in whom 50% of all abdominal masses are renal in origin. The most common renal abnormality detected on antenatal screening is hydronephrosis picked up at the 18–20 weeks of gestation scan. When defined as an APD > 5 mm antenatal hydronephrosis was detected in 100 of 18,766 antenatal ultrasound scans or 0.59% of pregnancies. However, in approximately half of these patients the postnatal ultrasound will be normal. The likelihood of significant pathology increases with increasing size of antenatal hydronephrosis, such that if the APD was more than 20 mm, then the majority would require surgery or long-term follow-up; of those with an APD of 10–15 mm, half will have a significant abnormality, and of those with APD < 10 mm, only 3% have an abnormality.

Another mode of presentation is where renal investigations are performed for suspected abnormalities in children with known multiple anomalies.

Investigations

The investigation for suspected or proven urinary tract dilatation aims to
1 demonstrate and document the nature and degree of dilatation;
2 assess renal function (on both sides);
3 define the abnormal anatomy.

Physical examination
Physical examination is aimed at detecting an abdominal mass (suggestive of obstruction or a large multicystic dysplastic kidney) or a palpable bladder.

Ultrasonography
Ultrasonography is the first investigation performed for suspected obstruction, and will not only demonstrate any abnormal anatomy but also may determine the likely cause. However, an ultrasound scan will not prove that a dilated system is obstructed, nor will it demonstrate function in the dilated system. Given its non-toxic nature efforts are continually being made to extend its role to hopefully replace other tests; hence, the use of Doppler ultrasound and resistive indices for obstruction and scarring and, contrast-enhanced ultrasound to demonstrate VUR (see Chapter 32).

Micturating cystourethrogram
A micturating cystourethrogram (MCU) is essential in the investigation of children with dilated upper tracts not only to exclude associated reflux but also to exclude distal obstruction, for example, posterior urethral valve in boys. The fervour with which one pursues an MCU will depend on the individual scenario; for instance, all newborn male infants with small thick-walled bladders and bilateral hydro-uretero-nephrosis must have an MCU. In contrast, a 7-year-old asymptomatic female sibling of a patient with VUR whose is found to have mild unilateral hydronephrosis may not have their clinical management altered by the result of an MCU and hence could be justifiably spared the trauma.

Renal isotope scan
Nuclear medicine or renal isotope scintigraphy may be useful in ascertaining differential renal function and even implied absolute renal function. Renal isotope scans are either static (DMSA), for demonstrating absolute renal parenchyma and detection of scars, or dynamic (DTPA or MAG-3). Dynamic isotope renography provides both differential renal function and evidence about obstruction or reflux. The interpretation of MAG-3 or DTPA excretion curves is prone to significant error and should be left to experts.

A MAG-3 scan can be used in the first few months of life when renal function is low (and DTPA scan is ineffective).

Intravenous pyelogram
Intravenous pyelography is used rarely today for the demonstration of function, but it is still an excellent investigation where it is essential to demonstrate the anatomy, particularly in duplex systems where both moieties are functioning.

Retrograde and antegrade pyelography
Both techniques are employed to demonstrate anatomy or obstruction where this is essential to the management of the patient.

MRu

MR urography is increasingly being employed as a non-toxic investigation for the determination of differential renal function as well as anatomical information.

PET

PET scanning, especially when combined with CT or MR, provides an excellent opportunity to locate the elusive upper pole of a duplex kidney in a young girl with urinary incontinence.

Pitfalls of investigations

The immaturity of the neonatal kidney presents difficulties in interpretation of functional tests in the first month of life. As the concentrating ability and total renal function is low in the neonate, it is likely that functional studies will give misleading results. For this reason, it is best to defer any functional study for at least 6 weeks post-term, although a MAG-3 scan can be used at this time. Isotope renography is further prone to errors caused by the level of patient hydration and the regions of interest drawn by the radiographer.

Aetiologic factors

Pelvi-ureteric junction obstruction

Pelvi-ureteric junction (PUJ) obstruction affects approximately 1 in 2000 children, is more common in boys and on the left side but may be bilateral in 20–25%. Partial obstruction of the PUJ is caused by intrinsic stenosis (75%), congenital kinking or a lower pole vessel crossing the ureter as it joins the renal pelvis (20%). If the obstruction is intermittent, there is good preservation of renal function in the early stages [Fig. 33.1]. Infection and progressive obstruction lead to loss of renal function unless severe blockage is relieved surgically. Occasionally, if progressive deterioration has been identified prenatally, early intervention is necessary after birth. However, less severe degrees of hydronephrosis in the newborn often resolve spontaneously. In a large series of babies with antenatal hydronephrosis, babies with APD < 12 mm rarely required surgery, those with APD > 50 mm all required surgery, and 25% of those with APD of 12–50 mm required surgery because of progressively increasing hydronephrosis or loss of function on repeated isotope renography.

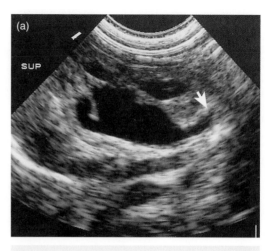

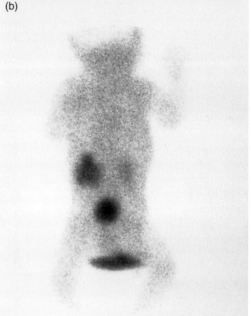

Figure 33.1 Postnatal ultrasonography examination in an infant with antenatal hydronephrosis, showing (a) PUJ obstruction (arrow) with pelvi-calyceal dilatation, but good preservation of renal parenchyma; (b) nuclear renal scan (DTPA) showing hold up at the pelvi-ureteric junction at 45 min.

Vesico-ureteric Junction (VuJ) obstruction

Any degree of ureteric dilatation seen on ultrasonography is abnormal as the ureter is a conduit for urine and not a storage vessel. A dilated ureter or megaureter (>7 mm) may be due to obstruction, reflux or a combination of both. Obstruction is usually secondary to a stenosis or valve in the lower ureter [Fig. 33.2]. Mild cases may resolve spontaneously, leaving a persistently dilated ureter that is no longer obstructed. A ureterocele is a cystic dilatation of the intravesical ureter that may be associated with a duplex kidney and usually requires endoscopic surgery to relieve the obstruction and improve drainage. More severe cases of ureteric obstruction may require surgical correction in the form of a ureteric reimplantation.

Vesico-ureteric reflux

VUR may present with a UTI and hydro-uretero-nephrosis on ultrasonography or may be found in 9% of neonates with antenatal hydronephrosis (see Chapter 32). Secondary PUJ obstruction due to increasing ureteric tortuosity and kinking may occur.

Posterior urethral obstruction

Posterior urethral valve affects 1 in 8000 newborns and accounts for less than 1% of antenatally diagnosed hydronephrosis. In males, epithelial folds running down from the verumontanum in the posterior urethra form a membrane or 'valve' that impedes the flow of urine with back pressure on the bladder, ureters and kidneys. When the obstruction is severe, intrauterine renal failure occurs with fetal death *in utero*, or death soon after birth from Potter syndrome. Less severe obstruction allows the fetus to survive, but if the problem is not detected early, septic complications from UTI and metabolic abnormalities caused by renal failure soon occur. The majority of boys are detected or suspected on antenatal ultrasound. The postnatal features include a thick-walled, palpable bladder and a poor urinary stream in a newborn male infant. The diagnosis is confirmed on MCU [Fig. 33.3]. Fetal intervention is often considered, but is seldom appropriate, and if it has any role, it is probably beneficial to lung development in severe oligohydramnios rather than for preserving or improving renal function. Up to a third of boys with a posterior urethral valve will develop renal insufficiency or end-stage renal failure.

Neurogenic (neuropathic) bladder

Neurogenic bladder causes hydronephrosis in a number of ways. Patients may have a functional bladder neck obstruction from sphincter dysfunction with upper tract dilatation secondary to high intravesical pressure. Many patients with neurogenic bladder have reflux secondary to the neuropathy, which further exacerbates the upper tract dilatation.

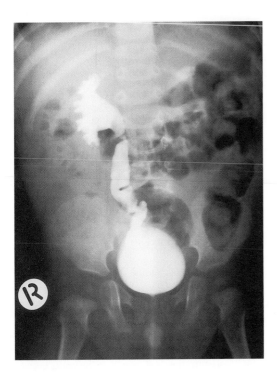

Figure 33.2 Right vesico-ureteric junction obstruction. Note the dilated ureter right down to the bladder.

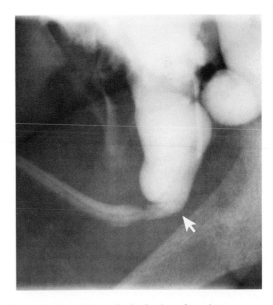

Figure 33.3 Posterior urethral valve (membrane) seen on a lateral view of the urethra on MCU (arrow). Note reflux into a megaureter, massive dilatation of the posterior urethra and a urethral catheter.

Double ureters and kidneys (duplex system)

Congenital duplex kidneys may develop hydronephrosis of either part of the duplex system. The upper moiety is usually the more abnormal [Fig. 33.4], and the dilatation is caused by dysplasia or distal obstruction (from ureterocele;

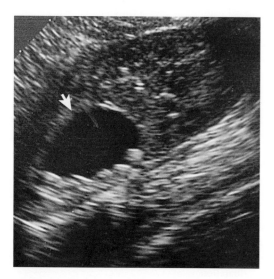

Figure 33.4 Duplex kidney with dilated upper moiety (arrow) on ultrasonography.

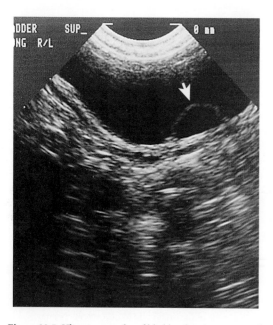

Figure 33.5 Ultrasonography of bladder showing ureterocele (arrow) in the same patient as Fig. 33.4.

Fig. 33.5), or an ectopic position of the ureteric orifice (e.g. in the bladder neck). Ectopic ureteric insertion is often associated with dysplasia in a very poorly functioning upper renal moiety. Dilatation of the more normal lower moiety may be caused by PUJ obstruction, or be associated with high-grade VUR.

Stones (urolithiasis)

Rarely in children, a renal or ureteric calculus may cause an acute obstruction resulting in hydronephrosis.

Management of obstructive lesions

It is best to divide the investigation and management of hydronephrosis into two age groups: those presenting in the neonatal period and those presenting later.

Antenatal hydronephrosis

Not all hydronephrosis on antenatal examination turn out to be significant. In fact, approximately half do not have any abnormality detected on postnatal investigation and are labelled as having had transient hydronephrosis. However, when hydronephrosis is detected antenatally, it is important to follow it throughout pregnancy. If other urinary tract abnormalities are detected on scanning, this would suggest that the hydronephrosis is pathological. Increasing hydronephrosis with oligohydramnios is also pathological, suggestive of low urine output with a posterior urethral valve. The more severe the hydronephrosis, the more likely there will be a pathological cause: most cases with antenatal APD < 10 mm will either be normal or have VUR whereas PUJ obstruction is more likely if the APD > 15 mm.

Despite lack of good randomised evidence of benefit, most urologists/nephrologists commence all neonates with antenatally diagnosed hydronephrosis on prophylactic antibiotics from birth while awaiting full evaluation, as there is significant risk of severe UTI developing in these children. They usually receive Trimethoprim 2 mg/kg at night.

Preliminary investigations should include a careful clinical evaluation to exclude abdominal masses, and inspection of the perineum to detect clinically obvious abnormalities, such as prolapsing ureteroceles.

All children with antenatally diagnosed hydronephrosis should undergo a postnatal ultrasound examination and an MCU within the first week. It is important that the ultrasound scan is not carried out too early (<48 h) as the neonate is relatively oliguric at this stage and ultrasonography may underestimate the severity of the dilatation. The ultrasound scan will confirm the degree of hydronephrosis [Fig. 33.1] and an MCU will exclude distal obstruction or VUR, which accounts for 10% of hydronephroses in the antenatal period.

Functional evaluation is of limited value at birth because of the relative immaturity of the kidney, it is best to defer a renal DTPA scan until the baby is six weeks old. A DMSA of MAG-3 nuclear scan, however, can be very useful in this period, as this shows up any functioning renal tissue.

Except for a posterior urethral valve, definitive treatment can be deferred in most cases until full evaluation of the degree of obstruction is completed. A significant number of apparent neonatal PUJ obstructions improve spontaneously. However, severe obstruction in the neonatal period will require early surgery.

In posterior urethral valves, the bladder is drained by urethral or suprapubic catheter. The metabolic and septic complications are treated before endoscopic resection of the valves is performed. The patient's creatinine is allowed to reach its nadir prior to undertaking surgery to ablate the valve, relieving the obstruction.

Children with severe obstruction usually have gross hydronephrosis on postnatal ultrasound scan. The kidney is tense and usually palpable. A DTPA scan may show a non-functioning kidney, but if the DMSA scan shows an appreciable amount of renal cortical tissue, early repair will lead to significant recovery of renal function.

Management of older children with lesions

In the older child, the preliminary investigations should always include a renal ultrasound and dynamic renography to determine function, drainage and possibility of obstruction. An MCU may be indicated especially if surgery is planned. Unless renal function is severely impaired (<10%), surgical relief of the obstruction should be undertaken. Where there is minimal function, the kidney should be removed [Fig. 33.6], and this can be done laparoscopically.

Percutaneous nephrostomy

This is a useful emergency measure to drain an obstructed kidney, particularly in the presence of infection. In a sick child with pyelonephritis, it leads to rapid clinical improvement, as well as significant improvement in renal function. Percutaneous nephrostomy also allows evaluation of overall function and delineation of the anatomy by antegrade pyelography.

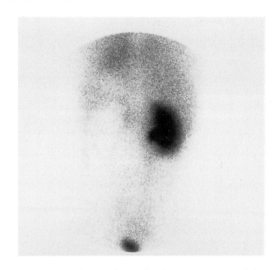

Figure 33.6 Nuclear renal scan showing no function on left side at 5 min (image taken from behind).

Pyeloplasty

The standard operative procedure to relieve a pelvi-ureteric obstruction is an Hynes-Anderson pyeloplasty. This requires excision of the narrowed segment and anastomosis of the spatulated ureter to the renal pelvis. The functional results of this operation are good, but these kidneys may retain their dilated appearance permanently. Laparoscopic pyeloplasty is gaining popularity, but the long-term results are not yet known. Attempts at endoscopic management of PUJ obstruction in children have had limited success and have not been widely undertaken given the success of the open pyeloplasty.

Total nephrectomy

Nephrectomy may be considered where the back pressure from obstruction has destroyed the kidney, which usually has a function of 10% or less. A poorly functioning kidney will not prevent the need for dialysis were the patient to lose the other kidney, and carries with it a significantly increased risk of sepsis and hypertension.

Partial nephrectomy

Duplex kidneys draining into an ectopic ureter or ureterocele (secondary to ureteric stenosis) are similarly likely to be very poorly functioning and a potential source of recurrent infections. Again, if these moieties provide less than 10–12% of overall renal function they are treated by partial nephrectomy and excision of the ectopic duplicated ureter.

Obstructed megaureters

Where the obstruction is at the uretero-vesical junction, excision of the stenotic segment, and reimplantation of the ureter into the bladder, is the accepted treatment, with good results. In small infants, a temporary stent may be placed endoscopically across the VUJ to relieve the obstruction and removed after 6 months. In our limited experience this may obviate the need for early reimplantation; however, long-term follow-up is required.

Key Points

- Hydronephrosis diagnosed antenatally is common, and often resolves, but all babies need immediate investigation at birth.
- Prophylactic antibiotics are widely recommended to prevent urosepsis while postnatal assessment occurs.
- Surgery is required for severe and/or progressive obstruction, especially if renal function is compromised.

Further reading

Elder JS (2003) Management of antenatally detected hydronephrosis. In: Puri P (ed) *Newborn Surgery*, 2nd Edn. Arnold, London, pp. 793–808.

Filmer RB, Spencer JR (1990) Malignancies in bladder augmentations and intestinal conduits. *J Urol* **143**: 671–678.

Jayanthi VR, Koff SA (2006) Upper tract dilation. In: Stringer MD, Oldham KT, Mouriquand PDE (eds) *Paediatric Surgery and Urology. Long-term Outcomes*, 2nd Edn. Cambridge University Press, Cambridge, pp. 533–539.

Peters CA, Bolkier M, Bauer SB, *et al.* (1990) Urodynamic consequences of posterior urethral valves. *J Urol* **144**: 122–126.

Woodward M, Frank D (2002) Postnatal management of antenatal hydronephrosis. *BJU Int* **89**: 149–156.

34

The Child with Wetting

Case 1

A 6-year-old girl presents with severe day and night wetting and urinary tract infections (UTIs). She can have dry days and her symptoms are worse with infection.

Q 1.1 What is the relation between UTIs and wetting?

Q 1.2 How would you investigate this case?

Q 1.3 Discuss further treatment.

Case 2

A 7-year-old girl presents with continuous mild wetting (a few drops leak out every few minutes) every day without fail, and no other symptoms.

Q 2.1 Of what condition is this a classic history?

Q 2.2 How is this diagnosis confirmed by investigation?

Q 2.3 What treatment is required?

Case 3

A 4-year-old boy presents with severe wetting day and night. When his doctor examines the lumbosacral spine, he finds a previously undiagnosed anomaly.

Q 3.1 Discuss the 'hidden' variants of spinal dysraphism that may be missed in the neonatal examination and present at a later age with wetting.

Q 3.2 Why does the further investigation of these anomalies become much more difficult and costly if not performed in the first few months of life?

Q 3.3 How does the management of major neuropathic incontinence differ from other types of incontinence?

Urinary incontinence is the most common disorder of the urinary tract in childhood. It causes immense distress to both the patient and the parents. Childhood urinary incontinence forms a spectrum of disease ranging from benign self-limiting nocturnal incontinence to neuropathic incontinence with potential renal impairment. Fortunately, the majority of children do not have any underlying pathology and will achieve dryness even without treatment. Despite these reassuring facts, most families seek medical attention because of the stress and anxiety associated with urinary incontinence. Initially help is sought from family doctors, continence advisors or paediatricians. Surgeons tend to see those patients who have overt neurological signs or who have failed previous therapeutic intervention.

Jones' Clinical Paediatric Surgery, 6th edition. By Hutson, O'Brien, Woodward and Beasley. Published 2008 by Blackwell Publishing, ISBN: 978-1-4051-6267-8.

Development of continence

The bladder (together with the urethra and pelvic floor) has two main functions, namely, the storage of urine at a low pressure and the emptying of urine at a socially appropriate time. These functions are achieved because of the viscoelastic properties of the interlacing network of smooth muscle fibres in the bladder wall and the integration, within the brain, of both somatic and autonomic nervous systems that are relayed both to and from the bladder. In infants, who void approximately 20 times a day, micturition is a reflex act coordinated in the pons. Over the next 2 years, the frequency of micturition reduces to around 11 times a day – mainly due to increases in bladder capacity. It is around this time that children also begin to recognise symptoms of bladder fullness. By 3 years of age, children have some conscious control and most have daytime control with occasional accidents. Most children are dry by day and night by the age of 4 years.

The attainment of voluntary control of micturition is dependent on a maturation of communication between the pontine micturition centre, the pontine storage centre, and the cerebellum, which receives sensory input from the bladder and pelvic floor, the basal ganglia and the frontal lobes. This development allows the socially appropriate inhibition of reflex voiding and the initiation of micturition at any stage of bladder filling.

Definitions

Previous confusion around urinary incontinence can be attributed to inappropriate use of terminology such as 'diurnal incontinence,' which has been used to mean either isolated daytime or both, day- and night-time incontinence. The International Children's Continence Society (ICCS) has published standardised definitions and terminology that are descriptive, unambiguous, neutral and in line with adult terminology. The emphasis is on describing and quantifying the patients' symptoms rather than attempting to pigeon-hole patients in subgroups [Table 34.1]. The ICCS terminology is relevant in patients over 5 years of age and/or those who have attained bladder control.

Prevalence

Urinary incontinence is a major healthcare problem said to affect 10 million Americans, of whom 85% are women. Occasional daytime urinary incontinence has been reported in about 10% of 11-year-old British school children (7% of boys and 16% of girls). The prevalence decreases with age, with incontinence reported by 3%

of 15- to 16-year-olds (1% of boys and 5% of girls). However, less than half of these patients have wetting of sufficient severity or frequency to seek treatment.

Nocturnal enuresis has been reported in 15–20% of 5-year-olds, 5% of 10-year-olds and 1–2% of 15- to 16-year-olds. Boys are more commonly affected than girls. Less than 3% of children will have an organic cause for their bedwetting. However, 25% will have daytime symptoms in addition to their bedwetting.

Assessment

Surgical assessment of children with urinary incontinence is directed towards the diagnosis or exclusion of an organic aetiology such as abnormal anatomy or neuropathy. This is usually possible based on history and physical examination with little need for aggressive investigation.

History

A full medical history is required to document the nature of the urinary incontinence, such as timing, frequency and pattern, periodicity, severity, precipitating factors, associated urinary symptoms of urgency or dysuria. A detailed voiding history should also be taken looking at the frequency/urgency of micturition, nature of urinary stream (i.e. continuous/intermittent, strong/weak), and any withholding manoeuvres such as crossed legs, squatting with the heel pressed into the perineum (Vincent's curtsey) or holding the penis. An assessment of fluid intake should be made with emphasis on the volume and nature of fluids. Patients should be asked about the bowel habit as constipation predisposes to UTIs, which may precipitate or exacerbate incontinence. The success or failure of previous treatment strategies should be recorded.

Table 34.1 ICCS recommended terminology for patient symptoms

Storage symptoms	
Increased voiding frequency	Consistently voiding eight times or more a day
Decreased voiding frequency	Voiding three times or less in a day
Incontinence	Uncontrollable leakage of urine, which may be continuous or intermittent
Urgency	The sudden and unexpected sensation of an immediate need to void
Voiding symptoms	
Hesitancy	Difficulty initiating micturition
Straining	Application of abdominal pressure to aid micturition
Intermittency	Micturition that is not a continuous stream but rather as several discrete spurts
Weak stream	The observed ejection of urine with a weak force

A detailed past medical and social history is also important, such as previous UTIs and major events within the family (parental separation/death, birth of new sibling, moving home, changing school, etc.), as these will impact on bladder function. The history should also include pre- and perinatal events such as birth trauma, neonatal hypoxia, prematurity and seizures that are associated with voiding disorder. The impact of wetting on both the child and the parents, their reactions to it and the family dynamics should be noted.

The most difficult part of taking a history is getting reliable and accurate details of the voiding pattern, fluid intake, frequency and severity of incontinence. This information is most reliably obtained by asking the parent/child to complete a detailed intake and output diary or bladder diary. Clearly longer periods are associated with reducing compliance and incomplete recording. The minimum for detailed fluid intake and output is 48 h.

Clinical examination

Physical examination is aimed at detecting organic disease. In addition to a routine physical examination, which should include blood pressure measurement, specific attention should be paid to examination of the abdomen looking for a palpable/enlarged bladder from which urine may be expressed. An expressible bladder is strongly suggestive of underlying neurological disease, especially if associated with severe faecal loading. The spine should be inspected and palpated to find subtle evidence of occult spinal dysraphism such as hairy patch, cutaneous haemangioma, sinus or a lipoma. The sacrum should be palpated and buttocks examined to exclude sacral agenesis. A limited neurological examination looking at gait, lower limb symmetry, calf muscle wasting, foot deformitiy, tone, power and lower limb sensation together with lower limb reflexes and the presence or absence of clonus must be carried out. Perineal sensation and ano-cutaneous reflex must be assessed.

The genitalia must be examined for evidence of skin excoriation consistent with incontinence and to detect anatomical abnormalities such as meatal stenosis, epispadias and pathological phimosis in boys and labial adhesions, epispadias, urogenital sinus and rarely ectopic ureter in girls.

Investigations

Urinalysis and urine culture though rarely positive are routinely undertaken to look for evidence of UTI and to screen for renal disease. For a child with monosymptomatic nocturnal enuresis analysis of osmolality of the first urine voided in the morning together with overnight urine volumes may help to direct therapy.

A plain abdominal film is not often indicated and is unlikely to yield usable information on the urinary tract, but it may provide information about faecal loading or occult spinal abnormalities.

Ultrasonography provides a simple, non-invasive, inexpensive look at the urinary tract. It may detect evidence of neuropathic bladder with a thick-walled bladder (>3 mm in distended bladder, >5 mm in empty bladder) or upper tract hydro-uretero-nephrosis, suggestive of high-pressure urine storage. It may also detect evidence of duplication, which in girls may herald an ectopic ureter as the cause of continuous urinary incontinence. Assessment of bladder volumes both pre- and postmicturition may reveal significant (>10% of estimated bladder capacity or 25 mL) postvoid urine residuals which may indicate outlet obstruction, underlying neuropath or may influence therapeutic options.

In patients with functional incontinence uroflowmet is the simplest and the most commonly performed ur dynamic investigation. Patients void into the urofl apparatus, which measures the volume of urine voi over time and plots the result as a graph of volume ver time. From this study one can comment on the shap the flow curve and hence the nature of the urinary str It may be a normal smooth bell-shaped curve; the tened plateau curve seen in outflow obstruction; the cato or irregular flow curve seen in patients incoordination between the sphincter and bladder o interrupted flow pattern seen with patients with detr failure who void by abdominal contraction. The con ter will also produce a number of parameters that des the curve of which the most useful are the voided ume, voiding time and maximum flow rate, for normograms are available to tell whether the flow within the normal range or not. In paediatric urol practice the uroflow assessment typically consists of voids with ultrasound scan of postvoid residual. recent addition of pelvic floor surface electromyogi to uroflow assessment facilitates the easier detecti bladder sphincter incoordination.

Formal urodynamic assessment or cystomet undertaken in a very small proportion of patie whom a clinical diagnosis has not been made, who failed medical therapy, those with a proven or susp neuropathy or those patients with high-risk bladde example, posterior urethral valve. Correctly perfo cystometry requires the simultaneous measureme intravesical and intra-abdominal pressure, togethe

pelvic floor electromyography while filling the bladder at rates close to physiological filling with x-ray contrast, under image intensifier screening. It is a time-consuming, intimidating test fraught with potential misinterpretation and should only be carried out by experienced personnel in a dedicated setting.

Conditions

The simplest and most valid classification, based on onset, is into 'secondary,' which refers to children who have previously been dry for 6 months, or 'primary' for those who have not. Subdivision into patients with nocturnal or daytime urinary incontinence is also valid, but remember that one in four children with nocturnal incontinence will also have some daytime symptoms.

Nocturnal urinary incontinence or nocturnal enuresis

It is best classified as 'monosymptomatic' for those children without any other urinary symptoms and 'non-monosymptomatic' for who have concomitant daytime symptoms.

Daytime urinary incontinence

Classification of daytime symptoms is more problematic as there is a great deal of overlap: the ICCS advocates symptom description with reference to incontinence, voiding frequency, voided volume and fluid intake. There are some recognised patient subtypes that are still clinically applicable.

Functional urinary incontinence
Overactive bladder or urge syndrome

This replaces the older term of 'bladder instability' and is probably responsible for more than 80% of the children with non-organic daytime urinary incontinence. The critical feature is that of urgency, but urinary incontinence, increased frequency of micturition and reduced voiding volumes may also be present. The symptoms usually worsen as the day goes on. Patients may have identified triggers such as cold, running water, sports or carbonated/caffeinated drinks, which will induce detrusor contraction and imminent urinary incontinence which may be averted by one of several withholding manoeuvres – classically squatting with the heel of one foot pressed into the perineum – Vincent's curtsey. Most patients will resolve spontaneously with final resolution often precipitated by moving away from home to live independently as young adults. Only 2–3% of the patients are affected in adult life.

Dysfunctional voiding

Dysfunctional voiding occurs when there is a failure to relax the pelvic floor/external sphincter during bladder contraction. This results in a staccato stream with variable urine flow and usually does not result in complete bladder emptying. Girls are almost exclusively affected. UTIs are almost universal and approximately 30% have vesico-ureteric reflux. These patients also often suffer quite severe degrees of constipation and have therefore been labelled dysfunctional elimination syndrome. These patients are believed to represent the severe end of those with the urge syndrome who having relied so heavily on voluntary pelvic floor contraction to prevent incontinence that they are now unable to relax during micturition.

Underactive bladder

Previously referred to as 'lazy bladder,' these patients rely on increased abdominal pressure to void, and do so with an interrupted urinary stream, and are prone to large postvoid residuals and recurrent UTIs. It is believed to result from bladder decompensation in patients with prolonged dysfunctional voiding.

Voiding postponement

Typically these patients are infrequent voiders who defer voiding due to either pleasurable distractions; for example, computer games/television (younger children) or due to some behavioural disturbance or psychological co-morbidity. The patients will often void to completion and may or may not suffer from urgency.

Giggle incontinence

A rare condition principally affecting girls who void to completion when giggling/laughing. These patients typically lack other symptoms. It does not tend to resolve, but patients adjust their lifestyle to enable to avoid provocative situations.

Structural urinary incontinence

There are a number of anatomical abnormalities that may predispose one to urinary incontinence.

Epispadias/exstrophy

A congenital malformation of the lower urinary tract that, if the epispadias extends sufficiently proximally

through to the bladder neck, will result in incontinence. The diagnosis of bladder exstrophy is obvious and often detected antenatally, as is epispadias in a boy. More subtle degrees of epispadias may be missed in a female patient unless the perineum is specifically examined.

Persistent urogenital sinus

This failure of embryological separation of the urethra and vagina may be associated with an incompetent sphincteric mechanism.

Ectopic ureter

In girls with duplex kidneys, the ureter that drains the upper moiety may enter the urinary tract in an ectopic position, which, if below the bladder neck or into the vagina, will result in constant low-flow urinary incontinence. This does not happen in boys as the ectopic ureter always enters the urinary system above the level of the external sphincter.

Bladder outlet obstruction

The most common cause of this is a posterior urethral valve in a boy. Nowadays the majority of boys with valves are detected prenatally, but prior to the advent of antenatal ultrasonography, a third of the patients would present late with urinary incontinence, and a minority still do.

Neuropathic bladder

This may be present in a patient with known neuropathy such as myelomeningocele, or those at high risk of neuropathy such those post surgery for anorectal malformations or pelvic tumours, or in those with a history of spinal trauma. It may also occur in patients with previously undetected neuropathy as in spina bifida occulta, tethered spinal cord, diastematomyelia or sacral agenesis. These patients may present in any number of ways, and their detection is based on a high index of suspicion and appropriate investigation.

Management

The management of children with urinary incontinence depends on the aetiology of their incontinence. For those with a structural cause surgery may be appropriate, and in the case of ectopic ureter, curative. For all other patients the main thrust of treatment is supportive and educational as the majority will resolve spontaneously even without intervention.

Urotherapy

Urotherapy is the general term for all forms of non-surgical, non-pharmacological treatment of lower urinary tract malfunction. It has a large number of components including

1 Education – by providing parents and children with an explanation of how the normal urinary tract functions, the natural history and likely progression of their condition.

2 Voiding education (bladder retraining) – this involves teaching the patient correct voiding posture (mainly applicable to girls). Girls need to sit in a comfortable position with their feet resting on the floor or a step and their hips abducted to open up their perineum/pelvic floor. Voiding needs to occur in a relaxed, unhurried manner. For patients with large postvoid residual urines then initiation of 'double voiding' may be appropriate (voiding is attempted again a few minutes after completion). Girls need to wipe in a backward direction after micturition. Patients need to be taught to avoid postponing micturition or implementing withholding manoeuvres. A programme of regular, timed voids with an initially short interval, that is progressively increased until a normal pattern of five to six voids a day is attained.

3 Lifestyle education – patients are advised regarding the avoidance/management of constipation and appropriate fluid intake.

4 Support – regular and intensive follow-up and support is critical to the success of any urotherapeutic strategy.

More aggressive forms of urotherapy are available and becoming more prevalent [Table 34.2].

Pharmacotherapy

The management of urinary incontinence is a billion dollar industry, with a huge array of medications and appliances available, although many are not licensed for use in children. Bladder emptying is under the control of excitatory parasympathetic fibres that originate in the sacral segments of the spinal cord and act via muscarinic receptors. Currently five different subtypes of muscarinic

Table 34.2 Specialised urotherapies available

- Pelvic floor training by physiotherapist
- Biofeedback, for example, pad and bell bedwetting alarm
- Electrical stimulation (transcutaneous or with implanted electrodes)
- Intermittent catheterisation

receptors (M1 to M5) have been identified. In the bladder, as in most tissues, there is a heterogeneous population of receptors with a predominance of the M2 subtype
and a smaller population of M3 receptors (ratio of 3:1).
Despite this, it is the M3 receptors that are primarily and
directly responsible for bladder contraction. M2 receptor
stimulation indirectly facilitates bladder contraction by
inhibiting sympathetic-mediated detrusor relaxation.
Most drug therapies are directed at reducing detrusor
overactivity with a number of potential pharmacological
targets [Table 34.3].

Table 34.3 New potential drugs for urinary incontinence

- Muscarinic receptor antagonists (oral Oxybutinin,
  Tolterodine, Trospium chloride, Solifenacin, Darifenacin)
- Vanilloid receptor antagonists (intravesical,
  e.g., Capsaicin, Resiniferatoxin)
- Botulinum toxin (injected into detrusor muscle
  endoscopically)

Key Points

- Wetting is common and stressful but rarely needs surgery.
- Clinical assessment aims to identify the surgical causes
  needing referral.
- The mainstay of treatment for functional wetting is
  education, bladder training, laxatives and anticholinergics.

Further reading

Kaefer M (2006) Disorders of bladder function. In: Grosfeld
    JL, O'Neill JA Jr., Fonkalsrud EW, Coran AG (eds) *Pediatric
    Surgery*, 6th Edn. Mosby Elsevier, Philadelphia,
    pp. 1805–1816.
Swithinbank LV, Brookes ST, Shepherd AM, Abrams P (1998)
    The natural history of urinary symptoms during adoles-
    cence. *BJU* **81**(Suppl. **3**): 90–93.

35

The Child with Haematuria

Case 1

A recently circumcised baby is noted to have a spot of blood on the tip of the penis after micturition.
Q 1.1 What is the likely problem?
Q 1.2 How is it treated or prevented?

Case 2

'Red water' is passed after a 3-year old falls off a chair onto the side of a toy box. Physical examination reveals a fullness in the upper abdomen on the left.
Q 2.1 What is the differential diagnosis?
Q 2.2 What is your plan of management?

Macroscopic haematuria is very uncommon in children with a reported incidence of less than 0.2%. It usually causes such alarm that the child is brought early for medical attention. Confirmation of the presence of red blood cells should be obtained, because haemoglobinuria, ingested dyes and plant pigments, occasionally can be misleading. Because of the potential causes, frank haematuria should be investigated promptly. Unfortunately, haematuria has often ceased by the time the child is examined, and the decision to investigate the child may be based solely on the observations of the parents or colleagues.

Microscopic haematuria has been detected in 0.5–1.6% of asymptomatic school children, and its presence should be confirmed on repeat testing. Isolated microscopic haematuria persists beyond 6 months in less than 30% of the patients.

History, physical examination and urine microscopy will yield a diagnosis in majority of the patients. The causes are many, and in some the diagnosis is readily made [Table 35.1]. Urine infection accounts for 50% of cases, perineal irritation (10%), trauma (7%), acute nephritis (4%) with stones, coagulopathy and tumours among the other rare causative factors. Twenty-five per cent of renal tumours, potentially the most worrisome cause, present with haematuria, but account for less than 0.7% of all cases of frank haematuria in children. There are usually other signs such as a palpable mass [Table 35.1].

Hydronephrosis and other malformations of the upper urinary tract often present with haematuria. It is seldom

Table 35.1 Plan of investigation of a patient with haematuria

1 Cause obvious or readily determined	
Renal mass	Overt glomerulonephritis
Bleeding disorders	Urinary tract infection
Hereditary haematuria	Meatal ulcer

2 Cause apparent on simple radiological investigation	
(a) Plain film	Urinary calculi
(b) Renal ultrasound	Hydronephrosis and hydroureter
	Cystic or malformed kidneys
(c) MCU	Vesico-ureteric reflux
	Vesical diverticulum
	Urethral polyp

3 Cause obscure without resort to more extensive investigation	
(a) Endoscopy	Urethral membrane
	Vesical diverticulum
	Vascular anomalies
(b) Retrograde pyelography	Small benign neoplasms of ureter or pelvis
(c) Renal biopsy	Atypical nephritis
(d) Selective renal arteriography	Vascular anomaly

Jones' Clinical Paediatric Surgery, 6th edition. By Hutson, O'Brien, Woodward and Beasley. Published 2008 by Blackwell Publishing, ISBN: 978-1-4051-6267-8.

the sole presenting feature, and the clinical findings, examination of the urine and renal ultrasound or nuclear scan, usually make a diagnosis possible.

History

Frequency, dysuria, abdominal pains and fever point to a urinary tract infection: and injuries severe enough to damage the kidneys, ureter or lower urinary tract nearly always will present with an obvious history of trauma.

A history of a recent sore throat or skin lesions suggestive of streptococcal infection will be present in most of those with glomerulonephritis.

Pain on micturition and a few drops of blood at the end suggest urethral abnormality or meatal ulcer.

Severe colicky loin pain radiating to the groin and preceding the haematuria is very suggestive of ureteric colic associated with the passage of a renal calculus.

A detailed family history will yield information suggestive of familial causes such as an inherited coagulopathy or an association with familial deafness (Alport's disease).

A history of frank haematuria occurring at the end of micturition in adolescent boys is consistent with a diagnosis of posterior urethritis.

Clinical examination

Physical examination is rarely helpful in determining the cause of haematuria. In boys who have been circumcised recently, the first thing to look for is a meatal ulcer. In these boys, appropriate local measures will prevent unnecessary investigation. Occasionally, haematuria is seen in boys with phimosis after attempted forceful retraction of the foreskin. The abdomen should be palpated for the presence of a renal mass and the skin should be examined to look for a rash suggestive of either systemic lupus erythematosis or Henoch-Schönlein purpura.

Hypertension may point to chronic glomerulonephritis, and a palpable mass in the loin will focus attention on three conditions – hydronephrosis, Wilms' tumour and neuroblastoma – which are considered in greater detail in Chapter 25.

Investigations

Microscopy and culture of a midstream or catheter specimen of urine is the basis of diagnosis. Granular and cellular casts or persistent proteinuria in addition to 'Glomerular' red cells, will lead to the diagnosis of glomerulonephritis, while pyuria and bacteriuria indicate infection as the cause of bleeding.

Phase contrast microscopy may show crenated and dysmorphic red cells to distinguish atypical focal glomerular lesions from lesions elsewhere in the urinary tract, which tend to give rise to more uniform red cell patterns.

Sterile pyuria accompanied by haematuria raises the possibility of a tuberculous infection.

If MSU and physical examination do not reveal the cause of haematuria more detailed investigation is warranted including blood tests for U+E, creatinine, pH, albumin, ASOT, C3, C4, immunoglobilins, ANF, anti-DNA antibodies, FBC and clotting factors and urine tests for protein–creatinine ratio and calcium–creatinine ratio.

Plain radiographs

In selected patients, a plain x-ray may reveal a calculus in the urinary tract or a renal soft tissue mass.

Renal ultrasonography

Except in children with meatal stenosis or readily demonstrable glomerulonephritis, a renal ultrasound scan is necessary in every case. Ultrasonography may reveal a urinary calculus, a hydronephrotic kidney or a renal mass, which may be either a tumour or an inflammatory condition of the kidney – xanthogranulomatous pyelonephritis. CT scan and radioisotope studies will help to differentiate the two.

Micturating cystourethrogram

A micturating cystourethrogram (MCU) will exclude vesical or urethral diverticula or urethral polyps. A plain x-ray prior to the MCU may show a calculus.

Endoscopy

In some patients with haematuria all investigations so far are normal. Cystoscopy may be undertaken next, preferably while haematuria is present, although this may be difficult in children, for bleeding is often of short duration. Occasionally cystoscopy reveals a vesical cause, for example, a small haemangioma or a diverticulum not shown in an MCU or a urethal cause, for example, urethral membrane or posterior urethritis.

Renal biopsy

Most children with 'idiopathic' or 'essential' haematuria have histological evidence of a focal type of glomerulonephritis in which haematuria is precipitated by physical effort or by an intercurrent infection. Biopsy is not required routinely, but does have a place when haematuria is persistent or severe and all other investigations have not yielded a diagnosis. Children with persistent microscopic haematuria, proteinuria, hypertension or a family history of renal disease may warrant renal biopsy.

Arteriography/MRI

When haematuria is too persistent and severe to be explained by atypical focal glomerulonephritis, and the renal ultrasound, MCU, cystoscopy and renal biopsy are all normal, renal arteriography or MRI may be needed occasionally to exclude the exceptionally rare vascular anomalies of the renal or ureteric vessels. This may also facilitate therapeutic intervention for conditions such as A–V fistulae.

Treatment

Haematuria is a symptom that leads to a variety of diagnoses, and the treatment of these conditions depends on the diagnosis (see related chapters).

Key Points
- Haematuria in children is rare but causes parental alarm.
- Histology is important to determine cause.
- Renal ultrasonography is essential to exclude serious renal lesions (stone, obstruction, tumour, inflammation).

Further reading

Milford DV, Robson AM (2003) The child with abnormal urinalysis, haematuria and/or proteinuria. In: Webb N, Postlethwaite R (eds) *Clinical Paediatric Nephrology*. Oxford University Press, Oxford, pp. 1–28.

Pan CG (2006) Evaluation of gross hematuria. *Pediatr Clin North Am* **53**(3): 401–412.

Trauma

36 Trauma in Childhood

Case 1

A 10-year-old boy is brought to the emergency department 35 min after being knocked off his bicycle at an intersection. Eye witnesses saw the child bounce off the car onto the road. The boy was unconscious on arrival, cyanosed and shocked.

Q 1.1 What are the priorities in initial assessment and management?

Q 1.2 What is a secondary survey?

Q 1.3 Could there be a simple explanation for the loss of consciousness?

Case 2

Ian is a 4-year-old who fell over in the backyard (no adult witnesses); he has a jagged puncture wound in the palm of his right hand.

Q 2.1 How would a deep visceral (nerve, tendon, arterial) injury be excluded?

Q 2.2 What management is required to prevent anaerobic infection?

Trauma is the commonest cause of death in the paediatric population over 1 year of age. (In the age group of less than 1 year, congenital abnormalities, prematurity and SIDS are the commonest causes.)

The 'trimodal distribution' of trauma death was first described in 1983:

1 Immediate (minutes): major vascular or neurological insult.

2 Early hours ('golden hour'; 1–2 h post injury): 35% of deaths, secondary to brain, abdominal or chest injury.

3 Late (days to weeks): 15% of deaths, from brain death, multiorgan failure and/or overwhelming sepsis.

The majority of the immediate deaths are not remediable to medical intervention and prevention of these injuries affords the best opportunity to reduce this mortality. There has been a dramatic reduction in trauma mortality over the last decade particularly due to improvements in car safety and restraints. Many of the early deaths are potentially preventable with airway, ventilation and circulation intervention. This produced the concept of the 'golden hour' where there is the opportunity to prevent early deaths with immediate and appropriate resuscitation, that is, primary survey A, B, C, D.

It is important to remember that whilst trauma is the commonest cause for deaths in childhood, the majority of paediatric trauma results only in minor injury, but may be associated with long-term morbidity that stretches into adulthood; here again injury prevention is the best strategy.

Injury prevention

There are three ways to lessen or prevent childhood injury

1 Education of parents and children about potential accident situations.

2 Minimisation of injury in the actual accident, for example, use of car restraints or cycling helmets.

3 Limitations of injuries sustained after the accident, for example, by first aid techniques. This requires an effective transport system, which allows early, accurate assessment of injuries by trained personnel and rapid resuscitation prior to transport to an appropriate institution.

Mechanism of injury

In paediatrics it is particularly important to obtain a detailed history of the accident in order to ascertain the likely injuries and particularly if non-accidental injury is

Jones' Clinical Paediatric Surgery, 6th edition. By Hutson, O'Brien, Woodward and Beasley. Published 2008 by Blackwell Publishing, ISBN: 978-1-4051-6267-8.

to be considered. Often, it is the ambulance personnel who provide valuable information relating to the time and mechanism of the accident.

Adult studies have supported that particular mechanisms may be associated with major trauma:
- prolonged extraction time (>20 min);
- motor vehicle accidents: at high speed (>60 km/h);
- ejection from the vehicle.

These factors predict that a child may have a major, but as-yet undetected injury, and this must be taken into account during assessment.

The top causes of paediatric minor trauma are illustrated in Table 36.1.

Table 36.1 The causes of accidents in children

Accident	Percentage
Falls	62
Bicycle accidents	12
Traffic accidents as pedestrians	9
Traffic accidents as passenger of motor vehicle	7
Other	10

Initial assessment and management

In assessing the injured child, many steps are accomplished simultaneously; for example, while conducting a rapid assessment of a patient's respiratory, circulatory and neurological status, the history and the events relating to the injury are obtained.

It is particularly important when considering the paediatric population to nurse the child if possible with a primary carer present. Ensure that you explain in simple language to the child what you are doing. Always provide adequate analgesia, and if possible, for an alert child, use distraction therapy and involve the carers as this will be an extremely frightening and anxiety-provoking situation for the child and family.

Establishing priorities

The Early Management of Severe Trauma course (instituted by the Royal Australasian College of Surgeons) has developed a set of priorities, which apply to adults and children.

In summary, patient management consists of a rapid primary survey and resuscitation of vital functions, followed by a more detailed secondary assessment; then stabilisation and transfer to definitive care centre.

The primary survey: 'A, B, C's'

During the primary survey, life-threatening conditions are identified and treatment instigated immediately:
1 A – Airway maintenance with cervical spine control.
2 B – Breathing and ventilation.
3 C – Circulation with haemorrhage control.
4 D – Disability: neurological status. Do not forget the glucose.

Extensive discussion of paediatric trauma resuscitation is beyond the scope of this book, but guidelines exist in Advanced Paediatric Life Support (APLS) and Advanced Trauma Life Support (ATLS) (see recommended reading).

During the A, B, C assessment, once problems are identified, immediate intervention is taken.

Airway
- Check that the child's airway is open whilst protecting the C-spine.
- Ensure that an infant is in a neutral position and not flexed due to the large occiput.
- A jaw thrust should be used to open the airway.
- Clear the airway with gentle suction under direct vision.
- An oropharyngeal airway may be required to maintain airway if necessary.

Breathing
- Assess the effort, efficacy, effect of breathing.
- Apply oxygen 10 L/min.
- Breathing adjuncts as necessary – bag and mask-endotracheal intubation.
- Monitor saturations/respiratory rate.
- Consider orogastric tube to prevent gastric dilatation.

Circulation
- Assess-heart rate/blood pressure/capillary refill/mental status.
- Establish two large bore intravenous cannulae rapidly.
- Intraosseous needle insertion if unable to gain access in 60 s.
- If circulation inadequate – 20 mL/kg normal saline bolus.
- Ongoing circulatory support – if third bolus is required, use O-negative blood.
- Ensure cross-matched sample sent early.
- Ensure platelets and FFP and cryoprecipitate available if on-going circulatory support required.
- All fluids should be warmed.
- Arrange early surgical consult.

- Consider hidden sources of bleeding: head, chest, abdominal, pelvis and femur.
- Establish haemorrhage control.

Children will compensate for hypovolaemic shock with tachycardia and vasoconstriction. Hypotension will not occur until more than 30% of circulatory volume is lost. Hypotension is a preterminal sign in paediatrics.

Note: Tachycardia may be a response to fear and pain or a normal anxiety response.

Disability

Assess mental state using the AVPU or the paediatric Glasgow coma score
- AVPU
  - A Alert child
  - V Responds to voice
  - P Response to pain (equivalent to GCS < 8)
  - U Unconscious
- Glasgow Coma Scale [Table 36.2]. Paediatric-specific charts
  - Eye-opening
  - Verbal response
  - Motor response
- Documentation of pupillary response and size
- Do not forget the glucose.
- All children undergoing resuscitation should have a glucose level checked and be provided with normal maintenance fluids of dextrose and saline.

Trauma Radiology
- CXR
- C-Spine lateral
- Pelvis – if the child is awake, orientated with no other distracting injuries and there is no clinical suspicion of a pelvic fracture then this x-ray may be omitted.

Monitoring
- Ensure continuous monitoring of all parameters. If any changes occur the primary survey should be repeated.

Secondary survey

The secondary survey begins after the primary survey (A, B, C) has been completed, and the resuscitation phase (management of other life-threatening conditions) has begun. It is a comprehensive examination top-to-toe and front-to-back (including log roll) examining all orifices, with full documentation of all injuries with instigation of first aid management. Ensure that you explain to the child and carers what you about to do and keep the child warm during exposure.

In paediatrics a rectal and vaginal examination are not routine and should only be performed once if deemed necessary by the appropriate specialist.

Analgesia
For all children involved in trauma it is likely be extremely anxiety-provoking experience and they should be nursed:
- With parents or primary carer in attendance to provide support.
- In a paediatric-focused environment – toys and distractions provided.
- Provided with adequate analgesia
  - for example, morphine IV 0.1 mg /kg.

Superficial soft tissue injuries

The basic management principles involve
- Providing analgesia
- Cleaning the wound
- Inspection and assessment
- Wound closure
- Dressing

The extent and severity of soft tissue injuries tend to be underestimated. It is important to take into consideration the mechanism of injury, that is, high velocity/penetrating/ is there a high risk of contamination?

The initial first aid management of any wound is irrigation and cleaning – sterile water will suffice.

Table 36.2 Glasgow coma scale (Paediatric) (see also Table 37.3)

Score	Eye opening	Verbal	or	Grimace response	Motor response
1	None	None			
2	To pain	Occasional whimper/moan		Mild to pain	Extension to pain
3	To voice	Inappropriate cry		Vigorous to pain	Flexes to pain
4	Spontaneous	Decreased verbal/irritable cry		Less than usual face movement	Withdraws
5		Alert babbles/words as normal		Spontaneous face movement	Localises pain
6					Obeys commands

For the injury itself, a full neurovascular assessment must be performed assessing movement, perfusion and sensation of all structures distal to the wound. The wound itself must be examined. In the paediatric population, it may be difficult to fully assess a wound without a general anaesthetic. However, it may be possible with the use of analgesic and sedative adjuncts to inspect a wound and avoid an unnecessary anaesthetic, that is, ALA (adrenaline/lignocaine/amethocaine), which is topical ointment when locally applied to a wound may have equal efficacy as Lignocaine infiltration, use of a sedative agent such as inhalation nitrous oxide or intravenous or intramuscular Ketamine. These agents must be given in a controlled environment by senior medical staff only.

Always involve senior colleagues or plastic surgeons in the assessment and management of any wound where
- There is neurovascular compromise.
- It is considered too large to close under local anaesthetic.
- A large degree of contamination has occurred – gravel or dirt can leave a 'tattoo' if not properly removed with scrubbing.
- There is involvement of the face or lip across the vermillion border and where a good cosmetic result is necessary.

These patients are best managed having their wounds surgically assessed, cleaned and closed under an anaesthetic.

Any wound where there is a risk of retained glass should have a soft tissue x-ray performed.

Wound closure

Superficial wounds can be cleaned and managed with a simple dressing. Simple small lacerations that are not under tension can be closed with either – a tissue adhesive 'Dermabond glue' or adhesive strips 'steristrips'. Other wounds will require surgical closure with sutures.

Specific injuries
The tongue
Despite initially vigorous bleeding and major deformity of the tongue contour, suture of the tongue is rarely needed. Most lacerations should be left to heal and remodel naturally. Infection of intraoral lacerations is rare. Consider referral to specialist for review if there is a full thickness injury or if there is a large flap.

The straddle injury
A slip on to the edge of the bath, bicycle bars or a fence may cause injury to the perineum. Where adequate assessment is not possible in the emergency room, children should be admitted for examination and definitive management under anaesthesia. In females, a straddle injury often causes a tear in the posterior fourchette, often with significant bleeding; minor splits do not require sutures. Injuries through the hymen need careful repair. Where a laceration has penetrated into the rectum, a colostomy for faecal diversion is required.

In boys, a straddle injury may tear the bulbar urethra and cause extravasation of urine into the scrotum and lower abdominal wall. A urethrogram demonstrates leakage of contrast and the need for catheter drainage of urine or primary urethral repair.

Antibiotics

The most important factor in the prevention of infection is in the use of primary first aid and cleaning and if necessary surgical debridement of extensive wounds. Antibiotics should be used when wounds are contaminated, but antibiotics are ineffective in the presence of dead tissue or foreign matter, and should never be relied upon to prevent infection in contaminated wounds.

Tetanus

Successful prophylaxis against clostridial infections rests upon the triad of: (1) immunisation; (2) antibiotics and (3) adequate surgical cleansing of wounds: removal of dead tissue, foreign material and blood clot.

Active immunisation
Tetanus immunisation should be part of routine childhood immunisation. Primary immunisation of infants is achieved with three doses of triple antigen (diphtheria, tetanus, pertussis) and booster doses at 4 and 15 years.

The new vaccination schedule recommends that the 1-yearly tetanus booster is no longer required up until the age of 50 years, provided the primary series of three vaccinations plus two boosters has been given.

It is important to be aware of the current schedule of childhood immunisations.

Passive immunisation
Tetanus immunoglobulin is available for the passive protection of individuals who have sustained a tetanus-prone wound, and those who have received less than three doses of tetanus vaccination.

Tetanus-prone wounds

Types of wounds likely to favour the growth of tetanus organisms include
- Compound fractures.
- Deep penetrating wounds.
- Wounds containing foreign bodies (especially wood splinters).
- Wounds complicated by pyogenic infections.
- Wounds with extensive tissue damage (e.g. contusions or burns).
- Any wound obviously contaminated with soil, dust or horse manure (especially if topical disinfection is delayed more than 4 h).
- Re-implantation of an avulsed tooth is also a tetanus-prone event, as minimal washing and cleaning of the tooth is conducted to increase the likelihood of successful re-implantation.

Wounds must be cleaned, disinfected and treated surgically, if appropriate.

Child abuse and neglect (Box 36.1)

Whenever an injured child attends for treatment, clinicians have a duty of care to exclude child abuse.

Incidence

The incidence of intentional injury is difficult to determine, but it is probably far higher than is generally realised, and has been estimated to be from 0.3% to 3.0% of all injuries in childhood. Infants and children less than 3 years of age are particularly vulnerable.

Clinical features

Certain clinical signs and other features may raise the index of suspicion of abuse and point to the need for a closer examination of the psychosocial climate of the patient and family. The social and psychiatric aspects are often more important than the trauma itself, but lie outside the scope of this book.

Some key features are as follows.

History
- The history is variable but may be quite reasonable and acceptable
- Mechanism is not in keeping with the child's developmental age
- Story is inconsistent between the care givers/historians
- The version may change
- Child may implicate an adult

Examination
- The injuries present do not fit the history given of the 'accident'
- Pattern of bruising unlikely accidental on abdominal wall/scapula area
- Linear bruises
- Torn frenulum
- Bite marks consistent with adult-sized-teeth
- Retinal haemorrhages
- Fractures of different ages
- Rib fractures

Investigation

Consider coagulation studies and a full blood count.

It is important to x-ray all bones where a clinical fracture is suspected. Investigations into suspected child abuse will involve a bone scan. A bone scan will identify 'hot spots' which may suggest underlying fractures. In children less than 1 year old, a skull x-ray should be taken because the bone scan may be unreliable in determining a skull fracture. Often a full skeletal survey will also be performed.

Diagnosis

This depends to a large degree on an awareness of the possibility that serious injuries in young children may not be accidental. Thus, it is important that where there is some suspicion of non-accidental injury, the child is admitted to hospital for assessment by the child protection unit.

Box 36.1 Observations suggestive of child abuse

1 Bizarre scars, scabs, weals, circumferential abrasions on the limbs and hemispherical bite marks.
2 Multiple retinal haemorrhages.
3 Periosteal thickening of long bones in unusual areas.
4 Symmetrical burns or scalds in unusual areas.
5 Multiple insect bites and/or infestations; for example, pediculosis.
6 Abnormal behaviour of the child in hospital; for example, withdrawal or stark terror alternating with effusive affection.
7 An abnormal attitude of the parents to the injury. This varies considerably; for example, lack of affect, indifference, panic, guilt or belligerence. Their reactions may conceal an appeal for help.
8 An apparently unrelated developmental abnormality: handicaps, both physical and neurological, that make the child 'different' can be associated with them becoming objects of abuse.

Table 36.3 Champion Trauma Score

Score	Respiratory rate (breaths/min)	Respiratory effort	Systolic BP (mm Hg)	Capillary return(s)	Glasgow coma scale
5	–	–	–	–	14–15
4	10–24	–	>90	–	11–13
3	25–35	–	70–89	–	8–10
2	>35	–	50–69	<2	5–7
1	<10	Normal	<50	>2	3–4
0	None	Shallow/retraction	No pulse	Nil	–

Table 36.4 Paediatric Trauma Score

Score	Body weight	Airway	Systolic BP (mm Hg)	CNS	Skeleton	Skin
+2	>20	Normal	>90	Awake	None	None
+1	10–20	Controlled	50–90	Obtunded/LOC	Closed fracture	Minor wound
−1	<10	Unmaintainable	<50	Coma/decerebrate	Open/multiple fracture	Major/penetrating

Management

The full management and treatment of non-accidental injury is beyond the scope of this text. The basic plan of management is to ensure the diagnosis and appropriate treatment of the child's injuries. Ensure that the child is managed in a place of safety and comfort. Always ensure early involvement of senior colleagues and the local government child protection unit.

Trauma scores and injury severity scores

There are various scoring systems, which exist to allow the quantification of the magnitude of single or multiple injuries, for example, Champion Trauma Score and Paediatric Trauma Score. These scores can be a useful predictor of outcome and allow comparison of groups of trauma patients.

Injury severity score

The Injury Severity Score (ISS) is based on the extent of tissue injury, which changes little following the initial insult. The ISS indicates increasing severity of injury on a scale from 0 to 75. Severe injury is defined by an ISS greater than 15.

Champion trauma score

To quantify the severity of trauma of different types, a numerical value is assigned to five physiological parameters: systolic blood pressure, respiratory rate, respiratory effort, capillary refill and GCS. The sum of the assigned values is the trauma score. On a 0–16 range (where 16 is the least injured) [Table 36.3], a trauma score less than 13 is an indication for transfer to a major trauma centre.

Paediatric trauma score

This quantifies the severity of multiple injuries in children to enable speedy triage and dispatch to an appropriate institution. It measures six different parameters: patient weight, patency of the airways, systolic blood pressure, neurological state, cutaneous wounds and the extent of bony injury. Each parameter is scored −1, 1 or 2, with low scores indicating severe trauma [Table 36.4].

There are three categories of mortality risk: Paediatric Trauma Score (PTS) greater than eight should have no mortality; PTS 8–0 has increasing mortality and PTS less than 0 has 100% mortality.

Key Points

- Systematic response to trauma (primary survey A,B,C,D; resuscitation, secondary survey, definitive treatment) saves lives.
- Airway, breathing and circulation are paramount for survival.
- Secondary survey needs comprehensive top-to-toe and front-to-back examination.
- Penetrating wounds need examination under anaesthesia (LA/GA) to exclude important visceral injuries.
- Surgical debridement (removal of dead tissue, foreign bodies and blood clot) is essential to prevent anaerobic infection.

Further reading

Lukish JR, Eichelberger MR (2006) Accident victims and their emerging management. In: Grosfeld JL, O'Neill JA Jr., Fonkalsrud EW, Coran AG (eds) *Pediatric Surgery*, 6th Edn. Mosby Elsevier, Philadelphia, pp. 265–274.

APLS Advanced paediatric life support the practical approach, 4th Edn. 2004 December, Blackwell Publishing.

ATLS Advanced Trauma Support/EMST Emergency Management of Severe Trauma, 7th Edn. Published by American College of Surgeons.

37   Head Injuries

Case 1

An anxious mother brings her 6-year-old son to the emergency department after he fell off the fence.
Q 1.1 Which children should be referred to the emergency department after a head injury?
Q 1.2 Which children should have a CT scan after a head injury?

Case 2

The air ambulance brings a 4-year-old boy who was hit by a car at 70 km/h when he ran on to a busy street. He has been unconscious since the accident (20 min).
Q 2.1 What are the principles of management of a child with a severe head injury?

Case 3

A 4-year-old child falls out of a tree 2 m to the ground, striking his head. There is a 5 min loss of consciousness. There is a boggy scalp haematoma on the left side and the child is pale, drowsy and confused with a thready, rapid pulse, complaining of headache and has a sluggish dilated left pupil and right-sided limb weakness.
Q 3.1 You are the medical officer who receives the child. What is your diagnosis?
Q 3.2 What urgency do you place on the child?
Q 3.3 What management do you propose?

Case 4

A 6-month-old baby presents with a history of falling out of a pram. Skull x-rays show a large fracture.
Q 4.1 What would lead you to suspect that a head injury was non-accidental?

Case 5

A 6-year-old boy falls over at school, hitting his head on concrete. He cannot remember the accident.
Q 5.1 What is concussion?

Traumatic brain injuries (TBI) are the leading cause of morbidity and mortality in children in the developed world. Head injuries account for one of the most frequent causes of emergency department admissions. Most children recover spontaneously but about 10% of children suffer from sequelae such as changes in behaviour, impaired intellectual performance and post-traumatic epilepsy. Prompt resuscitation to restore adequate circulating volume, oxygenation and blood pressure is necessary to prevent secondary brain injury. Careful and frequent neurological examination along with appropriate neuroimaging is vital if the many reversible aspects of head injury are to be treated and the outcome optimised.

Determinants of injury

The pattern of head injuries in childhood is similar to that in adults, but there are some important differences related to the nature of the injury and the physical characteristics of the child's skull and brain.

The most frequent causes of injury are accidents in the home including falls, playground injuries, sporting accidents, pedestrian or bicycle related injuries, motor vehicle accidents and non-accidental injuries (NAI). NAI resulting from child abuse occur mostly in the 0–4 years age group and is the commonest cause of severe head injury in this age group.

The vault of the skull in children is thin and pliable and capable of much greater deformation than in adults. The increased elasticity permits more energy to be absorbed by the skull. This dampens the acceleration or deceleration of

Jones' Clinical Paediatric Surgery, 6th edition. By Hutson, O'Brien, Woodward and Beasley. Published 2008 by Blackwell Publishing, ISBN: 978-1-4051-6267-8.

the head after impact and reduces the concussive effects. Children can tolerate blows of considerable severity without immediate loss of consciousness. The increased skull elasticity also causes local indentation resulting in Pond's depressed fracture. A child's skull can sustain considerable distortion without fracture, but when the limit is reached, the fracture that results is often extensive and frequently of the 'bursting' type. The skull sutures do not close until the fourth year, so that marked diastasis of the sutures may follow bursting injuries.

At the point of maximal distortion a fracture line may lacerate the underlying dura, pushing brain tissue out through the fracture. In the subsequent days and weeks the pulsations of the underlying brain may cause this brain herniation through the skull defect to progressively enlarge [Fig. 37.1] resulting in further widening of the fracture. This will produce what is called a growing fracture of childhood, which requires operative repair.

Children more frequently present with diffuse injury and cerebral swelling with resultant intracranial hypertension compared to adults. Children as a group survive TBI more often than adults and tend to have better functional outcomes than adults. This is believed to be due to the plasticity of the paediatric brain.

Mechanisms of brain injury

Sudden acceleration/decceleration of the head causes shearing of axons which constitute white matter tracts.

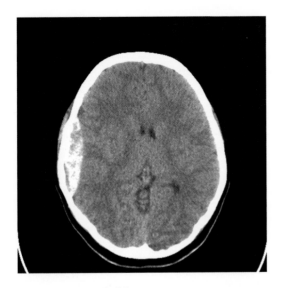

Figure 37.1 Growing skull fracture.

This results in diffuse parenchymal and vascular injuries. The clinical manifestation of this insult can vary from a transient loss of conciousness, called concussion, to profound and persisitent neurological deficits or death resulting from diffuse axonal injury (DAI).

Direct impact against the calvarium and brain causes coup injuries such as parenchymal petechiae, contusions, intraparenchymal haematomas and extra-axial haematomas such as extradural and subdural haematomas. Sometimes the viscoelastic brain rebounds within its rigid confines and results in contrecoup injuries on the side opposite the impact.

Penetrating injuries to the brain can produce cerebral lacerations and damage to the cerebral vessels.

Pathophysiology of TBI

All of the aforementioned brain injuries constitute primary brain injury. Subsequent to the primary insult, a cascade of biochemical and vascular events, collectively called secondary brain injury, is set into motion, which results in further compromise of the cerebral blood flow producing cerebral ischaemia and cytotoxic damage. These occur due to cerebral oedema, disturbed cerebral autoregulation, release of excito-toxic neurotransmitters and calcium entry into cells causing cell death. To date no effective pharmacological intervention has been successful in preventing or mitigating the effects of secondary injury. However secondary insults such as raised intracranial pressure from hydrocephalus, haematomas, hyperthermia, dyselectrolytaemia, hyperglycaemia, hypotension, hypoxia and seizures should be anticipated and treated promptly and aggressively to improve the outcome of head injuries.

General management of head injury

Recently NICE (National Institute of Clinical Excellence) in the UK has set out guidelines to identify those patients who need referral to the emergency department in a hospital [Table 37.1]. The principles of management of a child with a head injury include the fundamentals of trauma resuscitation with restoration of adequate airway, oxygenation and circulation being of the utmost importance [Table 37.2]. Following this, the establishment of the level of consciousness according to the Glasgow Coma Scale (GCS) [Table 37.3] and identification of focal neurological deficits is carried out. In certain cases, a CT scan of the head is required [Table 37.4]. Some types of head injury raise suspicion of child abuse [Table 37.5].

Table 37.1 Indications for referral to hospital after head injury in children

1 GCS < 15 at any time since the head injury
2 Any loss of consciousness as a result of injury
3 Any focal neurological deficit
4 Any seizure since the injury
5 Persistent headache since injury
6 Any suspicion of a skull fracture or penetrating head injury
7 CSF leak from ear or nose
8 Multiple injuries in association with head injury
9 Suspicion of non-accidental injury or poor social circumstances
10 Amnesia for events before or after the injury

Characteristic injuries

Skull fractures
Linear skull fracture
Linear fracture results from low-energy blunt trauma over a wide surface area of the skull. It runs through the entire thickness of the bone and, by itself, is of little significance except when it runs through a vascular channel, venous sinus groove or a suture. In these situations, it may cause epidural haematoma, venous sinus thrombosis and occlusion, and sutural diastasis, respectively.

Depressed fractures
Depressed skull fractures result from a high-energy direct blow to a small surface area of the skull with a blunt object such as a golf club. A depressed fracture may be open or closed [Fig. 37.2]. Open fractures have either an overlying skin laceration or the fracture runs through the

Table 37.2 Principles of management of a child with a severe head injury

1 Airway, breathing, circulation must be secured
2 Adequate resuscitation
3 Accurate neurological assessment
4 Investigation with CT scan
5 Prevention of secondary brain injury
   • Correction of hypoxia and hypercapnoea with intubation
   • Initial hyperventilation to reduce intracranial pressure
   • Replacement of blood volume to maintain adequate cerebral perfusion pressure
   • Urgent surgery to remove mass lesions
   • Anticonvulsants, antipyrexial treatment and antibiotics for compound injury
   • Intracranial pressure monitoring and continued ventilation and sedation in an intensive care unit
   • Vigorous control of intracranial pressure with sedation, paralysis, CSF drainage, decompressive craniectomy

Table 37.3 Glasgow Coma Scale (paediatric)

Score	Eye opening	Verbal response	or	grimace response	Motor response
1	None	None			
2	To pain	Occasional whimper/moan		Mild to pain	Extension to pain
3	To voice	Inappropriate cry		Vigorous to pain	Flexes to pain
4	Spontaneous	Decreased verbal/irritable cry		Less than usual face movement	Withdraws
5		Alert babbles/words as normal		Spontaneous face movement	Localises pain
6					Obeys commands

Note: The paediatric version of the Glasgow Coma Scale is scored between 3 and 15 with 3 being the worst and 15 being the best. It is composed of 3 parameters: best eye response, best verbal or grimace response, best motor response as described.

Table 37.4 Indications for CT scan after head injury

- GCS < 13 at any point since injury
- Suspected open or depressed skull fracture
- Any sign of basal skull fracture (haemotympanum, panda eyes, Battle's sign, CSF otorrhoea)
- Post-traumatic seizure
- Focal neurological deficit
- More than one episode of vomiting
- Amnesia for greater than 30 min of events before impact. Assessment of amnesia not possible in children <5 years old

Table 37.5 Indications of suspected non-accidental head injury in a child

Suspicious, inconsistent story

History of previous injuries

Multiple cutaneous bruises of different ages

Bilateral retinal haemorrhages

Acute subdural haemorrhage and brain swelling on CT scan

Chronic subdural haemorrhage

Bilateral skull fractures

Old fractures of long bones and ribs

Evidence of malnourishment

Subdued behaviour

Fear

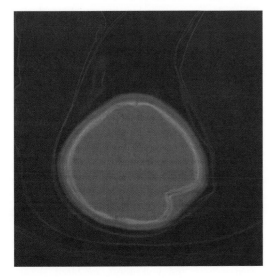

Figure 37.2 Depressed fracture of the skull.

paranasal sinuses and the middle ear structures, resulting in communication between the external environment and the cranial cavity. Open fractures may be clean or contaminated. The indications for surgery are cosmesis, underlying intracranial haematoma requiring evacuation, suspicion of a dural breach with an open fracture or a dirty contaminated wound.

Basilar skull fracture

A basilar fracture is a linear fracture at the base of the skull. A common type of basilar fracture is the temporal fracture.

Temporal bone fracture is encountered in 75% of all skull base fractures. The two main subtypes of temporal fractures are longitudinal and transverse, classified according to the orientation of the fracture line in relation to the direction of the petrous temporal bone. Longitudinal fracture is the more common of the two subtypes (70–90%) and usually causes a haemotympanum with conductive deafness. Transverse fractures are more commonly implicated in seventh nerve palsies and sensorineural deafness.

Intracranial haemorrhage

Several types of intracranial haemorrhages can occur, including the following.

Epidural hematoma

Epidural haematomas are more common in teenagers than young children [Fig. 37.3]. These occur due to a direct blow to the skull with associated laceration of the dural arteries or veins (often by fractured bones) and sometimes by diploic veins in the skull's marrow. More often, a tear in the middle meningeal artery causes this type of haematoma. When haematoma occurs from laceration of an artery, blood collection can cause rapid neurologic deterioration.

Subdural hematoma

Acute subdural haematoma tends to occur in patients with injuries to the cortical veins or pial arteries in severe head injury usually following acceleration/deceleration. The mortality rate is high due to the associated severe brain injury.

Intracerebral haemorrhages

Intracerebral haemorrhages occur within the cerebral parenchyma secondary to lacerations or contusions of the brain. Injury to the larger, deeper cerebral vessels results in extensive cortical contusion.

Intraventricular haemorrhage

Intraventricular haemorrhage tends to occur in the presence of very severe TBI and is, therefore, associated with an unfavourable prognosis.

Subarachnoid haemorrhage

Subarachnoid haemorrhage may occur in cases of head injury caused by lacerations of the superficial microvessels in the subarachnoid space. If not associated with another brain pathology, this type of haemorrhage could be benign. Traumatic subarachnoid haemorrhage also may lead to a communicating hydrocephalus if blood products obstruct the arachnoid villi.

Coup and contrecoup contusions

A contusion is a bruise in the brain. A combination of vascular and tissue damage leads to cerebral contusion.

Coup contusions occur at the area of direct impact to the skull. Contrecoup contusions are similar to coup contusions but are located opposite the site of direct impact. This occurs when the force impacting the head is not only great enough to cause a contusion at the site of impact but is also able to move the brain and cause it to strike into the opposite side of the skull, which causes the additional contusion. The amount of energy dissipated at the site of direct impact determines whether the ensuing contusion is of the coup or contrecoup type. Most of the energy of impact from a small hard object tends to dissipate at the impact site, leading to a coup contusion. On the contrary, impact from a larger object causes less injury at the impact site since energy is dissipated at the beginning or end of the head motion, leading to a contrecoup contusion.

Concussion

A concussion is the most common type of TBI.

A concussion is caused when the brain receives trauma from an impact or a sudden momentum. Concussion is caused by deformity of the deep structures of the brain, leading to widespread neurologic dysfunction that can result in impaired consciousness or coma. A person may or may not experience a brief loss of consciousness. A person may remain conscious, but feel 'dazed' or 'punch drunk'.

Concussion is considered a mild form of DAI and is thought to be due to a transient arrest of axoplasmic function.

Diffuse axonal injury [DAI]

Diffuse axonal injury is a frequent result of traumatic high-speed acceleration–deceleration injuries and a frequent cause of persistent vegetative state in patients. DAI is widespread damage to the white matter of the brain and is produced by a shearing injury due to rotational forces. The injury to tissue is greatest in areas where the density difference is greatest. For this reason, approximately two thirds of DAI lesions occur at the grey–white matter junction such as parasagittal frontal lobe and basal ganglia and the others where the brain impacts against a rigid structure such as the tentorium or falx cerebri producing lesions in the corpus callosum or the cerebral peduncles. Characteristic CT findings in the acute setting are small petechial haemorrhages that are located at the grey–white matter junction, within the corpus callosum and in the brainstem. The result of shearing forces histologically is trauma to the axons. This focal alteration of the axoplasmic membrane results in impairment of axonal transport. Neuropathologic findings in patients with DAI include axoplasmic swelling, retraction balls, Wallerian degeneration and glial scars. This widespread disturbance in the white matter can produce a variety of functional impairments depending on where the shearing occurred in the brain. Clinically, these injuries may manifest as temporary or permanent brain damage, coma or death.

Non-accidental injury [NAI]

Non-accidental injury is defined as any form of physical injury where the injury is not consistent with the account of its occurrence or where there is definite knowledge or a reasonable suspicion that the injury was inflicted by any person having custody, charge or care of a child.

Non-accidental head injury or Shaken Baby Syndrome is a deliberate violent shaking of a young child. The forceful whiplash-like motion causes the brain to be injured due to acceleration–deceleration forces. Blood vessels between the brain and skull rupture and bleed. The accumulation of blood causes the brain tissue to compress while the shearing injury causes the brain to swell. This can cause seizures, lifelong disability, coma and death.

Suspected NAI in a child always requires urgent referral. Consider admission and/or referral to the local social services department according to local policy. A high index of suspicion is required to first diagnose and then manage these injuries appropriately.

Indicators of possible NAI are detailed in Table 37.5.

Cranial birth injuries

Injuries to the infant that result from mechanical forces (i.e. compression, traction) during the birth process are categorised as birth injuries. Most birth traumas are self-limiting and have a favourable outcome.

Most birth injuries of the skull and brain come from excessive or rapid deformation of the skull as it passes through the birth canal, or due to compression by obstetric forceps. Distortion may produce surface lacerations of the brain or tearing of superficial vessels, the large veins or dural sinuses.

Depressed fractures of the skull during birth may be due to 'natural causes', but most result from incorrect placement of obstetric forceps.

Extra-axial injuries

Cephalhaematoma

Cephalhaematoma is the commonest birth injury and seen most frequently after vacuum extraction. It is a sub-periosteal collection of blood secondary to rupture of blood vessels between the skull and the periosteum; suture lines delineate its extent. Most commonly parietal, cephalhaematoma may occasionally be observed over the occipital bone. The extent of haemorrhage may be severe enough to cause anaemia and hypotension, although this is uncommon. Usually, management solely consists of observation. Transfusion for anaemia, hypovolaemia, or both is necessary if blood accumulation is significant. Aspiration is not required for resolution and is likely to increase the risk of infection. The resolving haematoma predisposes to hyperbilirubinemia. Resolution occurs over weeks, occasionally with residual calcification.

Subgaleal haematoma

Subgaleal haematoma is bleeding in the potential space between the skull periosteum and the scalp galea aponeurosis. This space extends from the orbital ridges to the nape of the neck and laterally to the ears. Most cases result from vacuum extraction. The diagnosis is generally a clinical one, with a fluctuant boggy mass developing over the scalp. The swelling may obscure the fontanelle and cross suture lines (distinguishing it from cephalhaematoma). The swelling develops and spreads across the whole calvarium; its growth is insidious, and subgaleal haematoma may not be recognised for hours. Patients with subgaleal haematoma may present with haemorrhagic shock. Watch for significant hyperbilirubinaemia. In the absence of shock or intracranial injury, the long-term prognosis is generally good.

Management consists of vigilant observation over days to detect progression and provide therapy for such problems as shock and anaemia. Transfusion and phototherapy may be necessary.

Caput succedaneum

Caput succedaneum is a serosanguineous, subcutaneous, extraperiosteal fluid collection with poorly defined margins; it is caused by the pressure of the presenting part on the dilating cervix. Caput succedaneum extends across the midline and over suture lines and is associated with head moulding. Caput succedaneum does not usually cause complications and usually resolves over the first few days. Management consists of observation only.

Skull fractures

Fractures are rare and more commonly depressed than linear. The parietal and frontal bones are most frequently involved. Management is expectant and one needs to be aware of the possibility of a growing skull fracture [Fig. 37.1].

Intracranial haematoma

Bleeding into the subdural space or brain is uncommon in the newborn and the clinical picture varies according to the rate of bleeding, site and volume. The infant may show signs of obtundation, with a tense fontanelle and anaemia. There will also be signs of local pressure, for example, lack of movement or weakness of the contralateral limbs.

Subdural haematoma

Subdural haematoma is the commonest intracranial abnormality following birth trauma. It arises from torn bridging cortical veins usually occuring during malpresentations or forceps delivery. The collection develops slowly, giving the brain and skull time to adjust. The clinical signs are an enlarging and sometimes asymmetrical head, delay in reaching the normal milestones, irritability, developmental delay, failure to thrive and occasionally convulsions.

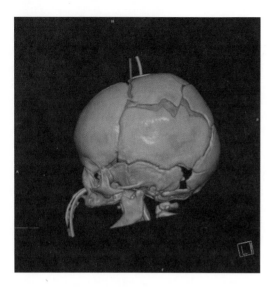

Figure 37.3 Extradural haematoma.

The diagnosis is confirmed by ultrasound or CT scan or by needle aspiration of the fontanelle. Repeated aspiration may be sufficient, but persistent reaccumulation will require either open drainage via small burr holes, or internal drainage by means of a shunt (subdural to peritoneal).

Extradural haematoma

Extradural haematoma is rare following birth trauma. It is usually associated with a skull fracture. It may present with an enlarging head, obtundation, seizures or occasionally with focal signs. It is diagnosed with an ultrasound or CT scan and management is conservative. If the mass effect worsens then needle aspiration rather than a craniotomy is preferable in this age group.

Sequelae of head injuries in children

Neurological

Although children show a surprising capacity for recovery after head injuries, they may suffer permanent disabilities as a result of the more severe injuries. Brain injury in the younger child may disrupt the development of intellectual and physical milestones and result in reduced intellectual performance and psychopathological sequelae. Brain injuries are known to produce attention deficit disorders, problems with memory and learning and deficits of psychomotor, linguistic and executive skills. Cognitive deficits particularly affecting memory disrupt learning ability and produce enormous educational difficulties. There is good correlation between injury severity as assessed by Glasgow Coma Scale and post-traumatic amnesia, and neurobehavioural outcome.

Focal deficits appropriate to the injured part of the brain may become permanent. The cranial nerves may also be permanently damaged.

Post-traumatic epilepsy is common after birth injuries, especially those which affect the temporal lobe. In older children, it occurs after compound depressed fractures of the vault associated with a laceration of the cortex, or following intracerebral haematomas.

CSF leak

CSF rhinorrhoea may result from a fracture of the base of the skull involving the frontal, ethmoid or sphenoid sinuses, whereas a fracture of the temporal bone may cause CSF otorrhoea and/or rhinorrhoea. Both types are initially treated conservatively. In about 70% cases of CSF rhinorrhoea and almost all case of CSF otorrhoea the leak stops spontaneously. Prophylactic antibiotics are not recommended because resistant organisms may develop and meningitis may still occur. If the CSF leak persists the communication with the exterior through a mucosal space is a potential source of meningitis and this may occur months or years later. A skull defect should be suspected when meningitis occurs after a head injury. The treatment of a CSF leak persisiting for more than 10 days after a head injury is an operative repair.

Further reading

Luerssen TG (2006) Central nervous system injuries. In: Grosfeld JL, O'Neill JA Jr., Fonkalsrud EW, Coran AG (eds) *Pediatric Surgery*, 6th Edn. Mosby Elsevier, Philadelphia, pp. 355–375.

Winn R (ed) (2003) Youmans Neurological Surgery. Saunders www.nice.org.uk;www.edc.gsph.pitt.edu/neurotrauma/thebook/book.html

38 Abdominal and Thoracic Injuries

Case 1

Jayden is a 7-year-old who fell off his bike. He was winded initially, but recovered within a few minutes. Several hours later he became pale and developed abdominal and shoulder pain.

Q 1.1 What is the likely diagnosis?

Q 1.2 Outline the management.

Case 2

A 3-year-old girl stepped on to the road and was hit by a car travelling at moderate speed. On arrival in the emergency department, her femur appears bent and vital signs suggest hypovolaemic shock and central cyanosis.

Q 2.1 What is your approach to the management?

Intra-abdominal injuries

The majority of abdominal injuries in children are due to blunt trauma. Penetrating trauma is rare. The commonest organs affected are the kidneys, spleen and liver. When the spleen and liver are torn, intraperitoneal bleeding occurs (haemoperitoneum). The injured kidney bleeds into the retroperitoneal space, and if the urothelium is disrupted, urine may extravasate into the retroperitoneal tissues as well.

A careful history of the accident will help predict the likely injuries. Knowledge of the mechanism of injury will provide clues as to the likely organs injured. For example, a bicycle handlebar injury to the left upper quadrant of the abdomen or to the lower chest is often associated with splenic trauma [Fig. 38.1].

Haemoperitoneum

Haemoperitoneum presents with signs of peritoneal irritation such as tenderness (often widespread) and a variable degree of reflex muscular rigidity (guarding). There may be accompanying signs of 'hypovolaemia', such as

Jones' Clinical Paediatric Surgery, 6th edition. By Hutson, O'Brien, Woodward and Beasley. Published 2008 by Blackwell Publishing, ISBN: 978-1-4051-6267-8.

tachycardia, cool peripheries and poor capillary return. Abdominal distension results both from the volume of blood in the peritoneal cavity and the swallowed air and ileus, which develops rapidly. Children are prone to acute gastric distension even after relatively minor abdominal trauma. This can produce symptoms such as pallor and cool peripheries, along with abdominal distension. These symptoms can confuse the abdominal examination, and consequently a low threshold should be given to inserting a nasogastric tube in acute abdominal trauma to allow a more reliable assessment of the abdomen. The use of a nasogastric tube is also important in helping to prevent aspiration of gastric contents (Mendelsohn syndrome).

Variations in posture and the time elapsed since injury result in wide variations in the distribution of signs of haemoperitoneum and the site of maximal tenderness. When the spleen is ruptured, the signs are usually maximal in the left upper quadrant with referred pain to the left shoulder tip. If the bleeding has occurred for some time or has been rapid, it is not unusual for signs to be more widespread, even occurring on the right side.

FAST (focused assessment with sonograph for trauma) ultrasonography in the emergency department is useful to demonstrate the presence of blood in the peritoneum. The use of ultrasound scans is widespread in adult trauma centres. However, in children the presence of blood is not an indication for surgical exploration, and often its

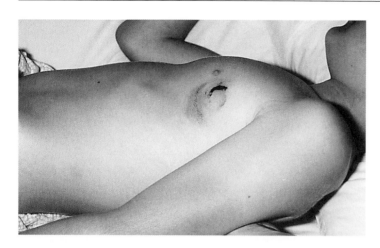

Figure 38.1 Handlebar injury with bruising over the lower ribs, which are so elastic the underlying spleen is torn without the ribs themselves being broken.

presence can be suspected clinically, and later proven with more definitive investigations, such as a CT scan. As discussed later, it is really the clinical signs, and ongoing deterioration, which indicate surgical exploration.

Radiological investigation

Many children with minor blunt trauma to the abdomen require no specific radiological investigation. CT with contrast remains the gold standard where serious abdominal injury is suspected (e.g. ruptured spleen, Fig. 38.2; liver, Fig. 38.3; or kidney) or in the case of an unconscious patient with multiple injuries where abdominal injury needs to be excluded. It should be noted that no patient with major trauma should be taken to CT for investigation unless he or she is stable. If stability cannot be achieved with resuscitation, it may be more appropriate for the patient to have an urgent laparotomy. The use of abdominal ultrasonography or IVP may be necessary in some patients.

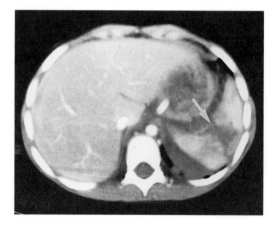

Figure 38.2 CT scan of upper abdomen showing a ruptured spleen (arrow).

Recognition of hypovolaemic shock

Shock is recognised in the child by tachycardia, poor peripheral perfusion and cool extremities. A systolic pressure of less than 70 mmHg can be an indication of significant hypovolaemia; however, blood pressure is age dependent, and this should be taken into account.

It must be remembered that, in children, blood pressure is not a good guide to hypovolaemia. It will remain stable in the face of significant blood loss (up 2/3 blood volume) and then decompensation occurs quickly. Deterioration in blood pressure therefore represents significant blood loss. Resuscitation should be instituted ideally before this occurs. The accurate measurement of

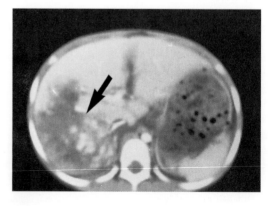

Figure 38.3 CT scan of upper abdomen showing a ruptured liver (arrow).

blood pressure in children also demands the use of a correct-sized cuff. As a general rule, the cuff width ought to be at least two-thirds of the length of the upper arm.

Non-operative management

Non-operative management is appropriate for most solid visceral injuries in children, provided they are kept under close supervision and are reassessed at frequent and regular intervals.

They are best managed in a facility with intensive care capabilities and with an experienced paediatric surgeon. Intensive care must include continuous nursing staff coverage, monitoring of vital signs at frequent intervals, and immediate availability of surgical personnel and operating theatres, should they be required. Nearly always, the bleeding stops and surgery is not needed.

Indications for surgery

Indications for surgical intervention for blunt abdominal trauma where injury to the spleen or liver is suspected include

1 Persistent unstable circulation and hypotension despite appropriate resuscitation. Initial resuscitation is with two boluses of 20 mL/kg of normal saline. If the child remains unstable following this, a surgeon should be contacted. A further 40 mL/kg of blood may then be given as two 20 mL/kg boluses. If the child fails to respond to this resuscitation, then surgical intervention to control the bleeding should be considered.

2 A proven or suspected gut perforation on clinical or radiological examination.

3 Severe, concomitant head injury in which an unstable circulation cannot be tolerated and where significant or ongoing intraperitoneal bleeding is suspected.

In splenic injuries requiring surgery, the spleen can be preserved by oversewing the tear ('splenorrhaphy') or by performing partial splenectomy, avoiding the significant risk of postsplenectomy sepsis that can occur when the entire spleen is removed. If the spleen has to be removed completely, the child should be given Pneumovax vaccine and commenced on long-term prophylactic antibiotics.

Diagnostic peritoneal lavage is not indicated in children because free blood in the perineal cavity *per se* is not an indication for surgery.

Haematuria

In all suspected intra-abdominal injuries, the presence or absence of blood in the urine must be established. Absence of haematuria virtually excludes a significant urinary tract injury except in the rare instance of a transected ureter, which is diagnosed by CT scan showing extravasation in the flank or loin, which should prompt further investigation or operative exploration.

Urethral injury should be suspected in pelvic fractures and straddle injuries with

1 frank blood appearing at the external urethral meatus;

2 inability to void spontaneously (particularly in the presence of a palpable bladder);

3 urine extravasation into the perineum.

In these patients, a urethral catheter must not be inserted blindly into the urethra, as this may convert a partial tear of the urethra into a complete transection. A carefully performed urethrogram must be obtained first to delineate the injury. Depending on the type of urethral injury, either primary surgical repair of the urethra or temporary urinary diversion, for example, suprapubic catheter, will be indicated.

Haematuria following relatively minor trauma suggests a predisposing factor, such as hydronephrosis or Wilms' tumour. All children with haematuria, even after trivial injury, need a renal ultrasound scan to exclude these underlying lesions (Chapter 35).

Extraperitoneal extravasation

The signs of extravasation of blood or urine usually develop more slowly and less dramatically than those of intraperitoneal haemorrhage; they are also more consistently localised and less variable.

Renal injuries

Because the kidney is involved frequently in blunt abdominal trauma, tenderness and muscular rigidity should be sought in the loin. However, a perirenal haematoma may cause localised tenderness and sometimes produce a mass which is palpable through the anterior abdominal wall.

When haematuria accompanies tenderness and rigidity in the loin, CT scan with contrast should be performed. This will distinguish between a contusion, which can be managed conservatively, and a rupture of the kidney with urine extravasation, which may require surgical exploration. Ultrasonography enables the renal injury to be monitored subsequently.

Early exploration – that is, within 3 days of injury – rather than a non-operative approach is advocated in major renal injuries. Delay in the recognition and management of injuries to the renal pelvis or parenchyma, which results in urine extravasation, is followed by severe inflammatory changes which prejudice attempts at conservation and later repair.

Bladder injuries

In extraperitoneal rupture of the bladder or membranous urethra, there are signs of extravasation of urine into the perineum, scrotum and suprapubic region.

When haematuria or urethral bleeding accompany signs of intraperitoneal or extraperitoneal haemorrhage in the lower part of the abdomen, a cystogram will establish whether the bladder is intact. However, if blood, as opposed to blood-stained urine, is seen at the urethral meatus, the catheter should be passed only after a carefully performed urethrogram has demonstrated that the urethra is intact.

Ill-defined intra-abdominal injuries

Apart from those patients with intraperitoneal haemorrhage, extraperitoneal extravasation or haematuria, there is a difficult group with ill-defined symptoms and signs which may persist for several days after the injury.

Many probably have minor contusions of the abdominal wall or the intestine or its mesentery. Non-operative management usually is justified in these cases. Sometimes, lap-belt deceleration injuries may cause severe trauma to the bowel wall when it is crushed against the sacral promontory. These injuries only become apparent after several days when the bowel perforates and peritonitis suddenly develops. The same type of trauma may also cause a periduodenal haematoma and pancreatic injuries, some of which may require surgical intervention. Severe lap-belt injuries with abdominal wall bruising ± lumbar bruise (hyperextension tear of lumbar ligaments/vertebral fracture) need immediate specialist referral.

Thoracic injuries

In contrast to their comparative frequency in adults, major thoracic injuries are not common in children. Most chest trauma in children is blunt. Penetrating thoracic injuries are extremely rare. Blunt thoracic trauma tends to form part of a composite picture of multiple injuries which may include cerebral, abdominal and peripheral trauma, any of which may be the predominant threat to life.

The child's chest wall is very compliant and allows energy transfer to the intrathoracic structures, frequently without any external evidence of injury and without fracture to the ribs. The elastic chest wall increases the frequency of pulmonary contusions and direct intrapulmonary haemorrhage. Consequently, pulmonary contusion is the most common significant thoracic injury in children. Tension pneumothorax or haemopneumothorax

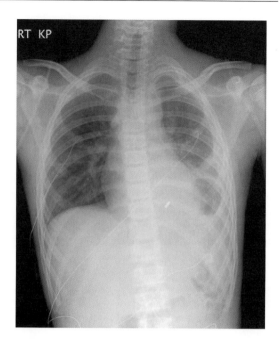

Figure 38.4 X-ray showing abdominal viscera in left hemithorax following crush injury and rupture of diaphragm.

are less common, but potentially lethal unless recognised and the tension relieved using intercostal drainage. Diaphragmatic rupture is extremely rare and may result from crushing of the torso and pelvis [Fig. 38.4]. Injury to the great vessels is rare in children, and reflects a lack of preexisting vascular disease and fewer high-speed injuries.

The diagnostic and therapeutic approach to chest trauma is the same for children as adults. Significant thoracic injuries rarely occur alone and are often a component of major multisystem trauma. Contusion of the lung and traumatic rupture of the diaphragm are unlikely to be recognised in the presence of multiple injuries unless a chest x-ray is taken. Pneumothorax, with or without haemothorax, may result from pulmonary contusion, and when of significant volume, should be relieved by an intercostal tube with an underwater seal.

Multiple fractures of the ribs are not common because of the elasticity of the thorax in children, and as a consequence, flail chest is rare. When the flail area is large enough to cause respiratory embarrassment, internal splinting by positive pressure ventilation is preferable.

When penetrating injuries occur, they may involve the heart and lungs, and the possibility of cardiac tamponade must be kept in mind.

Investigation and treatment

An x-ray of the chest should be taken in all cases of trauma with multiple injuries, in all thoracic injuries and in all patients with respiratory insufficiency.

A penetrating injury should be assumed to have caused injury to underlying viscera until the contrary is proven. The possibility of combined thoraco-abdominal injury should always be kept in mind.

Respiratory symptoms demand investigation and treatment which may include intercostal drainage, thoracotomy or tracheostomy, review by intensivists and possible ventilation and respiratory support in intensive care.

> ## Key Points
>
> - Bicycle handlebar injury may tear the spleen, and less commonly, the liver, kidney and pancreas.
> - Ruptured spleen causes significant haemoperitoneum, but bleeding nearly always stops without surgery.
> - Non-operative management is appropriate for most solid visceral injuries.
> - Haematuria after trauma needs investigation to document the status of the kidneys and urinary tract.
> - Blunt chest trauma leads to pulmonary contusions without rib fractures.

Further reading

Stylianos S, Pearl RH (2006) Abdominal trauma. In: Grosfeld JL, O'Neill JA Jr., Fonkalsrud EW, Coran AG (eds) *Pediatric Surgery*, 6th Edn. Mosby Elsevier, Philadelphia, pp. 295–316.

Stylianos S, Vitale MG (2006) Truncal trauma. In: Stringer MD, Oldham KT, Mouriquand PDE (eds) *Pediatric Surgery and Urology, Long-term Outcomes*, 2nd Edn. Cambridge University Press, Cambridge, pp. 936–946.

Wesson DE (2006) Thoracic injuries. In: Grosfeld JL, O'Neill JA Jr., Fonkalsrud EW, Coran AG (eds) *Pediatric Surgery*, 6th Edn. Mosby Elsevier, Philadelphia, pp. 275–294.

39 Foreign Bodies

Case 1

A mother notices her 12-month-old child put a small safety pin in his mouth and apparently swallow it. An x-ray shows it to be in the stomach. He is asymptomatic.

Q 1.1 Are any further investigations required?

Q 1.2 Is surgery to remove the pin indicated?

Case 2

A barefooted 8-year-old girl has trodden on a needle, which has broken, part of it remaining in the sole of her foot. A small puncture wound is seen, but the needle cannot be felt. It hurts her to walk on it.

Q 2.1 How is it best removed?

The young child's instinctive exploration and fascination with his or her environment can result in a wide range of foreign bodies lodging in a variety of places. Most are found in the alimentary tract; others may enter the aural or nasal cavities, the bronchial tree or be accidentally driven into the soft tissues. The location of foreign bodies tends to vary with the age of the child. Infants are more likely to ingest things into the alimentary canal, while older children who are active are more likely to experience puncture wounds.

Swallowed foreign bodies

In infants, oral exploration of the environment may lead to accidental swallowing of a variety of objects. Older siblings may feed the 'new baby' inappropriate hardware. Accidental swallowing may be precipitated by a fall or a slap on the back. At any age, a bone hidden in food (e.g. fish bone) may be swallowed. Ingestion of a foreign body occurs most commonly between 6 months and 4 years.

The vast majority of swallowed foreign bodies pass through the alimentary tract without a problem. With rare exceptions, objects that are first located below the diaphragm will pass naturally without hazard to the child.

The most common site (70%) of lodgement is in the oesophagus at the level of the cricopharyngeus muscle (the area between the clavicles on the x-ray). The other two sites of lodgement are mid-oesophagus and at the gastro-oesphageal junction.

Objects

The size of coins (the objects that are swallowed most often) determines whether they are likely to become impacted. Safety pins may stick in the oesophagus, but if they enter the stomach they will almost always be excreted without difficulty, even if open. Broken plastic toys are more dangerous, because they may be jagged or angular and their radiolucency may lead to delay in diagnosis. Hair clips ('Kirby-grips') pass easily as far as the duodenojejunal flexure, but may be too long and rigid to negotiate this flexure in children less than 7 years of age, and require endoscopy or laparotomy for their removal. In children more than 6 or 7 years of age, observation for up to 1 week is justified, although impaction at the duodenojejunal flexure should not be allowed to continue for more than 10–12 days.

'Button' or 'disc' batteries used in electronic toys, cameras and other electronic goods are particularly hazardous when swallowed. Their small size ensures their passage into the stomach, and the great majority pass through the alimentary canal uneventfully. Original button batteries were large and prone to oesophageal impaction. Buttons of today are smaller and much less likely to impact. Always be wary of old toys as these can have old

Jones' Clinical Paediatric Surgery, 6th edition. By Hutson, O'Brien, Woodward and Beasley. Published 2008 by Blackwell Publishing, ISBN: 978-1-4051-6267-8.

batteries that still can be hazardous if ingested. However, if there is any suspicion of ingestion, and any holdup occurs, an x-ray should be done to ensure the battery is out of the oesophagus. If the battery is seen in the oesophagus referral should be made for surgical endoscopic removal. Holdup in the oesophagus is hazardous because erosion and perforation can occur rapidly. The cause is thought to be related to discharge of current rather than breakdown of the battery. Even non-functioning batteries can discharge enough to erode through the oesophagus.

Beyond the stomach the battery will invariably pass. There has been concern in the past about deterioration and leakage from the battery with the possibility of absorption of battery contents. However, with modern batteries this has not been shown to be a concern. An x-ray after a week to show it has passed can be useful to reassure parents but, generally, no intervention is required even if it takes longer for the button to pass, as long as the child remains asymptomatic.

Prevention

It is important to ensure young children and infants have appropriate levels of supervision and that toys are age-appropriate to prevent accidental ingestion.

Clinical features

There may be no symptoms, and it is likely that innumerable small foreign bodies are passed uneventfully and unnoticed. In some cases, an attack of gagging, coughing or retching is reported by parents, which may then be followed by a reluctance of the child to eat or drink. This can then progress to oesophageal obstruction with symptoms of excessive drooling and dysphagia. Sometimes children are witnessed with something in their mouth prior to the onset of the symptoms.

If the accident has not been reported or observed, there may be a delay in the diagnosis and the first symptoms may be due to complications, for example, progressive dysphagia or dyspnoea caused by pressure of the swollen oesophagus on the trachea. In severe cases, the child may develop pain, swelling in the neck and fever, suggesting mediastinitis, and rarely a pneumothorax or pleuritic pain may be the first indication of perforation of the thoracic oesophagus by a foreign body. Rarely, the object can erode directly into the trachea or aorta; ulceration, mediastinitis and even an acquired tracheo-oesophageal fistula may occur. This may lead to a persistent cough or recurrent pneumonia if the fistula is into the trachea, and in the case of an aorto-oesophageal fistula, a child can get catastrophic haemorrhage.

Investigations

If the object is radio-opaque or unknown, radiographs of the head, neck, thorax and abdomen may be required, because a radio-opaque object may be located anywhere from the base of the skull to the pelvic floor. However, the site of the foreign body can also be indicated by the type of symptoms.

A radiograph will distinguish tracheal from oesophageal lodgement, for the maximum dimension of the trachea is in the sagittal plane, and that of the oesophagus is in the coronal plane [Fig. 39.1].

Some centres are now using metal detectors in emergency departments to detect metallic objects more accurately.

Radiolucent foreign bodies are more difficult to detect radiologically. In cases, where ingestion of a radiolucent foreign body is suspected and the patient is symptomatic, consultation with an ENT or general surgeon will be required to decide the next appropriate investigation, for example, a barium swallow.

Management

The vast majority of ingested foreign bodies do not need removal.

Located in oesophagus

Endoscopic removal is required for all objects impacted in the upper oesophagus. In the lower oesophagus, foreign bodies may pass with time and some people have advocated the use of medications to relax the lower oesophageal sphincter, such as Glucagon. Allowing time for the foreign body to pass can be appropriate where the impacted foreign body is not hazardous, for example, a food bolus obstruction. A button battery, however, should never be allowed to remain in the oesophagus, even if it is in the lower oesophagus.

Beyond oesophagus

Foreign bodies first located beyond the oesophagus have a good chance of being excreted without incident [Fig. 39.2]. Blunt objects small enough to enter the stomach will almost always be passed; the patient should return only if abdominal pain or vomiting occurs. Further radiographs are not usually indicated, but will show that the object has been passed, often unrecognised.

In general, where a blunt foreign body has been impacted without progress for 6 weeks, removal at laparotomy may be considered, even in the absence of symptoms.

Most sharp objects pass uneventfully and should be managed conservatively initially, although arrest and

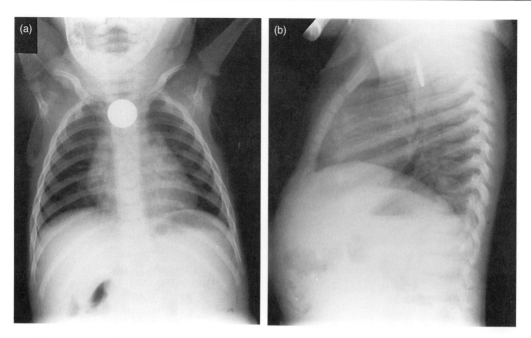

Figure 39.1 The orientation of a foreign body (e.g. coin) will distinguish tracheal from oesophageal lodgement. Here a chest x-ray shows a coin in the coronal plane characteristic of the oesophagus (a) antero-posterior view and (b) lateral view.

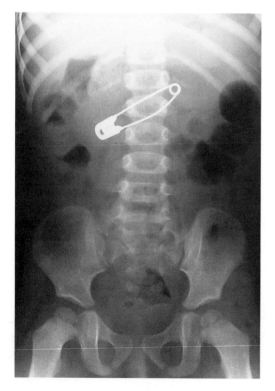

Figure 39.2 Abdominal x-ray showing a safety pin in the stomach. This should pass spontaneously.

failure to progress through the bowel may raise concerns of impending impaction, ulceration and perforation. If a sharp foreign body is being observed, for example, a nail or a pin, parents should re-present at any time the child develops an unexplained fever or sudden abdominal pain.

A bezoar is a conglomeration of hair (trichobezoar) or vegetable material (phytobezoar), which can be swallowed by children as a habit. The mass forms in the stomach or proximal gut and causes pain, vomiting or anorexia, malnutrition or unexplained anaemia. Less commonly, obstruction or perforation occurs. When x-ray studies indicate a mass of this kind, laparotomy and enterotomy are required.

Foreign bodies in the trachea and bronchi

Sudden onset of coughing, spluttering and gagging with a residual wheeze are suggestive of inhalation of a foreign body. The exact clinical picture varies with the size of the object, the site of lodgement and the time elapsed since the object was inhaled.

Large objects in the larynx or trachea produce obstruction which may be complete if they impact in the narrow glottis. Inspiratory stridor and respiratory distress with indrawing of the supraclavicular, substernal or intercostal areas indicate that the object is in the larynx or subglottic area.

Foreign bodies in the trachea or bronchus cause a wheeze and can produce clinical and radiological evidence of an overexpanded (emphysematous) lung because of a ball-valve effect of the foreign body. Objects impacted more distally may present with symptoms of chronic chest infection from lobar or segmental consolidation.

X-rays may demonstrate the object if it is radio-opaque. If it is radiolucent, as noted previously, segmental pulmonary collapse and lobar emphysema may be seen on the x-ray. Films taken in expiration and inspiration show air-trapping and assist in localising the presence and size of small radiolucent objects in the lungs, for example, a peanut.

In infants, respiratory symptoms such as acute dyspnoea, stridor or cough can occur when the object is impacted in the oesophagus. This is due to the dilated oesophagus pushing on the adjacent trachea. As previously noted, the orientation of the object on x-ray can identify the site of lodgement because the maximum diameter of the trachea is in the antero-posterior plane, compared with the transverse plane in the oesophagus [Fig. 39.1].

Management
Removal at endoscopy under general anaesthesia is required to remove foreign bodies. This may involve either a rigid or flexible bronchoscope. The foreign body may not always be easily seen because of mucosal swelling or infection. Organic material can also be very difficult to grasp. Mucosal abrasions and pulmonary changes caused by the foreign body, its complications or manipulations during removal, are indications for a course of antibiotics. The earlier the diagnosis and treatment, the less the likelihood of residual pulmonary or mucosal damage.

Special consideration
Great care needs to be taken with peanuts, which is why they should not be given to young children. Not only can they obstruct the bronchus, but the oil content can also produce a lipoid pneumonia which is known to develop rapidly.

Foreign bodies in the ear, nose and pharynx

In the ear
Unless there is a definite history, children with a foreign body in the ear present with a blood-stained discharge, irritation or deafness. Cooperation of the child is essential for the removal. Most may be removed with a good viewing instrument (auroscope) and illumination with a fine probe. However, if the first attempts fail it is appropriate to refer to ENT for a removal under sedation or anaesthetic.

In the nose
The child, who is usually between 2 and 4 years of age, presents with nasal irritation and obstruction, or a purulent discharge. The object can often be seen on direct examination or with an auroscope; very ocassionally, an x-ray may be useful. Prior to any procedure the nose should be treated with lignocaine spray and phenylephrine for anaestheic and to reduce local inflammation. In very small children, the foreign body sometimes can be blown out. This is achieved by asking the mother/carer to blow into the child's mouth and obstructing the other nostril. In older children, suction can be an effective method for removing objects, especially smooth round objects such as beads or buttons. Other methods involve the use of fine hooks or even a fine Foley catheter. If the child is not co-operative or the first attempts are unsuccessful, it is appropriate to involve the ENT surgeon or to use some form of sedation, such as ketamine, or occasionally an anaesthetic.

In the pharynx
The commonest object that gets lodged in the tonsil, the piriform fossa or the back of the tongue, is a fish bone. Subjective localisation is poor, and pain may be constant or felt only during swallowing.

After the fauces and pharynx have been sprayed with a local anaesthetic, the usual sites are examined with the aid of a spatula or a laryngeal mirror and proper illumination, and the object is removed with forceps.

Foreign bodies in the urinary tract

These are rare but most frequently involve the bladder – in girls in the preschool age group during play, or in boys during puberty, when objects may be introduced into the urethra. Sometimes a fragment of a ureteric catheter may break off and remain after surgery to the urinary tract. Any of these objects may cause infection, haematuria or pain, and may act as a nidus for the formation of a calculus.

Foreign bodies in the urinary or genital tract are removed by endoscopy.

Other foreign bodies

X-ray may help identify foreign bodies deep in the soft tissue if radio-opaque.

In the hand

Apart from superficial splinters, small objects may be driven into the palm, such as wood, plant spikes or metal. If it is unrecognised, a painless swelling may develop on the palm, with the foreign body sitting inside a fibrous capsule. Sometimes, however, infection may occur around the foreign body leading to an abscess that may ultimately drain, expressing the foreign body in the process. If the foreign body penetrates deep into the palm, it can go on to cause a deep web-space infection, with the potential for pus to track along the tendon sheaths.

Where a foreign body deep in the palm is suspected, exploration and removal under general anaesthetic is usually required. More superficial foreign bodies can sometimes be removed with sedation in the emergency department. However, prolonged attempts should be avoided, as this is distressing for the child and foreign bodies can sometimes be very difficult to identify in the absence of ideal surgical conditions.

In the lower limb

Nails, pins or needles driven into the foot or knee can be shown radiographically. When they are not visible through the skin, they are most easily and quickly removed under general anaesthesia and guided by an image intensifier.

Key Points

- Most foreign bodies that reach the stomach pass spontaneously.
- Sudden coughing with a residual wheeze is suggestive of an inhaled foreign body.
- Foreign bodies in the palm and sole should be removed under anaesthesia.

Further reading

Brown TCK, Clark CM (1983) Inhaled foreign bodies in children. *Med J Aust* **2**: 322.

Geddes NK, Raine PAM (1994) Respiratory obstruction, thoracic trauma and ingestion of foreign body. In: Raine PAM, Azmy AAF (eds) *Surgical Emergencies in Children: A Practical Guide*. Butterworth Heinemann, Oxford, pp. 193–219.

Jones PG (1963) Swallowed foreign bodies in childhood. *Med J Aust* **1**: 236.

Stringer MD, Capps SNJ (1991) Rationalising the management of swallowed coins in children. *BMJ* **302**: 1321–1322.

40 The Ingestion of Corrosives

Case 1

Chamel drank from an unlabelled soft drink bottle that she found in her father's garage. She immediately developed severe mouth, throat and epigastric pain and had difficulty swallowing. The fluid ingested was identified as caustic soda.

Q 1.1 What should be your initial first aid?

Q 1.2 What investigation should be performed in hospital? What major complication of this injury do you wish to prevent?

In children, swallowing corrosive fluids or solids nearly always is accidental, and the exploring toddler aged between 1 and 3 years is most often the victim. Symptoms of caustic ingestion include cervical and epigastric pain, irritability, excessive drooling, dysphagia and respiratory distress. However, about 20% present with no symptoms; in some, this is despite significant oesophageal injury.

Prevention

The most effective way to prevent such accidents is to keep all chemicals used in the home and garden out of reach of small children and in their proper containers. They should not be stored under the kitchen sink or in unlabelled containers.

Pathology

The oesophagus is the most common organ seriously injured by corrosive ingestion. Extensive or circumferential oesophageal burns may lead to severe strictures that cause dysphagia within weeks of injury.

Burns of the buccal mucosa, soft palate or tongue suggest that the oesophagus has been damaged as well.

Mucosal injury and oedema of the larynx occurs in 15%, and can be life-threatening, requiring intubation or tracheotomy.

Jones' Clinical Paediatric Surgery, 6th edition. By Hutson, O'Brien, Woodward and Beasley. Published 2008 by Blackwell Publishing, ISBN: 978-1-4051-6267-8.

First aid

1 If ingestion has just occurred, wash off any excess corrosive material from the lips and skin, using plenty of water.

2 Immediately dilute any corrosive in the mouth, oesophagus or stomach by giving cold water or milk to drink. Do not attempt to use an 'antidote' acid or alkali because the corrosive may have been identified incorrectly, and the chemical antidotes themselves may cause damage.

3 If ingestion of corrosive was not witnessed or confirmed by an adult, always assume it has occurred if the lips or mouth are blistered or if the toddler is drooling excessively and unable to swallow saliva.

4 Where the nature or composition of the corrosive is uncertain, consult the Poisons Information Service by telephone. Induce vomiting with ipecac syrup only if directed by a poisons service.

5 Send a sample of the corrosive agent with the child when transferring to hospital if identification has not been made with certainty.

6 All children should be sent to the nearest paediatric surgical centre as soon as possible after ingestion.

Definitive management

An oesophagoscopy at 24 h is necessary in corrosive ingestion whenever injury to the oesophagus is suspected. This will determine the severity of oesophageal injury, and hence the need for prophylactic treatment to reduce the likelihood of subsequent oesophageal stricture formation.

Where there is no damage to the oesophageal mucosa on oesophagoscopy, no treatment is required.

Patchy oedema of the intact oesophageal mucosa is regarded as the minimal degree of burn and is not likely to cause a stricture. No treatment is required and the patient may leave hospital as soon as normal feeding is re-established. A white mucosal slough or circumferential ulceration is more serious and may lead to a stricture. In these patients, antibiotics are given to limit the effects of secondary infection. Steroids may diminish the extent of fibrosis, although their value is uncertain. Oesophagoscopy and dilatation of the oesophagus is performed under general anaesthesia in children with extensive and deep oesophageal burns. This procedure is usually commenced 2 weeks after the initial injury.

If the mucosa has healed and there is no evidence of narrowing, treatment is discontinued. If there are abnormal findings at 2 weeks, treatment is continued for a further 6 weeks. Where there is worsening dysphagia and the stricture cannot be dilated effectively by bouginage, segmental resection and anastomosis may be required. Occasionally, an extensive resection and replacement of the oesophagus is inescapable; but in the long term, the best

oesophagus is the patient's own, and prolonged bouginage is justified to avoid an extensive oesophagectomy.

Key Points

- Oesophageal injury may be prevented by rapid dilution of corrosive by drinking cold water or milk.
- Ulcers on lips or inside mouth suggest oesophageal burn – confirmed by drooling saliva.
- Oesophagoscopy at 24 h determines severity of burn and treatment required.

Further reading

Gorman RL, Khin-Maung-Gyi MT, Klein-Schwartz W, *et al.* (1992) Initial symptoms as predictors of esophageal injury in corrosive ingestions. *Am J Emerg Med* **10**: 189.

Millar AJW, Namanoglu A, Rode H (2006) Caustic strictures of the esophagus. In: Grosfeld JL, O'Neill JA Jr., Fonkalsrud EW, Coran AG (eds) *Pediatric Surgery*, 6th Edn. Mosby Elsevier, Philadelphia, pp. 1082–1092.

Vergauwen P, Mouin D, Buts JP, et al. (1991) Caustic burns of the upper digestive and respiratory tracts. *Eur J Pediatr* **150**: 700.

41 Burns

Case 1

During your intern year, you are rotated to a rural base hospital. At 5 p.m. an 18-month-old boy is rushed into the emergency department after tipping hot tea on to himself 10 min earlier. The tea was just boiled and no milk had been added. The area of scald estimated with a Lund–Browder chart is 15%.
Q 1.1 What are the principles of management prior to transfer to the regional burns unit next morning?

Case 2

Jeremy is a 6-month-old infant brought to your clinic with red, weeping lower legs and feet after being scalded by a hot bath.
Q 2.1 What is the likely mechanism of injury?

Case 3

William and Ali are brought to the emergency department after they poured petrol on a campfire. Their faces are blackened and their hair and eyebrows are singed.
Q 3.1 Why might the oximeter show falling oxygen saturation?

The severity of a burn injury depends on the size and depth of burn, and its anatomical site. A burn may be caused by heat, electricity, radiation, chemical agents or friction. Burns caused by heat may be due to hot liquids, commonly referred to as scald injury. Dry thermal injury can occur from flames or contact with hot surfaces. The care of a burned child requires the services of a multi-disciplinary team and may extend over many years. A burned child has a rapidly progressive illness: within a short time, a healthy, alert, adventurous youngster may be in danger of losing his life. He will suffer pain and anxiety, and may develop lifelong physical and psychological scars.

Prevention

Most burns in children are due to scalds: are self-inflicted; are twice as common in boys (usually toddlers); and occur at home, mostly in the kitchen or bathroom. The child at greatest risk therefore is the male toddler, in the kitchen, while under the care of a parent who is preparing

or drinking a hot beverage. Flame burns occur mainly in adolescent boys playing with fire, most commonly matches and flammable fluids.

Prevention of burns rests on three main approaches:
1 *Education*, of both children and adults, concerning potential dangers and the need for continual vigilance. Current government programmes stress to the public that injuries to children can be prevented by (a) supervising them; (b) separating them from the hazard; (c) reducing the hazard or access to it and (d) removing the hazard. It is hoped that by introducing such programmes, the incidence of burn injury will be reduced: in the last 25 years, the frequency of burns has declined by 50% in the State of Victoria.
2 *Design*, for example, improvements in clothes, heating appliances, guards on stoves, temperature regulators in hot-water systems.
3 *Legislation*, for example, government (legal) control of fireworks, nightwear materials and design regulations.

When visiting a home, the family doctor is in a unique position to prevent burning accidents by warning the parents of specific hazards. These include the ability of young children to reach tabletops and overhanging saucepan handles on stoves, hot water in bathrooms, old-model radiators and unguarded fires, loose cotton nightwear and access to flammable liquids.

Jones' Clinical Paediatric Surgery, 6th edition. By Hutson, O'Brien, Woodward and Beasley. Published 2008 by Blackwell Publishing, ISBN: 978-1-4051-6267-8.

Treatment

Early, competent assessment of the burn is essential. The child should be admitted to a burns unit when there is

1 full-thickness skin-loss, >5% total body-surface area;

2 more than 10% of the total body surface has been burned;

3 inhalation injury has been sustained;

4 when important areas are involved, for example, face, hands, buttocks and genitalia;

5 poor social circumstances and probable maltreatment.

Treatment requires a team approach involving a surgeon, anaesthetist, social worker, school teacher, dietitian, physiotherapist and other paramedical therapists, all of whom confer and work together to ensure that the child is healed and back at home as soon as possible. The phases of treatment are summarised in Table 41.1.

First aid

First aid involves limiting the extent and severity of the burn. The child must be removed quickly from the source of injury: flames are smothered, by water if at hand; clothing should be removed immediately, especially with a scald; the whole body or limb should be cooled with water for 20 min. Ice or iced water is dangerous because it may cause general hypothermia or local ischaemia, and thus is contraindicated in children.

Transportation

In major burns, transport to a hospital is to be arranged, and intravenous fluids (e.g. Hartmann's solution) should be commenced early if delay in transportation is likely. If intravenous fluids are not available, a saline solution can be given orally, in small amounts at first and, later, in increased volume if tolerated. Intravenous morphine is

Table 41.1 The management of burns in children

1. First aid
2. Transportation
3. Assessment
4. Resuscitation
5. Prevention and control of infection
6. Adequate nutrition
7. Wound care
8. Early excision of dead tissue with grafting
9. Minimisation of scars and contractures with pressure garments, splints, and so forth.
10. Psychological support and rehabilitation
11. Reconstructive surgery, if necessary

administered, and the child wrapped in a clean sheet and covered with a blanket to prevent hypothermia.

Assessment

The severity of the burn depends on the burn surface area, the depth of damage and the anatomical site involved, in particular the face, hands, feet or perineum. In children, the area and depth of the burn are mapped on a Lund–Browder figure chart [Fig. 41.1], which allows an accurate estimation of the area involved, according to age. Unless this estimate is charted carefully, the area of the burn may be overestimated and excessive fluids given.

A full-thickness skin burn (white, charred and painless) is usually obvious early, but partial skin loss may be superficial (erythematous, blistering and painful white slough) or deep (mottled, red and painless). The depth of partial skin loss may not be evident for 10–14 days, even to the trained eye.

Resuscitation

If shock is present or the burn area exceeds 15% of the body surface (less in a young child), intravenous fluids are required, along with morphine (0.05–0.1 mg/kg), given slowly over 3–5 min.

Fluids required during the first 24 h after the burn include

1 *Maintenance fluids*. In most children, burn injury maintenance fluids can be given orally and should initially be milk or a milk substitute. If oral intake is impossible, early

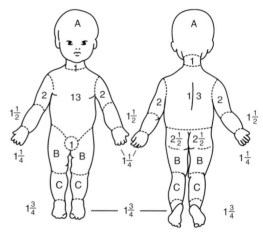

Figure 41.1 Method of estimating the extent of burned surfaces, allowing for differences according to age (after Lund and Browder [1944]). A is 10% at birth, decreasing to 4% in adolescence. B and C are 2½ in babies, increasing to 5% and 3½% respectively in adolescents.

nasogastric or nasojejunal feeding should be considered. If either of these methods fail, intravenous maintenance fluid should be given (*N*/2 saline in 5% dextrose according to weight). One-third the estimated daily requirement is given every 8 h.

2 *Resuscitation fluids*: 2–3 mL/kg body weight/1% burn surface are given, with one-half of the volume as colloid, for example, 5% normal serum albumin, depending on the severity of the burn and the remainder as Hartmann's solution. Half of the estimated volume is administered in the first 8 h and a quarter in each of the next two 8 h periods. The volume required in the second 24 h is approximately half that of the first 24 h.

The rate of intravenous fluid administration depends on the general condition of the child and an expected urine flow of 0.75 mL/kg/h, obtained via a catheter in the bladder. If the expected urine flow is not reached, the intravenous fluid rate is increased, and later decreased once shock has been controlled and urine output established. After approximately 3 days, a diuresis will occur and the serum electrolytes, urine osmolality and specific gravity will indicate the further requirements.

Blood transfusion rarely is required in the first few days after the burn, but is necessary when anaemia develops and when the burn is to be excised surgically and grafted.

The pH of the gastric juice is estimated regularly in severe burns, and antacids, H$_2$-antagonists, proton pump inhibitors and/or sucralfate are prescribed to prevent the development of stress ulcers.

Infection

Infection is the major cause of death following the initial burn injury. On admission, swabs are taken from the nose, throat, faeces and burned areas, but antibiotics are given only if there are specific indications. The major aim in treating burns patients now is to prevent infection, and it is thought that early enteral nutrition, which prevents translocation of gastrointestinal bacteria into the bloodstream, combined with early excision of the burned escar and the use of silver-based dressings, have all reduced the risk of both local wound infection and septicaemia.

Tetanus toxoid is given routinely.

Nutrition

Appropriate nutritional management of the severely burned patient is necessary to ensure optimal outcome. Initiation of early enteral feeding within 6–18 h post-burn improves nitrogen balance, reduces the hypermetabolic response, and also reduces immunological complications.

Young children with major burn injuries often require nasogastric feedings as they have difficulty meeting their nutritional goals with oral intake alone. The hypermetabolic response associated with severe burn injury results in high caloric and protein requirements to ensure optimal healing and outcome. The addition of trace elements and vitamins is also important for ensuring optimal healing of both injury and skin-graft donor sites.

Wound care

After cleaning the wound with an antiseptic, loose skin is removed and gross blisters punctured, leaving removal of blistered skin to a later date. Very superficial burns, for example, sunburn, can be left exposed or covered with a bland ointment, allowing a fine escar to form; this lifts when the underlying epithelium has healed. Erythematous weeping burns do well with a closed dressing (Vaseline tulle, or silicone coated, e.g., Mepitel®), which is left undisturbed beneath gauze and a firm crepe bandage for 5 days. The inner dressing can be left to separate spontaneously, the outer dressings being changed as necessary.

In burns of an indeterminate depth, the area is washed with a mild soap, and a nano-crystalline silver dressing, for example Acticoat®, is applied. These dressings can be left in place until review in 3–7 days.

Surgical treatment

The aim of surgery is to excise dead skin and apply split skin-grafts as early as possible. Early skin coverage prevents many problems, including infection, long hospitalisation, scar formation and psychological disturbances.

Full-thickness burns are treated as soon as the child has recovered from the shock phase. When a large area has been burned, the child is taken to the theatre twice a week for staged excision and grafting. If there is a lack of patient's skin, allograft skin from the Skin Bank can be used as a biological dressing, while awaiting re-epithelialisation of the donor sites.

Deep partial burns will heal in time from deeper cells remaining in the skin appendages, but may form ugly hypertrophic scars. As soon as such a burn becomes evident (which may take up to 2 weeks), the area is submitted to 'tangential' excision, down to a living base of skin matrix and then grafted.

Scars and contractures

Burn injuries, particularly deep dermal burns, are notorious for becoming hypertrophic and creating ugly scars. These will improve spontaneously but long-term pressure garments will accelerate their resolution, and are very worthwhile. Application of silicon and Hypafix® are valuable also.

Physiotherapy is employed from the time of admission, to assist movements of the chest, joints and muscles to achieve recovery of full function. Splints and pressure garments are tailored and may be needed for 6–12 months to prevent contractures and scars.

Psychological support and rehabilitation

Psychological support (ideally from parents, siblings and friends) is important during hospitalisation and rehabilitation, and may be required for some years. Guilt feelings in the child and parents are common. Discussion groups for parents, and burn support groups, should be available to help the child return to a normal life.

Reconstructive surgery

Contractures and scars can lead to functional disabilities and leave cosmetic blemishes. Surgical excision, inlay grafts and corticosteroid injections, may be required until adolescence is reached and active growth has ceased.

Key Points

- Burn severity depends on its size, depth and site.
- Early assessment, first aid and resuscitation is essential.
- Transfer to the regional burns unit all patients with full thickness burn >5%; total burn >10%; inhalation burn; face, hand or buttock burns; non-accidental burn.

Further reading

British Burn Association Recommended First Aid for Burns Scalds. *Burns* 1987, 13.

Chung DH, Sanford AP, Herndon DN (2006) Burns. In: Grosfeld JL, O'Neill JA Jr., Fonkalsrud EW, Coran AG (eds) *Pediatric Surgery*, 6th Edn. Mosby Elsevier, Philadelphia, pp. 383–399.

Lund CC, Browder NC (1944) The estimation of areas of burns. *Surg Gynecol Obset* 79: 352.

Monafo WW (1996) Initial management of burns. *New Engl J Med* 335: 1581–1584.

Orthopaedics

42   Neonatal Orthopaedics

Case 1

A 1-day-old baby, weighing 3.75 kg and born by a 'difficult' delivery, was not moving his right arm soon after birth. Examination revealed no deformities, but the baby cried when the arm was moved, or when lifted. Two weeks later a painless swelling was noted in the middle third of the right humerus.

Q 1.1 What is the swelling?

Q 1.2 What is the natural history?

Case 2

A newborn baby was unable to leave the neonatal nursery because of being generally unwell with signs of sepsis. On the tenth day, lack of normal kicking movements were noted in the left lower limb. There was a low-grade pyrexia and the white cell count, CRP and ESR were elevated.

Q 2.1 What might be seen on hip ultrasound?

Case 3

A baby boy weighing 4.65 kg was born by a shoulder presentation to a diabetic mother. There were no left shoulder or elbow movements but normal grasp reflex and finger movements.

Q 3.1 What is the likely diagnosis?

Q 3.2 What is the likeliest outcome?

Case 4

A newborn baby was noted to have both feet turned in to face each other immediately after birth. The father had had multiple operations for 'clubfeet' in childhood. On examination, it was found that the feet could be corrected to the normal position with gentle pressure from one finger.

Q 4.1 What is the likely diagnosis?

Q 4.2 What is the prognosis?

Case 5

In a country hospital, a newborn was noted to have both feet pointing upwards, lying along the lower tibia. The child was referred for an orthopaedic opinion, but the position improved before the consultation took place and then resolved without treatment.

Q 5.1 Is there a risk of other anomalies?

Case 6

A male infant was born with the right foot turned down and inwards. The foot felt stiff and could not be placed in a normal alignment. There was a strong family history of clubfoot.

Q 6.1 What is the treatment and likely outcome?

Parents may bring their child to an orthopaedic surgeon in the first month of life because something looks wrong (clubfoot, bowed tibia) or because something is not moving or working properly (brachial plexus palsy, birth

Jones' Clinical Paediatric Surgery, 6th edition. By Hutson, O'Brien, Woodward and Beasley. Published 2008 by Blackwell Publishing, ISBN: 978-1-4051-6267-8.

fracture). Alternatively, the paediatrician or orthopaedic surgeon may find something on examination of which the parent was not aware (developmental dislocation of the hip).

Newborn children have limited ways in which to respond to pain, be it from a birth fracture, osteomyelitis or a tumour. They often reduce or stop moving the limb, a condition known as 'pseudoparalysis'. The limb is not paralysed, but is held still because pain can be relieved by reducing or abolishing movements. The most common causes of 'pseudoparalysis' are fractures or infection.

Birth fractures

Birth fractures are quite common, with an incidence of 1–5 per 1000 live births, and they are usually found in large, healthy babies after a difficult delivery, especially by the breech. The most common sites are the clavicle, the humerus and femur. Fractures of the clavicle may not be diagnosed until a painless swelling is noted because of callus formation. Not all birth injuries are fractures; separations of the humeral and femoral epiphyses also occur and can be difficult to diagnose without a high index of suspicion and special imaging techniques such as ultrasonography. Most birth injuries heal quickly with simple splinting, and recover fully. Multiple fractures in a newborn suggest a bone fragility syndrome, such as osteogenesis imperfecta, or a generalised problem such as arthrogryposis multiplex congenita.

Neonatal musculoskeletal infection

Osteomyelitis and septic arthritis are difficult to distinguish in the neonatal period. The infection usually affects the end of the bone and the joint, and a better term is 'osteoarticular sepsis'. Infection in the neonate is the result of bacteraemia or septicaemia, and presents with non-specific signs of generalised infection rather than signs of a localised bone and joint infection. Diagnosis may be delayed, during which time the growth plate or joint may be destroyed, with resulting lifelong disability. A high index of suspicion is required in the neonate, with reduced limb movements and signs of sepsis. Fever may be absent or low grade.

The most common organism is *Staphylococcus aureus*, but a wide range of gram-positive and gram-negative organisms are recovered. Some are acquired from the birth canal. Identification of the organism from blood culture or joint aspirate is very important to direct antibiotic therapy appropriately.

The most important factor in prognosis is the interval between onset and intervention. Growth plates and joints can be destroyed quickly and quietly in the neonate. Joint aspiration is a diagnostic procedure, but once pus is identified, the affected joint must be drained by arthrotomy and splinted for comfort. For the hip, abduction splintage is used to prevent or treat septic dislocation.

Birth brachial plexus palsy ('Obstetric palsy')

A true paralysis of the upper limb may occur – usually in a large baby – and as the result of a difficult delivery. Injuries to the spinal cord are rare, and present as a partial or complete quadriplegia or paraplegia. A partial palsy of the upper limb is usually caused by a traction injury to the brachial plexus. The majority of injuries are neuropraxias, the nerve trunks are in continuity and 80% recover fully. As a general rule, a child who recovers elbow flexion by the age of 3 months will make a full recovery. These babies require careful evaluation at intervals to document recovery and to prevent secondary contractures and deformities by a simple program of stretching exercises. In particular, internal rotation contracture of the shoulder can be prevented more effectively by physiotherapy than by splinting.

Microsurgical repair may be helpful for those infants with complete tears to the roots of the brachial plexus, where there is little or no recovery.

Neonatal foot deformities

Most parents have a good idea of what a baby's foot should look like, and are anxious and distressed when they see a deformity. The majority of deformities are postural variations or 'packaging defects'. In the womb, the foot has been compressed in an abnormal position, either because the baby is large, the womb is crowded (twin pregnancy) or lacking in amniotic fluid (oligohydramnios). Soon after birth, when the baby has room to move, the posture improves and the appearance becomes normal. Occasionally, this process is sped up by a short period of stretching in a splint or cast, but surgery is not required. Postural clubfoot, metatarsus adductus and talipes calcaneovalgus, are good examples of packaging disorders.

In metatarsus adductus the foot curves inwards, especially the great toe, so that the sole of the foot has a 'bean' shape, but the hind foot is normal. The deformity is flexible and resolves rapidly, either with a short period of casting or spontaneously.

The foot in talipes calcaneovalgus [Fig. 42.1] has been lying along the tibia in the womb, the heel in a downward position, referred to as calcaneus, in comparison to the heel in an upward position of club foot, referred to as equinus. The deformity is flexible and corrects rapidly.

Postural clubfoot looks just like structural clubfoot, hence parental anxiety. However, the two conditions do

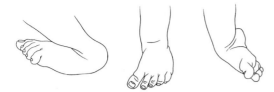

Figure 42.1 (a) Congenital talipes calcaneovalgus. The foot has been folded back against the front of the tibia, but there is no fixed deformity; (b) Metatarsus adductus; (c) Congenital talipes equinovarus (club foot): this can be postural (mobile) or structural (stiff).

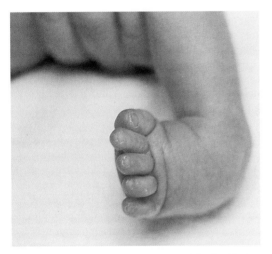

Figure 42.2 Congenital talipes equinovarus. The foot lies in a typical position and is rigid.

not feel in the least like each other. Postural clubfeet are soft and supple. Gentle pressure from an examiner's finger can place the foot in a normal position.

In contrast, 'manufacturing defects' are structural and require surgical correction. Clubfoot (talipes equinovarus) is a good example and is easily recognised because of the stiffness of the deformity when the examiner attempts to place the foot in the correct position [Fig. 42.2].

The incidence of clubfoot is about 1 per 1000 live births in Caucasians, 0.5 per 1000 in Asians but 5 per 1000 in Polynesians. It is more common in males, and is bilateral in about 40%. A family history is present, but both genetic and environmental factors are implicated. Clubfoot may be an isolated deformity, associated with conditions such as congenital hip dislocation, part of a syndrome or acquired because of neuromuscular disease. Serial casting by the Ponseti method, followed by splinting gives good

results in most clubfeet. A few feet will need surgical correction if non-operative treatment fails. The affected foot is usually smaller and the leg on the affected side shorter in unilateral cases.

Another important 'manufacturing defect' is congenital dislocation of the hip. This rarely presents in the neonate because the parents have noted something; rather, it is found thanks to a screening program.

Developmental dysplasia of the hip (DDH or CDH)

The preferred term is developmental dysplasia of the hip (DDH) rather than 'congenital dislocation of the hip' (CDH). This reflects two important features of the natural history of the condition:
• Not all cases are found at birth, some develop during the first year of life.
• Not all hips are dislocated; some have only a shallow or dysplastic acetabulum.

DDH covers a spectrum of hip dysplasia and instability, presenting from birth to early childhood. It is the result of both genetic and environmental factors, so that family history is a risk factor but so also is breech birth. According to diagnostic criteria, it affects 1–2 per 1000 live births, and is at least five times more common in females than males. Dysplasia usually refers to a shallowness or malformation of the acetabulum; subluxation to a partial displacement of the head of the femur from the acetabulum; and dislocation, to displacement of the head of the femur completely outside the acetabulum.

The condition is best diagnosed soon after birth by the use of tests of neonatal hip instability [Fig. 42.3], supplemented by the selective use of ultrasonography examination. Hip x-rays are of little value in the neonatal period because the femoral head is cartilaginous and hence invisible until the age of 4–8 months, when the ossification centre develops.

Ideally, the examination should be performed by an experienced examiner. In practice, DDH is uncommon and not every paediatrician or general practitioner (GP) is able to gain the necessary experience. The baby should be undressed, warm, relaxed and placed on a firm but comfortable surface. Offering a bottle, finger or dummy to suck can help.

The examiner holds the leg to be examined in the hand with the hip and knee flexed and the thumb on the inner side of the thigh over the lesser trochanter and the middle finger over the great trochanter. The right hand is used to

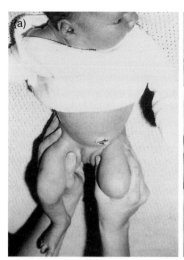
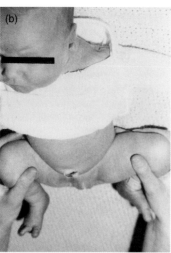

Figure 42.3 Developmental dysplasia of the hips. Ortolani's test: the thumbs are placed over the front of the hip joints (a) as both are fully abducted with the knees and hips flexed (b)

'clunk' or jerk, which may denote the hip entering or leaving the acetabulum (Ortolani test). Then, with the hip adducted, gentle downwards pressure is exerted to determine if the head of the femur is stable, or whether it may slip posteriorly out of the acetabulum (Barlow test).

A fine 'click' is not evidence of dislocation or instability, but the baby should be examined again. A 'clunk' as the hip enters the socket from a dislocated position is the most important finding and is an indication for immediate treatment. The unstable neonatal hip tends to dislocate in adduction and extension, and to reduce in flexion and abduction. Treatment is directed towards gently placing the hips in a position of abduction and flexion whilst allowing movement within a safe arc of motion. This is most efficiently and safely achieved by using a Pavlik harness [Fig. 42.4]. The progress of treatment is best monitored by careful repeated hip examinations, supplemented by ultrasound examinations, which can be performed whilst the harness is in place. Most hips will stabilise quickly and become normal. If the golden opportunity for early diagnosis and treatment is missed, operative treatment and a less satisfactory result are much more likely.

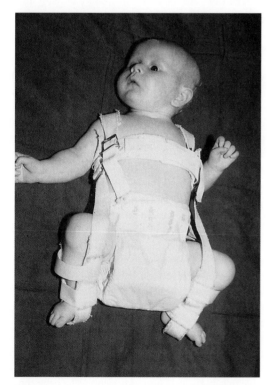

Figure 42.4 Pavlik harness. In the flexed and abducted position, the dislocated hip is held in the reduced position.

examine the baby's left hip and the left hand to examine the right hip.

The pelvis is steadied by the other hand and the flexed thigh is abducted and adducted, carefully feeling for any

Key Points

- Neonates hold painful limbs still, as if 'paralysed'.
- Fractures are common during difficult delivery.
- Fever and pseudoparalysis suggests osteoarticular sepsis.
- Brachial plexus traction injury at birth usually recovers (80%).
- The key to foot deformity at birth is whether it is mobile or stiff.
- Developmental dysplasia of the hip needs to be sought in high risk infants.

Further reading

Baxter A, Dulberg C (1988) Growing pains in children. *J Pediatr Orthop* **8**: 402–406.

Benson MKD, Fixsen JA, Macnicol MF (eds) (1994) *Children's Orthopaedics and Fractures*. Churchill Livingstone, Edinburgh.

Broughton NS (ed.) (1997) *A Textbook of Paediatric Orthopaedics*. WB Saunders Co., London.

Fraser RK, Menelaus MB, Williams PF, Cole WG (1995) The Miller procedure for flexible flat feet. *J Bone Joint Surg* **77B**: 396–399.

Glasgow JFT, Graham HK (1997) *Management of Injuries in Children*. BMJ Publishing group, London.

Griffin PP, Wheelhouse WW, Shiavi R, Bass W (1997) Habitual toe walkers. A clinical and EMG gait analysis. *J Bone Joint Surg* **59-A**: 97–101.

Hensinger RN (1986) *Standards in Pediatric Orthopedics*. Raven press, New York.

Kling TF, Hensinger RN (1983) Angular and torsional deformities of the limbs in children. *Clin Orthop Rel Res* **186**: 136–142.

Pirone AM, Graham HK, Krajbich JI (1988) The management of displaced extension type supracondylar fractures of the humerus in children. *J Bone Joint Surg* **70**(A): 541–650.

Rang M (1983) *Children's Fractures,* 2nd Edn. J.B. Lippincott Co, Philadelphia.

Staheli L (1990) Lower positional deformity in infants and children: a review. *J Pediatr Orthop* **10**: 559–563.

Steele JA, Graham HK (1992) Angulated radial neck fractures in children, a prospective study of percutaneous reduction. *J Bone Joint Surg* **74-(B)** : 760–764.

Svenningsen S, Terjesen T, Apalset K, Anda S (1990) Osteotomy for femoral anteversion. *Acta Orthop Scand* **61**: 360–363.

Wenger D, Maudlin D, Speck G, Morgan D, Leiber R (1989) Corrective shoes and inserts as treatment for flexible flat feet in infants and children. *J Bone Joint Surg* **71-(A)**: 800–810.

Wenger DR, Rang M (1993) *The Art and Practice of Children's Orthopaedics*. Raven Press, New York.

Williams PF, Cole WG (eds) (1991) *Orthopaedic Management in Childhood*, 2nd Edn. Chapman & Hall, London.

Kayes K, Didelot W (2006) Major congenital orthopedic deformities. In: Grosfeld JL, O'Neill JA Jr., Fonkalsrud EW, Coran AG (eds) *Pediatric Surgery*, 6th Edn. Mosby Elsevier, Philadelphia, pp. 2018–2032.

43 Orthopaedics in the Infant and Toddler

Jones' Clinical Paediatric Surgery, 6th edition. By Hutson, O'Brien, Woodward and Beasley. Published 2008 by Blackwell Publishing, ISBN: 978-1-4051-6267-8.

Case 1

A mother brought her 12-month-old child to her GP because he had just started to pull to stand, and she was worried that he had flat feet and bowlegs. Examination revealed a healthy toddler with symmetric bowing of the lower limbs: the gap between the knees when standing was 4 cm. There was no medial arch in the feet in the standing position.

Q 1.1 What is the likely outcome for this child?

Case 2

Jessica, an 18-month-old, presented because she was walking with in-toeing. She had a normal birth and developmental history but walked with both feet facing inwards and sometimes tripped. Examination revealed mild bowing and medial tibial torsion.

Q 2.1 What is the natural history and management?

Case 3

Susan presented at the age of 14 months with a limp. She was the first-born to a young mother who walked with a severe limp because of an arthritic hip. Susan had been born by breech delivery and was referred for an x-ray of her hips.

Q 3.1 What is the diagnosis?

Q 3.2 Could the problem be diagnosed earlier?

Case 4

John was brought to see his paediatrician because, at the age of 18 months, he limped on his right leg and when he ran his right arm was held stiffly with the elbow flexed. When examined, the muscles of the right arm and leg felt stiff when compared with the left, and the deep tendon reflexes were brisk.

Q 4.1 What is the likely problem?

Case 5

Bruce, aged 22 months, was collected from childcare by his mother who was told that he had been limping on his right leg. He was put to bed, but the next morning he refused to walk. He had a fever and was sore when his nappy was changed. His mother took him to his GP, who arranged admission to hospital.

Q 5.1 What might be wrong?

Q 5.2 What would a bone scan show?

Case 6

Mary, a 4-month-old, presented to her GP because of persistent crying and a swollen left thigh. She was a 'difficult' baby with feeding and sleeping problems. There were several bruises and abrasions.

Q 6.1 What is the diagnosis?

Q 6.2 What would x-rays show?

Case 7

Toby was well known at the emergency department of his local hospital. At the age of 20 months he had been seen three times with fractures of both his upper and lower limbs. On this occasion his blue sclerae were noted.

Q 7.1 What is the diagnosis?

Limp, or abnormal, gait are the most common reasons for orthopaedic referral in the infant and toddler. As children grow, there are rapid changes in the appearance and alignment of the lower limbs, such that the bowlegged toddler becomes a knock-kneed child, and eventually an adult with straight legs. Many toddlers who are referred to orthopaedic clinics are normal and have no specific disease or deformity. They are referred with a variation of normality, such as flexible flat foot, in-toeing, out-toeing, knock-knees or bowlegs. It is essential to recognise that there can be just as much parental anxiety in these circumstances as there is about a child with a definable pathological condition.

The general principles of the management of these children are as follows:

1 These conditions are common because they are normal variations.

2 A reasonable description of normal is the mean value of the measurement plus or minus two standard deviations. This is of value to surgeons, but not to parents.

3 These conditions generally resolve spontaneously and there is little evidence that intervention changes the natural history.

4 Overinvestigation of these children should be resisted.

5 Overtreatment should be resisted.

6 Within the large group of normal children with physiological variants, there are a small number with specific pathology. These children should be identified, investigated, diagnosed and treated appropriately.

The toddler with a symmetrically abnormal gait

Bowlegs

When the toddler first begins to walk the appearance of bowing is very common. It is frequently accompanied by some degree of internal tibial torsion and the one deformity accentuates the other. Bowing seems to be pronounced [Fig. 43.1].

Physiological bowing is symmetrical, not excessively severe, and improves with time. Measurement of the distance between the knees (the intercondylar separation [ICS]) in the standing child provides a simple means of follow-up to assess whether the condition is improving or not. Often this is all that parents require for reassurance. Night splints have been abandoned with the recognition that they do not influence the natural resolution of the condition.

Pathological bowing may be asymmetrical, is often more severe, and deteriorates with time. Causes of pathological bowing include Blount's disease, rickets, trauma and skeletal dysplasia.

In-toeing

In-toeing is one of the commonest presenting symptoms at paediatric orthopaedic clinics, because of the appearance and parental concern about long-term sequelae [Fig. 43.2]. Sometimes the concern is from the grandparents or a kindergarten teacher. There may also be a complaint that the child is clumsy or trips frequently. There is often a marked contrast between parent and child. The parent is anxious about the 'deformity', whereas the child runs around the consulting room in a carefree fashion, frequently not demonstrating nearly as much in-toeing as the parents claim is the case at home.

Internal tibial torsion

Internal or medial tibial torsion is very common in toddlers, and usually presents as in-toeing between 1 and 3 years of age. It is probably a 'packaging defect'; the result of intrauterine positioning. It frequently coexists with, and may be confused with, bowing of the tibia, physiological genu varum.

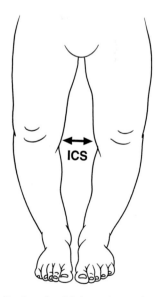

Figure 43.1 Bowlegs: the tibia has an outward curve and an inward twist (internal torsion), both of which accentuate the normal 'flat' appearance of the feet.

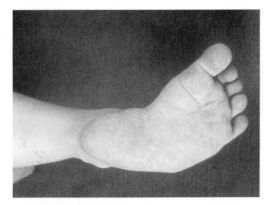

Figure 43.2 Metatarsus adductus. The mid-foot and forefoot are adducted, but the heel is normal.

The natural history is for spontaneous resolution. A number of orthotic devices have been used; principally boots on a curved metal bar with the feet turned outwards (Denis Browne splint). This is used as a night splint and is a potent cause of disturbed sleep and family distress. It may speed resolution of the deformity, but this has never been proven. Surgery is almost never required in normal children. In pathological conditions such as spina bifida it can be treated by derotation tibial osteotomy at the supramalleolar level.

The toddler with a painless, chronic limp

Developmental dysplasia of the hip
Developmental dysplasia of the hip (DDH) may present at walking age because of an asymmetric gait [Fig. 43.3]. At this age, the hip is not painful and does not cause an undue delay in walking. Bilateral hip dislocations may present even later than a unilateral dislocation because the deformity is symmetrical. The risk factors are the first-born female child, breech delivery, with a positive family history. In addition to the usual neonatal clinical examination of the hips, an infant with many risk factors should have an ultrasound examination of the hips in the neonatal period and an x-ray of the hips at 6 months. Delayed presentation leads to a high risk of arthritis in young adults.

Hemiplegia
The typical hemiplegic gait is a limp with a stiff, ipsilateral arm with a flexed elbow. Most children with hemiplegia have a brain lesion acquired in the perinatal period, but the mildly involved may not present until walking age.

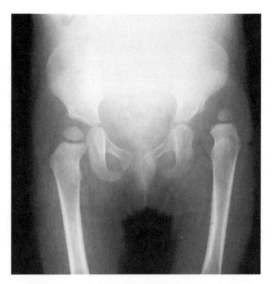

Figure 43.3 Congenital dislocation of the hip. X-ray showing permanently dislocated hip and poor acetabular development in an infant when the diagnosis was missed at birth.

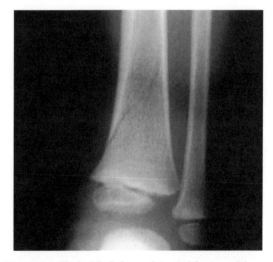

Figure 43.4 The 'toddler's fracture'. A spiral fracture of the distal tibia often presenting as a limp of unknown cause, which is difficult to see on x-ray.

Walking and running may unmask or accentuate the posturing in the upper limb.

Cerebral Palsy (CP) is the most common cause of physical disability in developed countries. It is classified according to the type of the movement disorder (spastic, athetoid, ataxic, mixed) and the distribution in the limbs (hemiplegia, diplegia, quadriplegia).

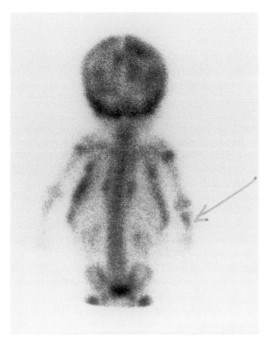

Figure 43.5 A Technetium bone scan is a sensitive means to detect occult fractures in child abuse. Note 'hot spots' in forearm (arrow) and ribs.

Toe-walking

When children are learning to walk, a short period of intermittent toe-walking is very common. It is then followed by a period of 'flat foot' strike, before the gait matures to the adult pattern, in which a heel strike is normal. In some children the period of toe-walking is prolonged and pronounced, causing parental concern and referral to the orthopaedic surgeon.

Differential diagnosis

The majority of these children are otherwise normal and are called 'idiopathic toe-walkers'. Pathological causes of 'toe-walking' are diplegic CP, muscular dystrophy, Charcot-Marie-Tooth disease and spinal dysraphism. Unilateral toe-walking is almost always pathological and the most common causes are hemiplegic CP and unilateral DDH.

Acute onset limping in the toddler

This is a common age for presentation of acute haematogenous osteomyelitis (AHO). Over a period of 12–48 h, the child develops fever, a limp, and then refuses to walk. A toddler's fracture of the tibia may present in a similar

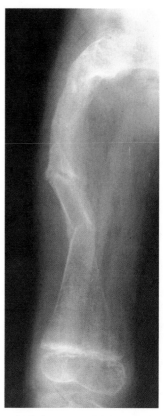

Figure 43.6 Multiple fractures and deformity of the femur in osteogenesis imperfecta.

manner because the fall or injury is not observed and the fracture may be difficult to see on x-ray [Fig. 43.4].

Fractures in the infant and toddler

It is difficult for a normal infant to sustain a femoral fracture. Infants cannot climb, they have limited mobility, and most accidental falls in this age group do not result in a fracture. The younger the child with any fracture, especially a femoral fracture, the higher is the incidence of child abuse. As many as 40% of femoral fractures in the under 12 month age group are caused by child abuse. A bone scan will detect any occult fractures [Fig. 43.5].

Most infants and children with fractures and an unconvincing history have been abused. However, a number may have fragile bones because of osteogenesis imperfecta, and a premature diagnosis of child abuse may cause irreparable harm [Fig. 43.6].

Further reading

Baxter A, Dulberg C (1988) Growing pains in children. *J Pediatr Orthop* **8**: 402–406.

Benson MKD, Fixsen JA, Macnicol MF (eds) (1994) *Children's Orthopaedics and Fractures.* Churchill Livingstone, Edinburgh.

Fraser RK, Menelaus MB, Williams PF, Cole WG (1995) The Miller procedure for flexible flat feet. *J Bone Joint Surg* **77B**: 396–399.

Glasgow JFT, Graham HK (1997) *Management of Injuries in Children.* BMJ Publishing group, London.

Griffin PP, Wheelhouse WW, Shiavi R, Bass W (1997) Habitual toe walkers. A clinical and EMG gait analysis. *J Bone Joint Surg* **59**(A): 97–101.

Hensinger RN (1986) *Standards in Pediatric Orthopedics.* Raven press, New York.

Kling TF, Hensinger RN (1983) Angular and torsional deformities of the limbs in children. *Clin Orthop Rel Res* **186**: 136–142.

Pirone AM, Graham HK, Krajbich JI (1988) The management of displaced extension type supracondylar fractures of the humerus in children. *J Bone Joint Surg* **70**(A): 541–650.

Rang M (1983) *Children's Fractures,* 2nd Edn. J.B. Lippincott Co, Philadelphia.

Staheli L (1990) Lower positional deformity in infants and children: a review. *J Pediatr Orthop* **10**: 559–563.

Steele JA, Graham HK (1992) Angulated radial neck fractures in children, a prospective study of percutaneous reduction. *J Bone Joint Surg* **74**(B): 760–764.

Svenningsen S, Terjesen T, Apalset K, Anda S (1990) Osteotomy for femoral anteversion. *Acta Orthop Scand* **61**: 360–363.

Wenger D, Maudlin D, Speck G, Morgan D, Leiber R (1989) Corrective shoes and inserts as treatment for flexible flat feet in infants and children. *J Bone Joint Surg* **71**(A): 800–810.

Wenger DR, Rang M (1993) *The Art and Practice of Children's Orthopaedics.* Raven Press, New York.

Williams PF, Cole WG (eds) (1991) *Orthopaedic Management in Childhood,* 2nd Edn. Chapman & Hall, London.

44 Orthopaedics in the Child

Case 1

Mary, a 4-year-old, was brought to see her GP because of in-toeing. Examination revealed that she walked with both feet and knees facing inwards by 20°. Her mother commented that she had been described as 'double jointed' as a child. Both had signs of generalised joint laxity.

Q 1.1 What is the diagnosis?

Case 2

Jacky, a 5-year-old, was brought to see an orthopaedic surgeon because of knock-knees. Examination revealed symmetric genu valgum with 6 cm between the ankles in the standing position.

Q 2.1 Is treatment required?

Case 3

Sara, a 6-year-old, was a keen gymnast and was noted to have 'flat feet'. Expensive orthotics were prescribed.

Q 3.1 Are these necessary?

Case 4

A 7-year-old boy falls out of a tree on to his outstretched hand. He presents shortly after with a very swollen, painful elbow and decreased radial pulse.

Q 4.1 Why is this important?

As children become older, parental anxiety about the appearance of their feet, legs and walking continues. As in the younger age groups, the majority of these children are also normal, but a different spectrum of problems is seen from those seen in the toddler. It may be rare to see DDH or cerebral palsy presenting for the first time in the child, but irritable hip, Perthes' disease [Fig. 44.1], osteomyelitis and septic arthritis are all seen.

As children become more adventurous in play and participate in sport, an increasing number and variety of fractures and epiphyseal injuries are seen.

Internal femoral torsion (Inset hips)

This is frequently seen in children between the ages of 3 and 10 years. The in-toeing is symmetrical. Parents complain that their children look awkward and trip

frequently, but the degree of disability is not great. The child often has signs of generalised joint laxity and may have associated features, such as flexible flat feet.

Examination reveals a characteristic shift of the arc of hip rotation inwards, hence the synonym 'inset hips'. A typical finding would be internal rotation of 80–90° and external rotation of 0–10°. This is the reason why the children can sit comfortably in the 'W' position [Fig. 44.2]. It is doubtful if sitting in this position causes the condition, but there is some evidence that habitually sitting in this posture slows down the natural tendency to spontaneous recovery.

In some children, correction of the in-toeing is accomplished by a compensatory tibial torsion. In these children, the feet no longer turn in, but in standing and walking the patellae are facing inwards or 'squinting'. This combination of deformities can look unattractive and gives the appearance of bowlegs.

Management

The natural history of the condition is for spontaneous resolution during the growing years. There is no evidence

Jones' Clinical Paediatric Surgery, 6th edition. By Hutson, O'Brien, Woodward and Beasley. Published 2008 by Blackwell Publishing, ISBN: 978-1-4051-6267-8.

259

that any form of exercises or orthotic devices influences the resolution. The condition can be treated surgically by means of external rotation osteotomy of the femur but the vast majority of children improve spontaneously and do not require intervention.

Knock-knees

Physiological genu valgum, or knock-knee deformity, is often seen in children between the ages of 3 and 8 years [Fig. 44.3]. The majority of children straighten spontaneously. The deformity is symmetrical, not excessive (e.g. gap between ankles on standing <10 cm) and improves with time. Pathological genu valgum is usually more severe, asymmetrical and increases with time. Causes include trauma (proximal metaphyseal greenstick fracture of the tibia or growth plate injury) rickets, skeletal dysplasias and congenital limb deficiencies.

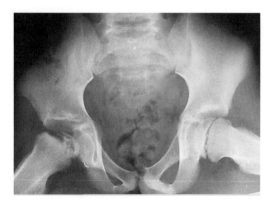

Figure 44.1 Typical x-ray appearance of Perthes' disease.

Management

There is no evidence that the natural history of the condition is affected by exercises, shoe inserts or night splints.

A small number of children with physiological genu valgum do not correct completely. The reasons to consider surgery are discomfort from 'knee-swishing' whilst running, concern about the appearance, and progression of the deformity in the pathological cases. In order to assess the degree and site of deformity, a standing x-ray of the lower limb should be obtained. Correction can be achieved by restricting growth in the distal femoral or proximal tibial growth plates on the medial side of the knee, using staples or screws. When the growth plates have already fused, osteotomy of the distal femur or proximal tibia is required.

Flat feet

Almost all infants have 'flat feet', and in the majority an arch will develop by the age of 6 years. The clinical findings of a flexible flat foot include absence of the medial longitudinal arch and a variable degree of hind foot valgus. When the child stands 'at ease', the only support to the medial arch is the interosseus ligaments and intrinsic muscles of the foot, which are not continuously active. When the child stands on tiptoe, the long flexor and extensor muscles are recruited into continuous activity. In the correctable flat foot, the medial longitudinal arch usually appears and the heel tilts into neutral or varus. This 'tiptoe test' can be used to explain the nature of the condition to parents and to reassure them that the internal structure of the foot is normal. In the flexible flat foot the medial arch is also reformed on weight bearing when the hallux is passively dorsiflexed. This is referred to as the 'toe-raising test of Jack'.

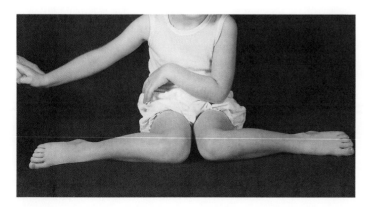

Figure 44.2 Internal femoral torsion (inset hips): the child can sit on the floor in the 'W' position.

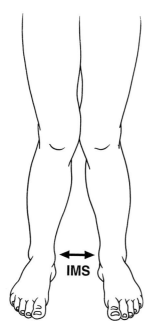

Figure 44.3 Knock-knees (genu valgum).

Pathological causes of flat foot include hypermobility syndromes and cerebral palsy.

Management

Most of the enthusiasm for 'treating' flat foot has probably been based on the observation that with use of any of the popular forms of treatment, the majority of children are noted to get 'better'.

Although shoe modifications and inserts do not change the shape of the foot in the long term, there is some evidence that orthotics may prolong the life of the shoe by decreasing deformation and wear. If excessive shoe wear and cost of replacements are important to the parents, or pain is a problem, the Helfet or UCBL heel cup or a simple medial arch support may be helpful. Expensive, custom-made orthotics are rarely, if ever, required.

In children with normal flexible flat foot, surgery is very rarely required.

Growing pains and night cramps

About 15% of children go through a period where they wake at night, crying because of pains in their legs. The child goes to sleep after an energetic day only to waken in pain and misery, but the following day all is well.

Presentation is often delayed until there have been many disturbed nights.

Clinical features

The child has no daytime pain and no limp. The pain at night is relieved by rubbing, heat and simple analgesics. Examination reveals no abnormalities.

Differential diagnosis

Night pains are a feature of osteoid osteoma, but this is always unilateral and often reasonably well localised. One cause of bilateral leg pains is leukaemia, which can be excluded in most children by a full-blood count. There are usually other features in leukaemia or an atypical story, so investigation is not necessary in all children with bilateral nocturnal leg pain.

Management

Full history taking and thorough examination excludes pathological causes and allays parental anxiety. Reassurance is very important, and fortunately, most parents can accept the situation. There may be a role for a programme of stretching exercises.

Fractures and epiphyseal injuries in the child

As the child becomes more adventurous in play and then active in organised sport, the incidence of musculoskeletal injuries increases dramatically. The weak link in the child's skeleton is the growth plate or physis. In children, epiphyseal separations are common, as are fractures of the long bones.

Specific soft tissue injuries, such as collateral ligament tears, are rare and the diagnosis of a 'sprain' in the child is frequently incorrect. A valgus force at the knee, which would result in a tear of the medial collateral ligament in an adult, is more likely to cause a separation of the distal femoral epiphysis in the child [Fig. 44.4]. The equivalent of an anterior cruciate tear in a child is avulsion of the tibial spine.

Non-specific, minor soft tissue injury is common in the child, including abrasions and bruising.

Fractures in children

Fractures are caused by forces applied to the skeleton, which result in failure of the bone under the applied load.

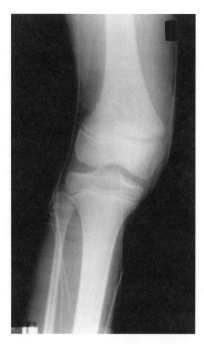

Figure 44.4 Valgus injury to the knee. In an adult, a tear of the medial ligament would be likely, whereas in this child the result is a Harris–Salter Type 2 separation of the distal femoral plate.

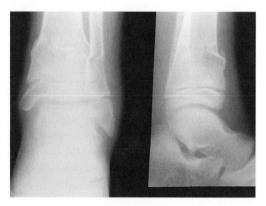

Figure 44.5 Children's bones may bend and buckle, as in this fracture of the distal tibia and fistula.

Because children's bones have different biomechanical qualities from adult bones, the patterns of failure are different. Children's bones may bend and buckle rather than breaking cleanly [Fig. 44.5]. Plastic bowing, buckle fractures and greenstick fractures are all incomplete fractures frequently seen in children but not in adults. Children's fractures heal more quickly than adult fractures, and recovery of function is also faster and generally more complete. Childrens' fractures are subject to a process of remodelling during further growth by which residual deformity may correct and function improve. Remodelling is faster and more complete in younger children and for fractures close to an active growth plate. Hence, residual angulation or displacement of distal radial fractures in younger children is well tolerated and there are few poor results in the long term. Fractures of the femur in children aged between 4 and 10 years are subject to 'overgrowth'. During the remodelling phase, which may last for more than 12 months, the hyperaemia results in faster growth of the injured limb compared with the uninjured limb. During the first year after fracture, this may amount to between 0.5 and 1.5 cm. With this in mind, femoral fractures in this age group may be allowed to heal with up to 1 cm of overlap or shortening, in the expectation that overgrowth will tend to make up the deficit and equalise the length of the lower limbs [Fig. 44.6].

In children, most fractures are isolated injuries caused by indirect forces
- in the upper limb, a fall on the outstretched hand;
- in the lower limb, a twisting injury, for example, roller skating.

These are usually closed injuries, with a good prognosis.

A small percentage of injuries are caused by direct violence, usually road trauma. These injuries are more likely to be multiple, severely displaced, open or compound, and have associated injuries to the head, spinal cord or abdomen.

Fractures in children are treated in many ways including cast immobilisation, traction, internal fixation and external fixation. The choice of management is based on an understanding of the risks and benefits of each type of treatment, with safety, efficacy and convenience being the most important factors.

Upper limb fractures

Fractures occur most frequently at the ends of the long bones but may be seen in the mid-shaft. The area next to the growth plate, the metaphysis, is especially vulnerable. In the upper limb, the most common injuries are fractures of the distal radial metaphysis, the diaphyses of the radius and ulna, and fractures around the elbow. Most fractures of the radius and ulna are managed by closed reduction and cast immobilisation for about 6 weeks [Fig. 44.7].

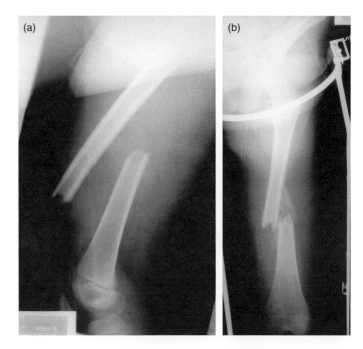

Figure 44.6 (a) Open fracture of the femur as a result of a fall from a tree. Note the gross displacement and shortening. (b) After wound care, reduction and traction, the fracture is healing in good position. Up to 1 cm of overlap is acceptable because of anticipated overgrowth.

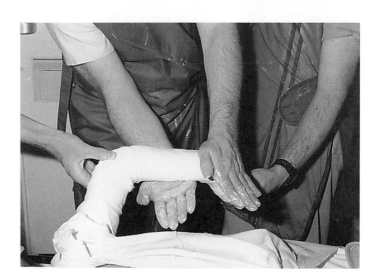

Figure 44.7 Treating fractures in children: moulding a plaster for a distal radial fracture.

Elbow fractures in children are common; there are many types, and a variety of management strategies are required. An accurate diagnosis is required which in turn requires good-quality antero-posterior (AP) and lateral x-rays, and a knowledge of the normal growth patterns of the elbow.

The most common of the more serious injuries is the supracondylar fracture of the distal humerus. This is a transverse fracture of the distal humerus, just above the growth plate, and is usually displaced backwards as the result of a fall on the outstretched hand [Fig. 44.8a]. The fracture displacement or subsequent swelling may result in vascular problems in the forearm and hand and Volk-man's ischaemia. Nerve palsies are also common. In the past, these fractures were usually managed by reduction and casting with the elbow flexed, but this increases the risk of Volkman's ischaemia. The preferred management

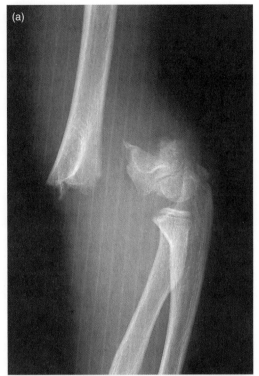

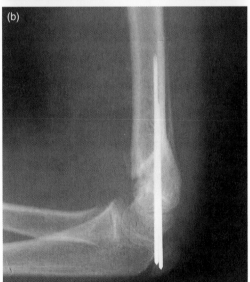

Figure 44.8 (a) Supracondylar frature of the humerus with gross displacement: the neurovascular structures are at risk. (b) The appearance after closed reduction and Kirschner wire fixation.

for displaced supracondylar fractures is now closed reduction and percutaneous fixation with Kirschner wires [Fig. 44.8b; Table 44.1].

Displaced fractures of the lateral condylar physis are Harris–Salter type 4 injuries and require open reduction and internal fixation. Fractures of the radial neck can usually be managed by closed reduction or an indirect percutaneous reduction with a Kirschner wire.

The Harris–Salter classification of growth plate injuries

There are many classifications of growth plate injuries, but that by Harris and Salter is the most popular and useful [Fig. 44.9]. The line of separation of the growth plate is identified on good-quality AP and lateral x-rays, looking for both horizontal and vertical components. Most injuries can be readily classified in to 1 of the 5 groups. Some complex injuries require further imaging including CT scans or MRI.

Type 1 and 2 injuries are the most common and are usually managed by closed reduction and cast immobilisation. Epiphyseal injuries heal very quickly and in Type 1 and 2 injuries, the prognosis is usually good. In Type 3 and 4 injuries, the growth cartilage and articular cartilage are both disrupted. Precise reduction is required (this usually means an open reduction) but growth disturbance is still a possibility. Partial growth arrest may cause a progressive angular deformity in the limb; a complete arrest results in progressive shortening.

Lower limb fractures

Fractures of the femur and tibia are common, and are usually classified according to the position of the fracture in the diaphysis; for example, the upper, lower or middle

---

Table 44.1 Features of arterial ischaemia in fractured limbs

1 Pain, severe and unremitting
2 Pallor of the digits with lack of capillary return
3 Paralysis with inability to move the digits – if full passive mobility produces pain, suspect ischaemia
4 Altered sensation

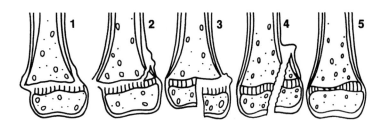

Figure 44.9 The types of growth- plate injury, as classified by Salter and Harris.

third. Femoral fractures can be managed by a wide variety of methods including traction, hip spica casts, internal fixation and external fixation [Fig. 44.6]. The method is chosen according to the age of the child, the fracture type and displacement, and the experience and preference of the surgeon. Younger children tolerate traction and casts very well. Open fractures and those associated with head injuries, tibial fractures and multiple injuries are better managed by internal fixation. Flexible intramedullary nails are the most widely used fixation devices. The time to healing is closely related to age: 2–3 weeks in the first year of life, 6–8 weeks in children and 8–12 weeks in teenagers. Remodelling and overgrowth have been referred to above.

Tibial fractures are very common but are usually more easily managed than femoral fractures. The majority are treated by closed reduction and cast immobilisation for 6–10 weeks. Displaced diaphyseal fractures carry a risk of compartment syndrome, and neurovascular monitoring is important for 48 h after injury. Tibial and femoral fractures cause a prolonged period of limping in most children because of weakness, stiffness and loss of confidence. Time and reassurance of parents is of more help than physiotherapy.

Key Points

- In-toeing needs no treatment if symmetrical.
- Knock-knee deformity is common between 3 and 8 years and usually needs no treatment.
- Custom-made orthotics are unnecessary in flat foot.
- Night pains in legs need full history and physical examination to exclude rare serious pathology and reassure parents.
- Fractures and epiphyseal injuries are much more common than 'sprains' or ligamentous injuries.

Further reading

Baxter A, Dulberg C (1988) Growing pains in children. *J Pediatr Orthop* **8**: 402–406.

Benson MKD, Fixsen JA, Macnicol MF (eds) (1994) *Children's Orthopaedics and Fractures.* Churchill Livingstone, Edinburgh.

Fraser RK, Menelaus MB, Williams PF, Cole WG (1995) The Miller procedure for flexible flat feet. *J Bone Joint Surg* **77**(B): 396–399.

Glasgow JFT, Graham HK (1997) *Management of Injuries in Children.* BMJ Publishing group, London.

Griffin PP, Wheelhouse WW, Shiavi R, Bass W (1997) Habitual toe walkers. A clinical and EMG gait analysis. *J Bone Joint Surg* **59**(A): 97–101.

Hensinger RN (1986) *Standards in Pediatric Orthopedics.* Raven press, New York.

Kling TF, Hensinger RN (1983) Angular and torsional deformities of the limbs in children. *Clin Orthop Rel Res* **186**: 136–142.

Pirone AM, Graham HK, Krajbich JI (1988) The management of displaced extension type supracondylar fractures of the humerus in children. *J Bone Joint Surg* **70**(A): 541–650.

Rang M (1983) *Children's Fractures,* 2nd Edn. J.B. Lippincott Co, Philadelphia.

Staheli L (1990) Lower positional deformity in infants and children: a review. *J Pediatr Orthop* **10**: 559–563.

Steele JA, Graham HK (1992) Angulated radial neck fractures in children, a prospective study of percutaneous reduction. *J Bone Joint Surg* **74**(B): 760–764.

Svenningsen S, Terjesen T, Apalset K, Anda S (1990) Osteotomy for femoral anteversion. *Acta Orthop Scand* **61**: 360–363.

Wenger D, Maudlin D, Speck G, Morgan D, Leiber R (1989) Corrective shoes and inserts as treatment for flexible flat feet in infants and children. *J Bone Joint Surg* **71**(A): 800–810.

Wenger DR, Rang M (1993) *The Art and Practice of Children's Orthopaedics.* Raven Press, New York.

Williams PF, Cole WG (eds) (1991) *Orthopaedic Management in Childhood,* 2nd Edn. Chapman & Hall, London.

45 Orthopaedics in the Teenager

Case 1

Kylie, a 12-year-old, was on holidays with her family. When she was on the beach in her swimsuit, her mother noticed that her shoulders were uneven and, when she bent forwards, the ribs on the right side were prominent. Although Kylie had no pain, she agreed to go for an x-ray of her back.

Q 1.1 What is the diagnosis?
Q 1.2 What did the x-ray show?
Q 1.3 What is the management?

Case 2

A 14-year-old boy presented at the emergency department for the third time in 6 weeks complaining of pain in his left knee, associated with limping. Symptoms were worse after basketball and relieved by rest. Blood tests and x-rays of the knee were normal and a diagnosis of sprained knee ligaments had been made. He had been prescribed anti-inflammatory medication and a knee brace. On this occasion, it was noted that his left hip lacked internal rotation and that the hip went into external rotation during flexion.

Q 2.1 What is the diagnosis?
Q 2.2 What investigations are appropriate?
Q 2.3 What is the management?

Case 3

Sue, a 14-year-old girl, presents with painful knees. There has been pain in the right knee, then the left, and currently both are sore. She has been seeing a physiotherapist for over a year with similar symptoms, including pain, giving way and clicking. Many sets of x-rays had been taken, and were reported as normal.

Q 3.1 What is the diagnosis?
Q 3.2 What investigations are appropriate?
Q 3.3 What is the management?

Case 4

Mary, a 13-year-old girl, complains of pain in her right knee for the past 8 weeks. The pain has been mild and intermittent, but has become more constant, keeping her awake at night. She had physiotherapy for a pulled muscle with some temporary benefit. She agreed to her mother's request to see her GP after she noted a lump on the inner aspect of her thigh, just above the knee.

Q 4.1 What is the differential diagnosis?
Q 4.2 What investigations are needed?
Q 4.3 What is the management?

The teenage years encompass the final period of skeletal growth leading to the closure of the growth plates. The adolescent growth spurt is relatively short but intense, a time of rapid growth in the length of long bones and remodelling of the skeleton to meet the needs of the young adult.

Evaluating musculoskeletal symptoms in teenagers can be difficult. Pain may be referred to the lower limbs from the back and hip pathology frequently presents with knee pain. Teenagers may conceal symptoms and signs from parents. A scoliosis may reach an advanced degree of deformity before being noticed by parents.

Scoliosis

Scoliosis means a lateral curvature of the spine and may be classified as structural or non-structural. Non-structural

Jones' Clinical Paediatric Surgery, 6th edition. By Hutson, O'Brien, Woodward and Beasley. Published 2008 by Blackwell Publishing, ISBN: 978-1-4051-6267-8.

curves have a cause outside the spine, the most common being a difference in leg lengths. Structural scoliosis is a complex, three-dimensional deformity of the spine, in which a rotational deformity is an important component [Fig. 45.1]. Idiopathic adolescent scoliosis is equally common in both sexes (minor curves are found in up to 4% of the population), but far more girls than boys come to surgery because their curves are more likely to progress. There is often a family history and curves may progress rapidly during the adolescent growth spurt. Scoliosis is recognised clinically by the 'forward bend test' and confirmed on x-ray. Curve progression should be monitored clinically and by measuring directly from the x-ray. Curves of less than 20° are unlikely to progress, curves of between 20° and 40° may be controlled by bracing, and curves of more than 40° may require surgical correction by spinal instrumentation and fusion.

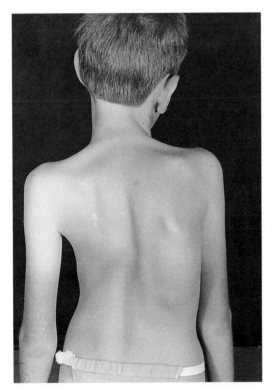

Figure 45.1 Scoliosis. There is a right thoracic scoliosis producing prominence of the right scapula and ribs due to rotation of the vertebral bodies. The left shoulder is lowered and the left waist is increased. The deformity of the spine and chest is more apparent on forward bending.

Slipped upper femoral epiphysis

Diagnoses such as 'sprains' and 'pulled muscles' can be dangerous. They lack precision and are often incorrect, a smokescreen for fuzzy thinking, wrong diagnoses and/or incorrect treatment.

There is only one growth plate that may fail under normal physiological loads, the proximal femoral growth plate. During the last 2 years of rapid growth that lead up to the closure of the growth plate, the upper femoral growth plate may slip, allowing posterior displacement of the femoral head in relation to the shaft [Fig. 45.2]. This process may occur in normal teenagers, but is more likely if the loads on the growth plate are increased (e.g. in obesity) or the growth plate is weakened by endocrine disorders, radiation or renal disease.

The time frame of the slipping dictates the clinical presentation. If the slip is acute (or unstable), the adolescent will have severe pain in the hip, will be unable to walk and all movements of the hip will be grossly restricted. The x-ray appearances are usually easily recognised, and ultrasonography of the hip will usually show a haemarthrosis, as well as the acute slip. However, if the slipping occurs gradually over a period of many weeks, the presentation can be much more difficult to recognise. The pain, which may be mild and intermittent, is often felt mainly or only in the knee. The adolescent can walk, but there may be an intermittent limp. There is usually a good range of hip motion except internal rotation, which is lost or restricted early in the slipping process, and eventually there will be a characteristic sign whereby the hip rolls into external rotation when it is flexed. Early chronic slips are often difficult to recognise on x-ray and the lateral view is the most sensitive projection. Delay in diagnosis of chronic slips is frequent because of failure to consider that knee pain may be referred from the hip, or because a lateral hip

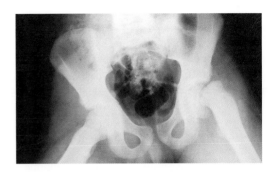

Figure 45.2 Slipped upper femoral epiphysis on x-ray.

x-ray is not done. Delay in diagnosis may result in continued slipping and a much worse prognosis. Such delays in diagnosis frequently lead to litigation.

Both types of slip require immediate operation. Chronic (stable) slips are pinned *in situ* to prevent progression, and have a good outcome if the degree of slip is not severe. The management of acute (stable) slips is more controversial and the outcome is uncertain. Reduction by traction followed by pinning may be the safest option but there is a significant risk of avascular necrosis and later degenerative arthritis.

Anterior knee pain

Knee pain is very common in adolescents and there are many causes. Most knee disorders are self-limiting and are managed by advice and reassurance. However, knee pain may be the presenting symptom of a limb- and life-threatening condition, such as an osteosarcoma. Not every patient with knee pain should have a bone scan or MRI. The history and examination are the primary tools to distinguish the serious from the trivial.

Anterior knee pain is a common clinical syndrome in adolescents, especially girls, with up to 30% affected. Pain is usually intermittent, is located around or behind the patella, and is made worse by exercise and relieved by rest and simple analgesics. It is often bilateral, but one side may be more symptomatic than the other.

Examination is usually unremarkable apart from patellar tenderness and crepitus. X-rays are normal but are done to exclude more serious pathology. Arthroscopic examination of the knee may reveal changes in the retropatellar cartilage, which are sometimes called chondromalacia. However, the relationship of these changes to pain is not clear. Some of the most painful knees are normal on arthroscopic examination, and the changes of chondromalacia may be present without pain. Anterior knee pain can be considered to be an overuse syndrome affecting the immature retropatellar cartilage, which is ultimately benign and self-limiting. It does not lead to arthritis or any other sequelae in later life.

Management is conservative: explanation, education and simple measures to control symptoms, including analgesics, restricting activities that provoke symptoms, hamstring stretching and quadriceps strengthening. Neither arthroscopic examination nor surgery should be advised routinely.

The differential diagnosis includes osteochondritis dissecans of the tibial tuberosity (Osgood-Schlatter's disease),

bipartite patella, meniscal tears, plica syndrome, patellar instability and referred pain from the hip.

Bone tumours

The principal symptoms of a bone tumour are pain and the presence of a mass or lump. Slow-growing bone tumours often present as a mass, with pain as a less prominent feature. The most common bone tumour is the benign osteocartilaginous exostosis, usually abbreviated to 'exostosis' [Fig. 45.3]. Exostoses are benign bone tumours that are usually solitary and are found near the ends of long bones because they originate from aberrant cartilage cells from the growth plate. Some children have multiple exostoses and this may be inherited as an autosomal dominant condition, 'hereditary multiple exostoses'. The bony lumps are noticed incidentally or after minor trauma. They grow slowly until skeletal maturity or a little later. Clinically and radiologically, they are benign in behaviour, although incomplete excision may lead to local recurrence. Excision is advised if the lumps are symptomatic or the diagnosis is in doubt.

A solitary bone cyst usually presents as a patholgical fracture of the proximal humerus or femur [Fig. 45.4]. Often the fracture stimulates healing of this benign lesion.

Painful benign bone tumours include osteoid osteoma and osteoblastoma. These are small tumours that present with night pain, characteristically relieved by aspirin. Diagnosis may be delayed because the tumours are small and are not always easily demonstrated on x-ray. Excision is usually performed by CT guidance using a trocar passed percutaneously into the nidus.

Malignant bone tumours usually present with well-localised pain, which is progressive, disturbs sleep and is

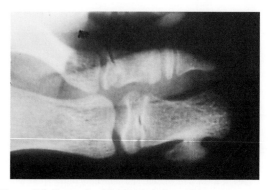

Figure 45.3 Exostosis of the distal phalanx of the great toe.

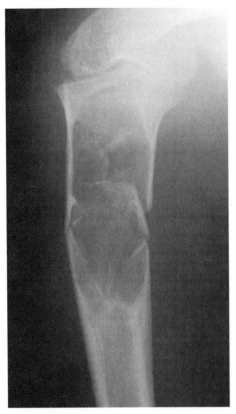

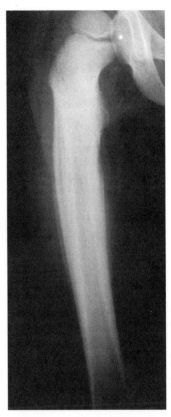

Figure 45.4 Solitary bone cyst of the humerus. Note the fractures of the thinned cortex.

Figure 45.5 Ewing's sarcoma involving the proximal half of the diaphysis of the femur, with layers of new bone and fusiform swelling of the soft tissue.

not easily or fully relieved by rest or analgesics. The rapidly growing ends of long bones are most likely to be affected, including around the knee (the distal femur and proximal tibia) and the proximal femur and the proximal humerus. The two most common primary malignancies of bone, osteosarcoma and Ewing's sarcoma [Fig. 45.5], are most common in childhood and adolescence.

Diagnosis and staging is achieved by imaging studies that may include plain x-rays, bone scans, CT and MRI followed by biopsy, in all cases. Although there are features that suggest malignancy on x-ray (e.g. bone destruction by the lesion, a large soft tissue mass and a marked periosteal reaction), these features can be mimicked by benign bone tumours, bone dysplasias and infection.

The prognosis for saving both life and limb in adolescents with primary bone tumours has improved dramatically with limb salvage surgery and chemotherapy. The tumour must be completely excised with a margin of healthy tissue, and the limb reconstructed, whenever possible, using a variety of techniques including bone grafts (autografts and allografts) and endoprosthetic replacement. Chemotherapy is usually commenced after the diagnosis has been established by biopsy but before the tumour excision surgery.

Key Points

- Scoliosis is common (4%) in both sexes, but is often more severe in girls.
- Structural scoliosis persists when 'touching the toes' (forward bend test).
- 'Knee pain' in adolescents is commonly referred from the hip (e.g. slipped upper femoral epiphysis).
- Pain around the patella is common in girls from overuse affecting immature retropatellar cartilage.
- A mass (with or without pain) in the limb needs urgent investigation for bone tumour.

Further reading

Baxter A, Dulberg C (1988) Growing pains in children. *J Pediatr Orthop* **8**: 402–406.

Benson MKD, Fixsen JA, Macnicol MF (eds) (1994) *Children's Orthopaedics and Fractures*. Churchill Livingstone, Edinburgh.

Fraser RK, Menelaus MB, Williams PF, Cole WG (1995) The Miller procedure for flexible flat feet. *J Bone Joint Surg* **77**(**B**): 396–399.

Glasgow JFT, Graham HK (1997) *Management of Injuries in Children*. BMJ Publishing group, London.

Griffin PP, Wheelhouse WW, Shiavi R, Bass W (1997) Habitual toe walkers. A clinical and EMG gait analysis. *J Bone Joint Surg* **59**(**A**): 97–101.

Hensinger RN (1986) *Standards in Pediatric Orthopedics*. Raven press, New York.

Kling TF, Hensinger RN (1983) Angular and torsional deformities of the limbs in children. *Clin Orthop Rel Res* **186**: 136–142.

Pirone AM, Graham HK, Krajbich JI (1988) The management of displaced extension type supracondylar fractures of the humerus in children. *J Bone Joint Surg* **70**(A): 541–650.

Rang M (1983) *Children's Fractures,* 2nd Edn. J.B. Lippincott Co, Philadelphia.

Staheli L (1990) Lower positional deformity in infants and children: a review. *J Pediatr Orthop* **10**: 559–563.

Steele JA, Graham HK (1992) Angulated radial neck fractures in children, a prospective study of percutaneous reduction. *J Bone Joint Surg* **74**(**B**): 760–764.

Svenningsen S, Terjesen T, Apalset K, Anda S (1990) Osteotomy for femoral anteversion. *Acta Orthop Scand* **61**: 360–363.

Wenger D, Maudlin D, Speck G, Morgan D, Leiber R (1989) Corrective shoes and inserts as treatment for flexible flat feet in infants and children. *J Bone Joint Surg* **71**(**A**): 800–810.

Wenger DR, Rang M (1993) *The Art and Practice of Children's Orthopaedics*. Raven Press, New York.

Williams PF, Cole WG (eds) (1991) *Orthopaedic Management in Childhood*, 2nd Edn. Chapman & Hall, London.

46   The Hand

Case 1

A 3-year old has a fixed flexion deformity at the interphalangeal joint of the thumb.
Q 1.1 What is the diagnosis?
Q 1.2 Is splinting indicated?
Q 1.3 Is surgery required?

Case 2

A 4-month-old child of a diabetic mother has weakness of the right arm. Hand movement
has recovered following a difficult vaginal delivery. However, elbow flexion and shoulder control
have not yet appeared.
Q 2.1 What is the diagnosis, cause (aetiology, pathology and anatomy) and treatment?

The results of reconstructive surgery of the hand in a child can be much better than for similar conditions in adults. Injuries should be repaired immediately. The correction of malformations is often completed in the first year of life, or at least prior to starting school. The stiffness that adults experience after upper-limb surgery is seldom a problem. The hand needs to be protected, immobilised and maintained in an elevated position until sufficient healing has taken place to allow the child to play and use the hand without restriction. A plaster slab or cast must be applied in such a way that the child cannot easily remove it. It must be comfortable and immobilise the hand, wrist and often the elbow in a safe position. In most cases, the tips of the digits should be able to be inspected to ensure that vascular compromise does not occur. Elevating the arm in a well-designed sling under the clothing is the best way of ensuring that the limb is protected. In a child, a plaster should be maintained for 2 weeks after simple suturing, 3 weeks after skin-grafting (e.g. syndactyly release), and almost 4 weeks following tendon surgery. Ongoing protective splinting may then be required.

Congenital anomalies

These are common and varied. A classification based on embryological aberrations is useful in describing and

Jones' Clinical Paediatric Surgery, 6th edition. By Hutson, O'Brien, Woodward and Beasley. Published 2008 by Blackwell Publishing, ISBN: 978-1-4051-6267-8.

recording malformations [Table 46.1]. Unfortunately, many unrelated conditions, such as trigger thumb, syndactyly, clinodactyly, and so on are classified as a failure of differentiation. Anomalies may be localised to the hand or be a local manifestation of a generalised condition, such as arthrogryposis multiplex congenita. Some deformities, for example, certain forms of syndactyly, are strongly familial; others are sporadic, with no known cause. Other associated congenital conditions should be looked for. Some are potentially lethal, such as when radial club hand coexists with cardiac and haemopoietic abnormalities.

Management

A child with a hand anomaly (congenital 'difference') may have functional and/or cosmetic impairment. They will, however, learn to use it with dexterity, provided certain basic anatomical elements are present that provide rudimentary pinch and/or grasp. The psychological effects on the parents need to be managed.

Syndactyly

This affects 1 in 2000 births and may be incomplete or complete (to the finger-tip) and simple or complex (fused bones). It may be part of a syndrome, such as Poland or Apert syndrome. Family history is positive in up to 40% of cases; inheritance is dominant but there is reduced expression and penetrance. Early surgery (in the first 6 months) is indicated when border digits, particularly the thumb, are involved, leading to growth disturbance in digits of unequal length [Fig. 46.1].

Table 46.1 Classification of malformations of the hand

Failure of formation	• Transverse congenital amputations • Phocomelia • Radial club hand • Cleft hand
Failure of differentiation	• Syndactyly • Clinodactyly • Camptylodactyly • Clasp thumb
Duplication	• Polydactyly • Triphalangeal thumb
Overgrowth	• Giantism • Macrodactyly
Undergrowth	• Hypoplasia • Brachydactyly • Symbrachydactyly
Constriction ring syndrome	• Intra-uterine amputations • Congenital constriction bands • Acrosyndactyly
Congenital	• Skeletal abnormalities (achondroplasia)

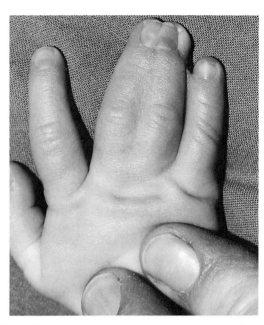

Figure 46.1 Syndactyly, complete and complex (fused) distal phalanges between ring and middle fingers, with simple and almost complete syndactyly between the ring and little fingers.

Clasp thumb

This may be due to a congenital trigger thumb caused by a swelling within the flexor pollicis longus tendon impinging on the fibrous flexor sheath. Alternatively, it may represent a weakness in the extensor muscles, which can be improved by splinting initiated in the first month of life. A deficiency of skin on the palmer surface may be improved by splinting but may need correction using skin flaps or grafts.

Trigger thumb

Trigger thumb is a common and often bilateral abnormality. It is sometimes identified at birth but is usually found in children up to 5 years of age. There may be a family history of this condition. The primary lesion is thickening in the flexor tendon of the thumb associated with narrowing of the tendon sheath at the metacarpophalyngeal joint [Fig. 46.2]. Once the affected digit is flexed, extension is restricted by impingement of the thickened tendon proximal to the narrowing. Usually children present with fixed flexion deformities of the interphalangeal joint. Clinically, the thickening in the tendon can be palpated at the level of the metacarpal head in the palm. Treatment involves longitudinal incision of the tendon sheath to allow full excursion of the thickened tendon through the area of narrowing. Splinting is not effective.

Distal arthrogryposis

This condition, which may be inherited, is associated with skin deficiency, underdeveloped flexure creases and weakness associated with underdevelopment of the musculature. The thumbs may be clasped and the digits ulnar-deviated. An intense program of splintage, initiated in the neonatal period, produces quite dramatic improvements.

Camptylodactyly

This condition affects 1 in 100 hands, and causes a flexion contracture, particularly of the proximal interphalangial joint of the little finger, and is due to an imbalance of anomalous muscles, tendons and fascial structures. In severe cases, the joint becomes deformed. The results of surgery are frequently disappointing but early aggressive splinting can be effective.

Clinodactyly

This condition affects 1 in 100 hands. Radial deviation, particularly of the little finger, is often due to a delta-shaped middle phalanx associated with an anomalous C-shaped cartilage growth plate. Resection during childhood of the abnormal cartilage bridging the radial border of the phalanx can allow the finger to grow almost normally.

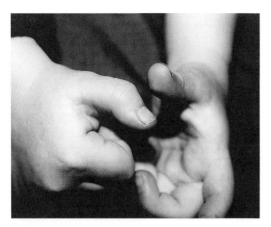

Figure 46.2 Right trigger thumb presenting as a fixed flexion deformity.

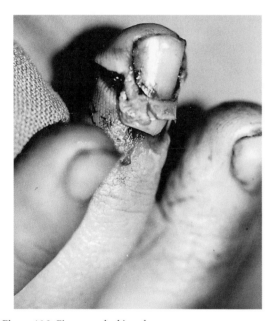

Figure 46.3 Finger crushed in a door.

Polydactyly

Radial (preaxial) polydactyly involving the thumb occurs in 1 in 1000 births, particularly in Asia. This condition is sporadic and unilateral, except when one of the duplicated thumbs is triphalangeal in which situation the condition is often bilateral and is inherited as an autosomal dominant condition. Ulnar (postaxial) polydactyly occurs in 1 in 300 in Africans, and in 1 in 3000 in Caucasians. This condition is often bilateral, inherited in an autosomal recessive pattern and may be part of a syndrome.

Symbrachydactyly

This is a sporadic unilateral condition with hypoplasia of the digits that are short and stiff (aplasia of bones and joints). In severe cases, the digits are represented by soft tissue nubbins. Microsurgical transfer of toes can significantly improve function in some patients. Others may benefit from free grafting of toe proximal phalanges into redundant soft tissues in the first 2 years of life.

Obstetric brachial plexus palsy

This is due to a traction injury associated with a difficult delivery frequently in babies weighing in excess of 4 kg. Injuries to the upper (C5, C6 $\pm$ 7) nerve roots or the upper ($\pm$ middle) trunk of the brachial plexus is known as Erb's Palsy. These improve in 90% of cases. If there is no recovery after 3 months, particularly if all nerve roots are involved, then exploration and reconstruction with nerve grafts should be contemplated within the first year of life. The results of reconstruction are far better than those achieved in adults with brachial plexus trauma.

Injuries to the hand

The repair of injuries to the hand differs little from that in adults, except that the results are generally better. Absorbable skin sutures should be used. Restoration of function is more rapid and more complete, and prolonged hand therapy is rarely necessary.

Failure to diagnose the extent of the injury when the child is first seen leads to unsatisfactory results and the need for later reconstruction. Subjective tests for nerve injuries are of little value and co-operation during a detailed examination is unlikely. Injuries to tendons and nerves may be overlooked until loss of function is noted by parents, weeks or months later.

Awareness of the likelihood of these injuries associated with lacerations of the hand is essential. Abnormal posture of the fingers with the hand at rest suggests possible tendon injury. Most injuries are cuts or crushing injuries. Any wound in a child that cannot be adequately examined, particularly if it overlies an important structure, must be explored under general anaesthesia. Any damage to tendons and nerves can be repaired primarily under ideal conditions. No matter how minor the injury, a full plaster and sling should be used to promote uncomplicated healing.

Injuries to finger-tips

Crushing and slicing injuries with loss of part of the finger-tip are common in childhood [Fig. 46.3]. In most crush injuries, the tissue remaining after judicious debridement and thorough lavage is viable. Any associated fracture of the distal phalanx should be reduced and in some cases pinned with a fine Kirschner wire. If possible, a portion of the tip of the finger should be left exposed so that the circulation can be observed in the early postoperative period.

In slicing injuries with skin-loss, some form of primary closure with a skin-graft or local flap may be indicated. In younger children, the cross-sectional area of the finger-tip is small, healing is rapid and the results of healing by second intention can be excellent. Amputations at the level of the mid-distal phalanx can often be microsurgically replanted, by anastomosis of preferably two blood vessels. More distal amputations or unreplantable crushed or avulsed parts may be, after de-fatting, replaced as a graft with moderate success.

Key Points

- Congenital hand anomalies may be complex and require sophisticated reconstruction, but prognosis for function is good.

- A toddler with a fixed flexion deformity of the thumb has 'trigger thumb', needing surgery.
- Injuries to the hand need absorbable sutures and plaster immobilisation.
- Lacerations may need exploration under GA to exclude tendon, nerve or vessel injury.

Further reading

Flatt AE (1994) *The Care of Congenital Hand Anomalies*. Quality Medical Publishing, St. Louis.

Johnstone BR, Duncan J (1998) Hand injuries in children. In: Conolly WB (ed) *Atlas of Hand Surgery*, Churchill Livingstone, New York, Ch. 21, pp. 135–146.

Smith PJ, Grobbelaar AO (1997) Congenital hand anomalies. In: Aston SJ, Beasley RW, Thorne CHM (eds) *Grabb and Smith's Plastic Surgery*, 5th Edn. Lippincott-Raven, Philadelphia, Ch. 80, pp. 959–973.

Tonkin MA (1997) Congenital deformities. In: Conolly, WB (ed) *Atlas of Hand Surgery*, Churchill Livingstone, New York, Ch. 33, pp. 267–277.

Chest

47   The Breast

Case 1

An 8-year-old girl presents with a slightly tender lump behind the left nipple, which has been present for 2 months. There is no growth spurt or menarche.
Q 1.1 What is the problem and its natural history?
Q 1.2 When is further investigation or surgery indicated?

Case 2

A 2-week-old baby has bilateral enlargement of the breast buds with milk production. The right breast is painful, red and tender.
Q 2.1 What is the diagnosis and treatment?
Q 2.2 What is the gender of the baby?

In the paediatric age group, there are no serious conditions involving the breast in either sex, but there are a number of minor conditions which may give rise to anxiety or inconvenience, and some of these require treatment.

Absent breasts and multiple nipples

Absence of the breast (amastia) is a rare, and usually unilateral, anomaly that is frequently part of a regional dysplasia that also affects the pectoral muscles and subjacent ribs (Poland syndrome; Chapter 48). Breast tissue with the absence of a nipple (athelia) can occur in ectopic sites such as accessory breasts.

Multiple nipples, which are also rare, can occur anywhere along a curved line in front of the anterior fold of the axilla. It is even rarer to have a supernumerary breast, which is usually in the axilla. These can be removed by surgery.

Neonatal enlargement

Galactorrhoea

Transplacental passage of lactogenic hormones may lead to hyperplasia and the secretion of breast milk in

Jones' Clinical Paediatric Surgery, 6th edition. By Hutson, O'Brien, Woodward and Beasley. Published 2008 by Blackwell Publishing, ISBN: 978-1-4051-6267-8.

newborn babies of either sex. The enlargement usually lasts a week if left alone, but attempts to empty the breast by massage will prolong and increase milk production. Unusually overactive secretion can be stopped within 24 h by oral oestrogens, but this is rarely necessary. The engorgement predisposes to infection, which is potentially serious although not particularly common.

Neonatal mastitis

If an abscess forms, it should be drained by a small incision placed peripherally (at the edge of the areola) in girls to minimise disruption of the canaliculi beneath the nipple. As the entire breast is no larger than the areola, extreme care is required to avoid unintentional mastectomy or physical damage to the breast bud. Damage to breast tissue may lead to breast deformity in adult life.

Precocious puberty

This is very uncommon, but may occur in girls as early as 12–18 months of age. Menstruation and bilateral hyperplasia of the breasts should always raise the possibility of an underlying cause, such as an ovarian (or adrenal) tumour or an intracranial lesion, but in the constitutional type, no cause is found and the possibility of dwarfism from excess production of oestrogens should be investigated.

Premature hyperplasia (Premature thelarche)

This is probably the commonest minor physiological aberration, and when unilateral, may present a diagnostic problem. The usual finding is the development of one breast in girls, sometimes as young as 5 years, though more commonly 7–9 years of age.

The presenting feature is a firm discoid lump 1–2 cm in diameter, situated symmetrically and concentrically beneath the nipple. It is initially symptomless and found accidentally, although it may become mildly tender, perhaps in part due to repeated palpation and to anxiety. There are no other signs of puberty, which develops at the normal time.

The clinical signs are so diagnostic that no confirmation by other means is required. This is not precocious puberty, for the menarche occurs at the normal age. The affected breast may return to normal, but the swelling commonly remains static and the same changes frequently appear in the opposite breast within 3–12 months: both then remain static without further increase in size until puberty. Reassurance and explanation are all that are required. Biopsy should not be performed, for it may damage the breast bud.

Pubertal 'mastitis'

This occurs in boys as well as girls. In girls, there is some tenderness, discomfort and a granular texture on palpation; and serous fluid can be expressed from the nipple. One breast is often affected more than the other. It is a temporary phase of development and no treatment is required.

In boys, the discoid, subareolar lesion as described in premature hyperplasia occurs in one or both breasts at about 12–14 years. No treatment is necessary.

Gynaecomastia

This occurs in several conditions, perhaps most commonly in a spurious form in obese preadolescents, when it is formed of fat alone. It may affect up to 20% of boys in early puberty, but eventually resolves spontaneously.

In thin boys, the possibility of a disorder of sexual development should be considered and requires close examination of the genitalia, chromosomal and hormonal studies, urethroscopy, biopsy of the gonads, or even laparoscopy (Chapter 10). The combination of gynaecomastia and small testes suggests Klinefelter syndrome.

Gynaecomastia may arise as a side effect of oestrogen therapy for some other condition.

In most cases, no cause can be found, and if the enlargement is of sufficient magnitude to cause embarrassment, simple mastectomy may be justified. The standard curved submammary incisions should not be used, for the scar may simulate the contour of a breast even after it has been removed. Preferably, a half-circle periareolar incision of the breast provides sufficient access to remove the breast tissue.

> **Key Points**
>
> - Premature thelarche without other signs of precocious puberty is common, and requires no treatment.
> - Neonatal lactation in response to maternal hormones resolves spontaneously, but predisposes to secondary infection.
> - Transient gynaecomastia is common in boys in early puberty (<20%).

Further reading

Brandt ML (2006) Disorders of the breast. In: Grosfeld JL, O'Neill JA Jr., Fonkalsrud EW, Coran AG (eds). *Pediatric Surgery*, 6th Edn. Mosby Elsevier, Philadelphia, pp. 885–893.

Dehner LP, Hill DA, Deschryver K (1999) Pathology of the breast in children, adolescents and young adults. *Semin Diagn Pathol* **16**: 235–247.

48 Chest Wall Deformities

Case 1

Bruce is a 10-year-old boy who is brought by his parents because of increasing concern about the appearance of his deformed chest, which is making him reluctant to socialise and play sport. He is embarrassed about his appearance and wants it corrected.

Q 1.1 Is the deformity significantly limiting his cardiorespiratory performance?

Q 1.2 What investigations are required?

Q 1.3 What advice would you give him and his parents?

Deformities of the chest wall often (but not always) appear early in life and are classified as follows:

1 Primary depression deformities of the sternum (funnel chest: pectus excavatum).

2 Primary protrusion deformities of the sternum (pigeon chest: pectus carinatum).

3 Deficiency deformities of the chest wall (e.g. Poland syndrome).

4 Failure of midline sternal fusion.

Aetiology

The deformity is a primary condition, except in a few of the protrusion deformities, where it may be secondary to chronic asthma, congenital heart disease, a massive lung cyst, diaphragmatic hernia or hydatid cysts of the liver. Extremely rarely depression deformities may be seen in Marfan syndrome, homocystinuria and congenital laryngeal stridor with inspiratory retraction.

A hereditary factor can generally be established, but is of mixed penetrance or recessive, and consequently may slip one or more generations.

Depression deformity (Funnel chest or pectus excavation)

Clinical features

Pectus excavatum (funnel chest) is four times as common as pectus carinatum (pigeon chest). It is more frequent in

males, and may be symmetrical or asymmetrical. These children are usually thin: muscular and ligamentous laxity is marked, and posture tends to be poor. The sternal depression is maximal at the sterno-xiphisternal junction, but may extend up the sternum to any level.

When most of the sternum is affected, the depression is shallow and the deformity may be described as the 'saucer' type. A localised depression is compatible with a well-developed upper chest, and the very localised 'funnel' may be referred to as the 'cup' type.

In asymmetrical lesions, the sternum is rotated, usually from right to left around its longitudinal axis, producing prominence of the costal cartilages on one side and recession of those on the other.

A shallow sulcus may extend laterally on each side from the sterno-xiphisternal junction, a sulcus which corresponds to the attachment of the diaphragm to the lower costal cartilages, that is, Harrison's sulcus. The costal margin on each side may become generally everted or protrude as a boss ('costal flaring'). Postural kyphosis is common, and scoliosis not infrequent.

The deformity may be of any degree of severity, from being barely detectable to one in which the lower sternum seems to almost touch the front of the vertebral column [Fig. 48.1].

A funnel chest may be present at birth, or become apparent at any age up to 16 years. There is a group of males in which it develops rapidly at about 15 years of age, when rapid growth in height is occurring.

When the deformity is severe at birth, there is paradoxical retraction of the sternum on inspiration. This ceases at about the age of 4 years and is replaced by orthodox respiratory movement of subnormal amplitude. In the

Jones' Clinical Paediatric Surgery, 6th edition. By Hutson, O'Brien, Woodward and Beasley. Published 2008 by Blackwell Publishing, ISBN: 978-1-4051-6267-8.

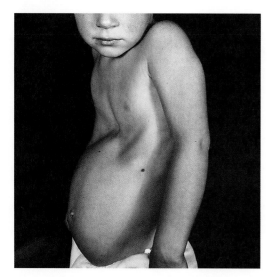

Figure 48.1 Depression deformity. An extensive deep depression centred on the xiphisternal junction. Note the lateral sulcus, in profile, on the right side.

great majority of cases there is a tendency for the deformity to progress until growth ceases, but in others, it becomes less severe.

Symptoms

These are largely related to psychological effects and occasionally to cardiac function.

Psychological features may become apparent from an early age. The child resents being 'different' and, when undressed for examination, brings the arms together to try to conceal the shape of the chest. Older children may refuse to go swimming for fear of becoming an object of attention. Comments from schoolmates may be unkind. The psychological effects can completely alter the child's personality and affect social development.

Diminished exercise tolerance is uncommon, and confined to those with the most severe deformities. Pain may be present but has no obvious organic basis. The deformity is not responsible for any supposedly increased tendency to respiratory infections.

The progression and severity of the condition, and its significance to the patient and his parents can best be assessed by serial examinations at yearly intervals, with photographs recording the deformity at each visit.

An x-ray of the chest is sometimes taken to demonstrate the position of the heart and to establish the distance of the sternum from the vertebral column.

Treatment

The deformity cannot be improved by any form of exercises or brace. Encouragement of participation in physical activity helps some children to become less self-conscious about lesser degrees of depression deformity. In selecting patients for surgical correction of the deformity, it is important that the patient wants to have the correction. Only in very severe cases is surgery indicated in the first decade of life.

Surgery is often performed as the child approaches puberty. In the classical sternochondroplasty, the chest cage is exposed through a transverse incision, with elevation of muscle flaps. The sternum is mobilised and the costal cartilages divided to correct the deformity. The corrected position of the sternum is maintained by struts (usually of steel) placed transversely behind the sternum. Alternatively, and more commonly, a 'Nuss' procedure is performed; this involves placing a curved metal strut behind the sternum using a minimally invasive technique. Both operations cause considerable discomfort and require continuous narcotic infusions postoperatively.

Protrusion deformities (Pigeon chest or pectus carinatum)

High protrusion

This may be associated with a deficiency deformity. The sternum is angulated forwards at the level of the third sternochondral junction, and below this point it recedes as a depression. There may be 'pinching-in' of the lower costal cartilages. The deformity tends to increase with age, and never regresses spontaneously.

The radiological findings are unique, for there is osseous fusion of all the synchondroses of the sternum, which probably occurs before the age of 1 year.

Surgical treatment is for cosmetic reasons and achieves excellent results. In less severe cases in girls, the decision to operate may be deferred until after puberty, for breast development may help to mask the deformity.

Low protusion

These may be secondary to intrathoracic pathology, particularly chronic asthma. In a few of those in whom it is a primary condition, there is a tendency to spontaneous improvement, which is usually apparent by the age of 8 years; otherwise, there is a general tendency for the deformity to increase until growth ceases.

The maximal protrusion is at the sterno-xiphisternal junction or a little higher, and there is usually some pinching-in of the lower costal cartilages [Fig. 48.2]. Prominence of the costal cartilages on each side near their junction with the sternum may be present, forming a median trough that, though locally depressed, is still part of the sternal protrusion. Rotation of the sternum producing an asymmetrical deformity is not uncommon.

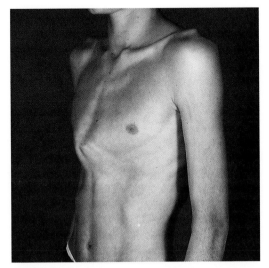

Figure 48.2 Low protrusion deformity maximal just above the sterno-xiphisternal junction.

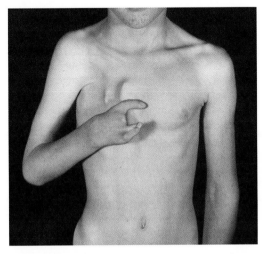

Figure 48.3 Deficiency deformity. Poland syndrome; absent nipple, areola and pectoral muscles with hypoplasia of the chest wall and syndactyly and symbrachydactyly.

Radiography is necessary to confirm the degree of protrusion and to exclude the presence of any intrathoracic condition which might be contributory. The symptoms are related entirely to the cosmetic defect, or to any underlying condition.

Treatment

Secondary deformities usually resolve spontaneously after elimination of the underlying cause. Many primary lesions also show a tendency to spontaneous improvement. In the first decade of life, repeated observation will indicate the trend. Many patients present for the first time after puberty.

Surgical correction is considered for patients with severe and/or progressive cosmetic deformity.

Deficiency deformities

In the usual type, the pectoral muscles are absent on one side and there is a variable degree of hypoplasia of the underlying ribs and costal cartilages. The third and fourth cartilages may be deficient anteriorly, with some paradoxical respiratory movement visible through the chest wall, although this is rarely of any clinical significance. All elements of the breast may be absent, but usually the nipple and areola are present. Hypoplasia of the upper limb on the affected side and syndactyly may occur (Poland syndrome; Fig. 48.3). The sternum in these patients may show a high protrusion deformity of cosmetic significance. The dominant problem, however, is the soft tissue deficiency.

Treatment

Surgery is only rarely indicated for filling in the bony chest wall deficiency or for correction of sternal protrusion. Muscular flaps, utilising the *latissimus dorsi* can be used to provide soft tissue bulk, to be followed in girls by augmentation mammoplasty. It is more difficult to replace absent tissues than it is to reorganise disordered tissues; despite this, much can be done to improve the appearance in these children.

Key Points

- Funnel chest is common in boys, usually idiopathic and maximal at the xiphisternum; symptoms are psychological.
- Funnel chest is treated, if required, in early adolescence by Nuss procedure (minimally invasive insertion of struts).
- Protrusion deformities may be secondary to thoracic disorder or deficiency deformity.

Further reading

Kandel J, Haller JA (1998) Chest wall and breast. In: Oldham KT, Colombani PM, Foglia RP (eds) *Surgery of Infants and Children: Scientific Principles and Practice.* Lippincott-Raven, Philadelphia, pp. 871–882.

Nuss D, Kelly RE Jr. (2006) The Nuss procedure for pectus excavation. In: Grosfeld JL, O'Neill JA Jr., Fonkalsrud EW, Coran AG (eds) *Pediatric Surgery*, 6th Edn. Mosby Elsevier, Philadelphia, pp. 921–930.

Shamberger RC (2006) Congenital chest wall deformities. In: Grosfeld JL, O'Neill JA Jr., Fonkalsrud EW, Coran AG (eds) *Pediatric Surgery*, 6th Edn. Mosby Elsevier, Philadelphia, pp. 894–920.

49 Lungs, Pleura and Mediastinum

Case 1

Jemma, a 3-year-old, became unwell with a viral upper respiratory infection. Forty-eight hours later, she became very sick with high fever, lethargy, cough and shortness of breath, eventually becoming cyanotic.

Q 1.1 What could be the problem?

Q 1.2 How is it best treated?

Case 2

Adrian is 16, athletic and tall for his age. He developed sudden severe chest pain and shortness of breath, not relieved at all by his usual asthma medication.

Q 2.1 What is the diagnosis and its management?

While the principles of diagnosis and treatment of pulmonary disease in children are similar to those of adults, there are additional aspects that need to be considered:

1 The respiratory passages are small and encroachment upon the lumen by exudate or oedema may cause obstruction of the airways.

2 The cough reflex is relatively ineffective at clearing mucus or exudate in infancy, and retention of secretions may have serious consequences.

3 Obstruction may allow infection to supervene and lead to patchy or lobar collapse.

4 Hypoxia develops rapidly in neonates and increased respiratory effort increases the consumption of oxygen; the vicious circle may culminate in respiratory failure.

5 Disturbances of intrathoracic pressure relationships are tolerated poorly and a tension pneumothorax may cause irreversible cardiorespiratory failure, particularly if there is pre-existing lung disease.

With few exceptions, for example, hydatid disease, operations on the lungs and pleura in childhood are of two kinds: the resection of pulmonary tissue and the provision of pleural drainage.

Resection, usually lobectomy, is required for a variety of developmental anomalies, including congenital lobar emphysema, hamartoma, sequestrated lobe, and sometimes

for bronchiectasis. Metastases from osteosarcoma or Wilms' tumour may also warrant resection.

Inhaled foreign bodies sometimes produce few symptoms, and the final diagnosis of an intrabronchial foreign body occasionally is made after resection of a diseased segment of lung.

Pleural drainage may be necessary in three conditions:

1 Pneumothorax, for example, neonatal pneumothorax (Chapter 4); traumatic pneumothorax (Chapter 38).

2 Empyema (see below).

3 Haemothorax, an unusual condition because of the rarity of major thoracic injuries in childhood.

Aspiration of the pleural cavity may be used diagnostically to obtain pleural fluid for microscopy and culture or occasionally as a preliminary step in providing immediate continuous drainage of an empyema by means of an intercostal catheter.

Staphylococcal pneumonia

This occurs usually as a complication of a viral infection of the upper respiratory tract [Fig. 49.1].

Diagnosis

Although x-rays make the diagnosis with a high degree of certainty, identification of the organism responsible is the absolute criterion. When *Staphylococcus aureus* is isolated from a throat swab or sputum, and typical changes are

Jones' Clinical Paediatric Surgery, 6th edition. By Hutson, O'Brien, Woodward and Beasley. Published 2008 by Blackwell Publishing, ISBN: 978-1-4051-6267-8.

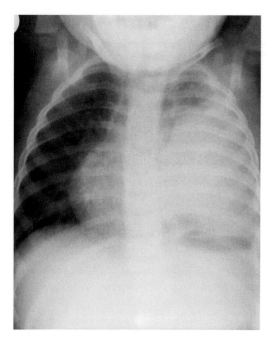

Figure 49.1 Staphylococcal pneumonia involving the left hemithorax.

present in lung radiographs, the diagnosis is at least presumptive. The development of a pleural complication and culture of staphylococcus from a specimen of pus from the pleural cavity confirm the diagnosis.

The diagnosis may be delayed at presentation because the clinical signs suggest upper respiratory tract infection, and the pathological changes initially may be confined to this area. Progression to pneumonia, may not be recognized immediately. The baby or young child may become worse rapidly for the following reasons:

1 Septicaemia, and a shock-like state of collapse.
2 An air leak under tension at one or more of three sites:
  • intrapleural (pneumothorax);
  • intrapulmonary (pneumatocele);
  • in the mediastinum (pneumomediastinum).
3 A collection of pus
  • intrapleural (empyema, or pyopneumothorax) when both pus and air are present;
  • intrapulmonary (single or multiple lung abscess).
4 Obstruction of the airways.

Treatment

Intravenous antibiotics are given, and until the results of culture and sensitivity tests are known, an effective combination is flucloxacillin and gentamicin. Serial x-rays are

obtained because of the rapid evolution of the pathological changes on radiology.

Complications and sequelae

Suppurative pericarditis, meningitis, septicaemia and osteomyelitis may complicate staphylococcal pneumonia, but are uncommon when appropriate antibiotics are given early and in adequate dosage. Empyema is the complication that is likely to require surgical intervention.

Empyema

The incidence of parapneumonic effusions and empyema appears to be increasing in many Western societies. It is more common in boys and during early childhood [Table 49.1].

Aetiology

Pleural effusions are usually unilateral and are a complication of acute bacterial pneumonia.

S. aureus is the predominant organism, but other causative pathogens include
• *Streptococcus pneumoniae*;
• *Haemophilus influenzae*;
• *Mycoplasma pneumoniae*;
• *Pseudomonas aeruginosa*.

Clinical presentation

There are two patterns of presentation:
1 The child who presents with symptoms of pneumonia (e.g. fever, cough, breathlessness, poor appetite, abdominal pain, lethargy and malaise) but is more unwell than would be expected with simple pneumonia alone. They often have pleuritic chest pain and decreased chest expansion on the affected side. There is dullness to percussion and reduced or absent breath sounds. The effusion is obvious on chest x-ray.
2 This occurs in a child with known pneumonia who does not respond to the usual and appropriate treatment. If a child remains pyrexial or unwell 48 h after admission and treatment with antibiotics, empyema should be suspected.

Outcome and prognosis

The majority of children have complete recovery and regain normal lung function but this may take many months.

Investigations

An erect plain x-ray of the chest demonstrates obliteration of the costophrenic angle and a rim of fluid around

Table 49.1 Definitions pertaining to pleural infection

Parapneumonic effusion	Pleural fluid that collects between the visceral and parietal pleura as a result of underlying infection (pneumonia)
Empyema	The presence of pus in the pleural space.
Exudative phase	The earliest phase in which the underlying pneumonia causes accumulation of clear fluid within the pleural space.
Fibropurulent phase	The second phase, where deposition of fibrin in the pleural space leads to septation and loculation. The fluid thickens ('complicated parapneumonic effusion') and contains many white cells.
Organisational phase	The final phase where fibroblasts infiltrate the pleural cavity. The intrapleural membranes become thick and non-elastic ('the peel'), which may prevent lung re-expansion and impair lung function

the lung ('meniscus sign'). On a supine film, there may be a homogeneous increase in opacity over the whole lung field. A lateral chest radiograph may sometimes assist in differentiating pleural from intrapulmonary shadows.

Ultrasonography provides information on the size and distribution of the effusion, and can differentiate free from loculated pleural fluid. It can also guide chest drain insertion or thoracocentesis, if required. Chest CT scans are not performed routinely.

Blood cultures are performed in all patients with parapneumonic effusions. Similarly, sputum, if available, should be sent for bacterial culture. There is no role for routine bronchoscopy.

Treatment

All children with parapneumonic effusion or empyema should be admitted to a tertiary paediatric centre.

Supplementary oxygen is administered if the PaO_2 is less than 92%. Intravenous fluids are provided if the child is dehydrated or unable to drink, and antibiotics are given intravenously. The severity of pleuritic pain means that many of these children need regular analgesia. Physiotherapy has not been shown to influence outcome.

Many small parapneumonic effusions will respond to antibiotics without the need for further intervention. However, effusions that are enlarging and/or compromising respiratory function in a pyrexial and unwell child need drainage. This can be done by chest tube drainage with introduction of fibrinolytics, or by surgical drainage and debridement. Chest tube drainage alone is usually ineffective.

Intrapleural fibrinolytics given through the chest drain have been shown to shorten hospital stay and may be used in early non-loculated disease, or for 3 days using 40,000 U/40 mL 0.9% saline for children aged 1 year or above, or 10,000 U/10mL 0.9% saline for children aged less than 1 year.

Early referral to paediatric surgeons is advantageous. There is a trend towards early surgical intervention, the main indication being where there is ongoing sepsis with a persistent or increasing pleural collection. In many centres, the initial approach is by a thoracoscopy approach (video-assisted thoracoscopic surgery [VATS]) to debride the fibrinous pyogenic material, break down loculations and drain pus from the pleural cavity, and to irrigate the pleural space with saline. If this is unsuccessful or disease is advanced, a mini-thoracotomy may be required to better debride the organising empyema. This usually involves a small posterolateral thoracotomy. A chest drain is left *in situ* to allow drainage of any residual fluid and pus. Surgery is more likely to be required when the empyema is longstanding or there is significant underlying lung pathology.

Pneumothorax

Clinical features

The clinical picture is determined by the age of the patient, the size of the pneumothorax, the presence or absence of tension and the nature of any underlying pulmonary disease [Table 49.2]. Symptoms include pain in the chest and dyspnoea.

Table 49.2 Causes of pneumothorax

1 Spontaneous, often teenager, from apical bleb
2 Rupture of subpleural abscess in staphylococcal pneumonia
3 Neonatal pulmonary disease for example, hyaline membrane disease
4 Rupture of subpleural emphysematous bulla; for example, asthma, cystic fibrosis
5 Traumatic, following chest wall injury (Chapter 38).
6 Perforation of oesophagus by ingested foreign body or during oesophagoscopy
7 Iatrogenic, or example, after paracentesis
8 Rupture of hydatid cyst
9 Postoperative, after thoracotomy

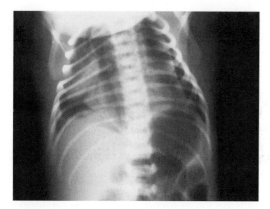

Figure 49.2 Neonatal pneumothorax. The tension pneumothorax has caused displacement of the mediastinum to the right with collapse of the right lung.

Table 49.3 Causes of pleural effusions

1 Pulmonary infection: acute (staph. pneumonia), chronic (TB)
2 Disturbed haemodynamics: cardiac failure, hypoproteinaemia
3 Malignancy: lung, pleura, mediastinum
4 Chylothorax: damaged and/or obstructed thoracic duct

Signs include displacement of the trachea to the contralateral side, and displacement of the apex beat. There is diminished movement of the chest wall, a hyper-resonant percussion note and diminished air entry on the side of the pneumothorax. In the typical 'spontaneous pneumothorax' of adolescence, there is sudden onset of symptoms, usually in a tall, athletic boy with no pre-existing illness.

X-rays are usually diagnostic [Fig. 49.2], but occasionally a huge cyst or unusual types of diaphragmatic hernia may look similar radiologically.

Treatment

Urgent relief of tension by needling or intercostal drainage with an intercostal chest tube is required. The underlying cause may require further investigation (usually by performing a CT scan of the chest). In 'spontaneous pneumothorax', the scan will often reveal apical cysts, and treatment involves thoracoscopic excision of the cysts. Pleurectomy is performed rarely.

Pleural effusion

The accumulation of fluids (pus, serofibrinous exudate, blood, chyle or transudate) in the pleural cavity occurs in a variety of conditions [Table 49.3].

The physical signs are usually unmistakable, but radiographs are necessary and may require careful interpretation to distinguish a pleural 'collection' from such conditions as hydatid cyst or neuroblastoma.

Paracentesis provides information on the nature of the fluid and material for cytological and bacteriologic examination, and indicates the necessity for further drainage.

Chylothorax

Chylothorax may occur spontaneously, or after thoracic operations where the thoracic duct has been injured. Some cases require aspiration or even thoracoscopy or thoracotomy. Replacing the fat content of the diet with medium-chain triglycerides, which are absorbed via the portal vascular system may control, or even cure, the condition: long-chain fats enter the lacteals and travel via the thoracic duct.

Bronchiectasis

Recurrent or chronic bronchitis is the most common precursor of bronchiectasis. This type of bronchiectasis tends to be widespread, although the disease is usually most marked in one area.

Infection associated with permanent collapse of one or more lobes of one lung may be the cause, but the bronchiectasis may remain 'dry'; that is, structural changes can be demonstrated by bronchography but symptoms and signs are minimal or absent if the affected area remains free of infection.

Other causes include pulmonary tuberculosis, hydatid disease and congenital weakness of the bronchial wall (bronchomalacia), cystic fibrosis and the inhalation of a foreign body. In healed tuberculosis, the bronchiectasis is usually 'dry', while in bronchomalacia and cystic fibrosis, dilatation of the bronchi is usually widespread and associated with copious sputum.

Clinical features

Physical signs may be diffuse, localised or even absent, according to the aetiology and the extent of the disease. Clinical assessment of the nature and amount of sputum, any interference with normal life and school attendance and the frequency of acute toxic episodes of pneumonitis should precede any investigations.

Bronchoscopy aims to confirm the diagnosis and determine the distribution and severity. A CT scan of the chest confirms its location. Culture of the sputum is a useful guide to chemotherapy, particularly during exacerbations of infection.

Treatment

Conservative treatment, with physiotherapy, postural drainage and antibiotics, is usually effective.

Lobectomy and/or segmental resection is required occasionally, and in localised disease, is curative. As a general rule, resection should be deferred until late childhood in case progressive disease in the remaining lobes of the lungs develops. When the bronchiectasis is more widespread, resection of a particularly diseased area may considerably improve the patient's well-being and reduce the amount of sputum produced, although some coughing may persist.

Congenital malformations

Congenital lobar emphysema and congenital cystic lung (Chapter 4) may present in older children, and there is no typical clinical pattern. Often recurrent respiratory infections lead to an x-ray examination of the chest and the diagnosis.

A CT scan may provide additional information, and fluoroscopy may demonstrate 'trapped air' in the lobe concerned, that is movement of the mediastinum towards the affected side during inspiration, and away from it during expiration.

Treatment involves removal of the affected portion of the lung.

Pulmonary sequestration

A sequestrated lobe is pulmonary tissue that does not have a normal communication with the bronchial tree, and it receives its blood supply from an anomalous systemic artery, usually from the aorta. It does not participate in the normal function of the lung and is prone to infection. Two types are recognised: extralobar and intralobar.

In extralobar sequestration, there is complete anatomical and physiological separation from the normal lung and the sequestrated portion may be above or below the diaphragm. This is sometimes seen in association with congenital diaphragmatic hernia. The arterial supply is from the aorta (above or below the diaphragm) or one of its branches (Fig. 4.3; Chapter 4).

In intralobar sequestration, the abnormal tissue is contiguous with normal lung which partially surrounds it. This type is almost always in the posterolateral portion of the right or left lower lobe. The blood supply comes from large direct branches of the aorta (75%) or from other thoracic or abdominal vessels (25%), and the venous drainage is through the pulmonary veins.

The sequestrated lobe may consist of a large cyst, multiple cysts, branching bronchi without cysts, or all three of these.

Clinical features

The diagnosis may be made on routine antenatal ultrasonography. At birth the infant may be asymptomatic. In children presenting beyond the neonatal period the usual history is of repeated episodes of pulmonary infection with signs confined to one area. Although the infection commonly subsides, acute suppuration may supervene. Subsidence of the acute phase leaves in its wake chronic suppuration with poor health, a persistent cough and sometimes low grade pleural pain. Haemoptysis occurs occasionally.

Chest x-rays show an opacity in the posteromedial part of one of the lower lobes or cystic spaces with or without fluid levels in a lower lobe. In the acute phase, the opacity increases in size and may produce mediastinal displacement.

Ultrasonography demonstrates the anomalous arterial supply, confirms the diagnosis, and is useful in planning the surgical approach.

Treatment

Resection is indicated because of the susceptibility to infection. Where acute infection has occurred, it is treated with antibiotics and the sequestration is resected during a quiescent phase.

The child with a mediastinal mass

A child may present with a mediastinal mass in one of two ways:
1 A symptomless mass demonstrated in a chest x-ray.
2 Symptoms caused by compression of mediastinal structures.

A symptomless mass

The thymus is large in infancy, and determining whether its appearance on chest x-ray is normal requires experience. Some radiographic techniques cause apparent enlargement.

A symptomless mediastinal mass may develop in the course of a generalised disease, for example, from enlarged hilar lymph nodes in leukaemia or Hodgkin's disease, or as metastases from a known malignant disease. Paravertebral and para-aortic masses of neuroblastoma may involve the mediastinum, often as the primary site but also as metastases from tumour elsewhere, for example, in the abdomen (Chapter 25).

Compression of mediastinal structures

In childhood, this is nearly always the result of a malignant mass, of which lymphosarcoma is the most common. Congestion of the veins of the head, neck and upper limbs from obstruction of the superior vena cava, wheezing, an unproductive or reverberating brassy cough and increasing dyspnoea are all ominous signs.

Lymphosarcomas usually arise in the anterior mediastinum in the region of the thymus, and x-rays usually show a large mass which extends laterally. The edges are irregular, rounded or ill defined; the tumour may extend into the pleura and cause a pleural effusion. The histological diagnosis can be made from cytology of the cells in the pleural effusion.

A neural crest tumour (neuroblastoma or ganglioneuroma) is the usual cause of a paravertebral mass: areas of both neuroblastoma and ganglioneuroma may be present

in a single tumour [Fig. 49.3]. Erosion of the ribs and extension into a vertebral foramen causing spinal symptoms are seen with infiltrating mediastinal neuroblastomas.

A ganglioneuroma is a benign tumour arising in a paravertebral gutter. It often grows through a vertebral foramen into the spinal canal, resulting in two solid elements connected by a narrow isthmus in the intervertebral foramen, a 'dumb-bell' tumour.

Thymomas are much less common and are difficult to distinguish from lymphosarcomas. They tend to grow slowly, to reach an even larger size, and to have a more distinct margin in x-rays of the chest.

Teratomas in the anterior mediastinum are very rare. They are cystic or solid, only occasionally malignant, and may extend laterally into one or other pleural cavity.

Bronchogenic cysts arise close to the trachea or the hilum of the lung; they usually contain air and many show a fluid level in x-rays. There may be a history suggestive of intermittent partial obstruction of one of the larger bronchi, and surgical excision is curative. This is often performed through a thoracoscopic approach.

Management

Compression of the trachea and/or bronchi may cause severe respiratory distress, sometimes precipitated by a supervening virus infection. When a chest x-ray shows a

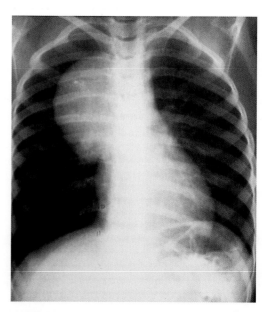

Figure 49.3 A mediastinal mass: in this case a neuroblastoma with calcification in the posterior mediastinum.

mediastinal mass, tracheostomy is usually of no assistance, for the obstruction is below the level of the suprasternal notch. Nasotracheal intubation may be necessary as an emergency. This situation is most commonly caused by a lymphosarcoma, and this presumptive diagnosis should be confirmed quickly by examination of the peripheral blood, the bone marrow or an accessible enlarged lymph node (or occasionally the mass itself). As with other malignancies, the stage of the disease will determine treatment. However, use of steroids and cytotoxic agents, even without a histological diagnosis, is justified in an emergency and brings dramatic relief. The prognosis for most types of lymphosarcoma is good.

Incidental chest x-ray presentation

Sometimes a mass is found incidentally on chest x-ray. Initial investigations should include

1 Examination of the peripheral blood for evidence of leukaemia.

2 Examination of the bone marrow for metastatic neuroblastoma.

3 Examination of the urine to determine the excretion of MHMA in a 24-h specimen.

4 A radiographic survey of the skeleton for metastases or sites of leukaemic infiltration.

5 A complete radiological assessment of the mediastinal mass, including oblique views, a barium swallow, tomography, myelography, computerised tomography and magnetic resonance imaging, as indicated.

In many instances, these investigations will give a good indication of the diagnosis, but surgical exploration may still be required to obtain material for a histological diagnosis or to determine whether the mass is removable.

Surgical excision is generally curative in conditions such as teratomas, duplication ('enterogenous cysts'), bronchogenic cysts and ganglioneuromas. In the latter, both thoracotomy and laminectomy, combined or in stages, may be required to remove both components of a dumbbell tumour.

Total removal of infiltrating primary neoplasms or extensive metastases in para-aortic lymph nodes is often impossible, but there is evidence that even incomplete removal may be of benefit in neuroblastoma, in which maturation to benign ganglioneuroma can occur, particularly in those arising in the posterior mediastinum.

The operative findings, the histology and the results of the preliminary examinations will determine the need for chemotherapy and radiotherapy.

Key Points

- Staphylococcal pneumonia may rapidly lead to air leak or empyema/lung abscess.
- Children with parapneumonic pleural effusion should be admitted to a tertiary paediatric centre.
- Spontaneous pneumothorax is common in adolescent boys.
- Chronic/recurrent bronchitis may lead to bronchiectasis.
- Chest x-ray should be done in recurrent respiratory infections to exclude underlying cause (congenital cystic lung, foreign body, tumour).

Further reading

Adzick NS, Farmer DL (2006) Cysts of the lungs and mediastinum. In: Grosfeld JL, O'Neill JA Jr., Fonkalsrud EW, Coran AG (eds) *Pediatric Surgery*, 6th Edn. Mosby Elsevier, Philadelphia, pp. 955–970.

Balfour-Lynn IM, Abrahamson E, Cohen G, et al. (2005) BTS guidelines for the management of pleural infection in children. *Thorax* **60**(Suppl 1): i1–i21. DOI: 10.1136/thx 2004.030676.

Puligandla PS, Laberge J-M (2006) Infections and diseases of the lungs, pleura and mediastinum. In: Grosfeld JL, O'Neill JA Jr., Fonkalsrud EW, Coran AG (eds) *Pediatric Surgery*, 6th Edn. Mosby Elsevier, Philadelphia, pp. 1001–1037.

Skin and Soft Tissues

50 Vascular and Pigmented Naevi

Case 1

The mother of an 11-year old is concerned about a few small brown flat moles that are slowly enlarging and becoming slightly nodular.
Q 1.1 Is it possible that any of these could be a melanoma?
Q 1.2 How should they be managed?

Case 2

A 2-month-old was born with a red spot on the left upper eyelid. This has progressively grown into a large red nodular lesion and partial ptosis is now present.
Q 2.1 What are the possible functional and cosmetic consequences?
Q 2.2 How should this be managed?

Vascular lesions

Cutaneous vascular malformations are common. Both haemangiomas and vascular malformations may occur as isolated lesions or as part of a syndrome with multisystem involvement.

Haemangiomas

Haemangiomas are the most common tumours of infancy and childhood. They have increased endothelial cell turnover and many mast cells, with a relatively predictable behaviour and life cycle. They occur in 12% of all 1-year-olds.

Capillary haemangioma (strawberry naevus)

These usually appear shortly after birth as a pale, pink or bright red spot or patch on the skin, the so-called herald spot. They may be ablated with laser treatment at this stage. The hallmark of these tumours is their rapid growth in infancy, which continues for 3–4 months [Fig. 50.1]. Gradual involution often begins at about 1 year of age, with a grey patch appearing centrally, and is usually complete by 6–8 years. A small amount of redundant atrophic telangiectatic skin and subcutaneous tissue may remain,

Jones' Clinical Paediatric Surgery, 6th edition. By Hutson, O'Brien, Woodward and Beasley. Published 2008 by Blackwell Publishing, ISBN: 978-1-4051-6267-8.

requiring cosmetic correction. Rarely, these lesions persist and involute later in life, or require excision. Multiple skin lesions may be associated with visceral involvement.

Cavernous haemangioma

Lesions with a deeper component in the subcutaneous tissue or muscle often have a more developed vasculature, and are less likely to regress completely. These 'cavernous haemangiomas' are composed of blood lakes that refill slowly after compression [Fig. 50.2].

Management of these lesions consists of accurate diagnosis and careful observation. Parents need reassurance during the normal rapid growth phase of the lesion. Problems of ulceration, bleeding and, rarely, infection occur secondary to minor trauma. These are best dealt with non-operatively. Bleeding is controlled with pressure unless it is profuse or recurrent. Early surgery is indicated when there is a functional or gross cosmetic impairment, and where partial or complete excision is possible. This is particularly true when the eyelid is involved as occlusion of the visual axis, for even a few weeks can produce an amblyopic eye [Fig. 50.3].

Rarely, these lesions may progress rapidly, with tissue destruction – the so-called wild-fire haemangioma. Multiple skin lesions may be involved with visceral involvement. Very large haemangiomas may also lead to high-output cardiac failure or a consumptive coagulopathy (Kasabach–Merritt syndrome) requiring alpha-interferon or steroid therapy and haematological support.

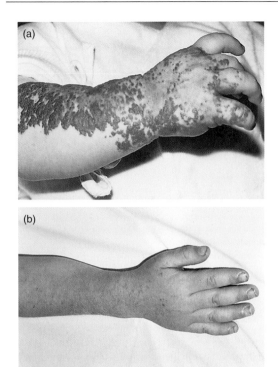

Figure 50.1 The common capillary haemangioma (a) shortly after birth; (b) at 4.5 years of age.

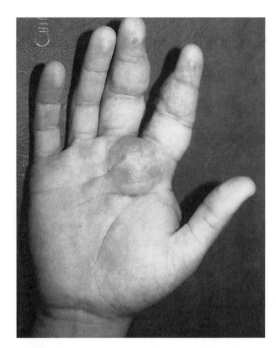

Figure 50.2 A cavernous haemangioma.

Pyogenic granuloma

Pyogenic granuloma is the other common 'cellularly dynamic' lesion. It may follow minor trauma to the face, and it grows rapidly, becomes ulcerated and friable, and bleeds readily. It is characterised by a central feeding vessel supplying a mass of new capillaries and an associated inflammatory infiltrate. Pyogenic granuloma is treated by excision, which should include the feeding vessel to prevent recurrence.

Vascular malformations

Regional vascular malformations, in contrast to haemangiomas, are composed of mature vascular elements and do not regress. They may be capillary, venous, arterial, lymphatic or a combination of these. High flow (arteriovenous malformations) may produce skeletal overgrowth, regional vascular steal phenomena and haemodynamic instability. They may progress with trauma, surgery, puberty, oral contraceptives and pregnancy. When these are potentially life-threatening, or have intolerable symptoms, wide resection, often with preliminary embolisation and complex reconstruction is required.

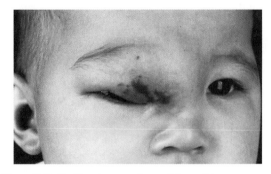

Figure 50.3 Capillary haemangioma of the eyelid. This lesion requires frequent assessment, as obstruction of the visual axis, for even a few weeks, will result in an amblyopic eye (Chapter 13).

Capillary malformations

Naevus flammeus medialis is the 'salmon patch' or 'stork's beak mark' seen on the nape of the neck in infancy. This lesion does not change with time. *The port wine stain* is a cutaneous capillary malformation. There is gradual darkening and hypertrophy of the lesion over a patient's life time. This lesion may be part of a syndrome, for example, the Klippel–Trenauney syndrome (limb overgrowth with lymphatic and venous anomalies), or the Sturge–Weber syndrome [Fig. 50.4] (lesions involving the upper face with possible congenital glaucoma and intracerebral involvement).

Current therapy centres on the use of lasers, with wavelengths selective for haemoglobin and rapid, short-duration target heating times. This coagulates the lesion while producing the least scarring in the skin. The results of treatment in children are better than those in adults.

Venous malformations

These compressible lesions often affect the limbs and may occasionally undergo thrombosis and contain phleboliths. They may show venous insufficiency and also may slowly expand. They can be managed with compressive garments, low-dose aspirin and sclerotherapy.

Telangiectasia

Telangiectasias may also be congenital and may be isolated or appear as part of a syndrome, for example, Rendu–Osler–Weber syndrome.

Lymphatic malformations

Malformations of the lymphatic system range from the small nodular lesions of lymphangioma simplex to large cervical cystic hygromas. These lesions represent malformations of various parts of the lymphatic system, from capillary lymphatics to ducts and sacs, and may also have

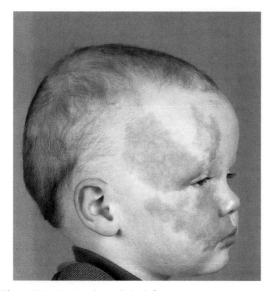

Figure 50.4 A port wine stain in infancy.

an element of venous ectasia. Lymphangiomas have a propensity to infection which must be treated with antibiotics. Well-defined lesions should be excised if possible. Cystic hygromas are usually located deep in the cervical and upper thoracic area, and may be associated with inflammatory and infectious complications. These should also be excised as completely as possible. However, they are not encapsulated, and are not confined by tissue planes [Fig 16.2].

Pigmented naevi

True pigmented naevi are melanocytic in origin.

Junctional naevus

Histologically, these naevi show clusters of melanocytes in the basal layers of the skin. They are flat brown or black spots clinically and normally persist throughout childhood. Junctional activity after puberty is a very slight risk for malignant melanoma. Malignant change is so rare that excision of these in childhood should be avoided unless they have particularly worrying features or if they are a significant cosmetic blemish.

Compound and intradermal naevi

A compound naevus has both junctional and intradermal components. Naevus cells bud off into the dermis where they proliferate and form a cluster of cells resulting in a raised palpable lesion. In later years, the junctional activity ceases and the lesions become mature intradermal naevi. They are believed to be benign with no risk of malignant transformation. Surgical excision is for cosmetic reasons.

Spitz naevi

The juvenile or Spitz naevus is usually reddish in colour, as melanin is less prominent. There is considerable junctional activity and spindle cells are present in the dermis. The presence of mitotic figures and atypical cells sometimes leads to confusion with malignant melanoma.

Congenital naevi

Congenital naevi are found in 1% of babies. They may be small (<1.5 cm), medium or large (>20 cm). These are histologically similar to acquired compound naevi and the cells form nests deep within the dermis in association with hair follicles and sebaceous glands. The giant naevus occurs in 1 in 20,000 babies, and covers a major segment of the body; for example, 'bathing-trunk' naevus [Fig. 50.5a]. Multiple smaller naevi may also be present in other areas,

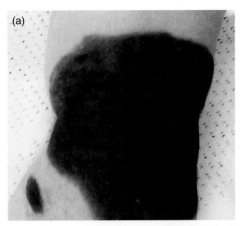
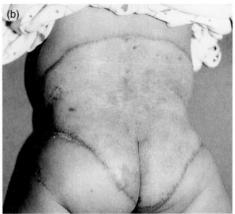

Figure 50.5 Giant hairy naevus (a) at 3 weeks of age; (b) following healing after removal using a sharp curette (and excision of the rim that failed to cleave off with the curette).

and there may be meningeal involvement. The giant naevus is largely intradermal, but may have a junctional component. The risk of malignant melanoma, mainly after puberty, is about 4% over a lifetime in large naevi and may be higher in giant naevi. With adolescents, the lesions tend to become more nodular and hairy.

Treatment is performed mainly for cosmetic reasons by excision and direct closure where possible, or reconstruction with flaps, with or without tissue expansion. In many instances, complete removal is impossible. In giant naevi, extensive skin grafting is best avoided. Early referral is essential, as many giant naevi can be dramatically improved by curettage in the first few months of life [Fig. 50.5b].

Halo naevi

A halo naevus occurs when melanocytes disappear from the periphery of a pigmented naevus. This is believed to be an immunological phenomenon, and lymphocytes are seen on histological examination. The naevus may disappear completely, leaving a pale patch of skin that later re-pigments.

Ephilis

An ephilis or freckle is a localised increase in epidermal pigmentation only. The melanocytes are normal in number.

Lentigo

A lentigo is a patch of increased numbers of melanocytes occupying the basal layer of the epidermis.

Blue naevi

A blue naevus consists of spindle-shaped melanocytes with large amounts of pigment in the deeper dermal layers. The presence of the dark pigment beneath the translucent epidermis produces the characteristic blue-grey colour. The 'Mongolian spot' found on the back and buttock of Asian and black infants, which fades with age, is a classic example.

Key Points

- Strawberry naevi have a characteristic growth and involution and rarely need treatment.
- Pyogenic granuloma may follow trauma to the face and is treated by surgery.
- Vascular malformations do not regress and may need a complex treatment plan best devised after referral to a regional 'vascular anomalies clinic'.
- Lymphatic malformations should be excised if possible.
- Pigmented naevi only very rarely are premalignant except for the giant naevis.

Further reading

Fonkalsrud EW (2006) Lymphatic disorders. In: Grosfeld JL, O'Neill JA Jr., Fonkalsrud EW, Coran AG (eds) *Pediatric Surgery*, 6th Edn. Mosby Elsevier, Philadelphia, pp. 2137–2146.

Klement G, Fishman SJ (2006) Vascular anomalies: haemangiomas and malformations. In: Grosfeld JL, O'Neill JA Jr., Fonkalsrud EW, Coran AG (eds) *Pediatric Surgery*, 6th Edn. Mosby Elsevier, Philadelphia, pp. 2094–2110.

Lorentzen M, Pers M, Bretteville-Jensen G (1977) The incidence of malignant transformation in giant pigmented naevi. *Scand J Plast Reconstr Surg* **11**: 163–167.

Mulliken JB (1990) Cutaneous vascular anomalies. (Vol 5) In: McCarthy JG (ed) *Plastic Surgery*, W.B.Saunders, Philadelphia, Chapter 66, pp. 3191–3274.

Mulliken JB (1997) Vascular anomalies. In: Aston SJ, Beasley RW, Thorn CHM (eds) *Grabb and Smith's Plastic Surgery*, 5th Edn._Lippincott-Raven, Philadelphia, pp. 191–203.

Orlow SJ (1997) Congenital melanocytic nevi. In: Aston SJ, Beasley RW, Thorn CHM (eds) *Grabb and Smith's Plastic Surgery*, 5th Edn. Lippincott-Raven, Philadelphia, pp. 127–130.

Swerdlow AJ, English JSC, Qiao Z (1995) The risk of melanoma in patients with congenital nevi: a cohort study. *J Am Acad Dermatol* **32**: 595–599.

Zarem HA, Lowe NJ (1997) Benign growths and generalized skin disorders. In: Aston SJ, Beasley RW, Thorn CHM (eds) *Grabb and Smith's Plastic Surgery*, 5th Edn. Lippincott-Raven, Philadelphia, pp. 141–160.

51 Soft Tissue Lumps

Case 1

A 1-year old has a non-hair-bearing patch of yellow, slightly raised and irregular skin measuring 2 × 3 cm on the scalp.
Q 1.1 How and when should this be treated?
Q 1.2 What may happen if it is not treated?

Case 2

A year ago a 13-year-old girl whose parents are from South Asia had her ears pierced. She now has 1-cm lumps at the sites of piercing.
Q 2.1 What is the diagnosis and how should this be managed?

There are many cutaneous and subcutaneous lesions that occur in childhood. Some of the more common are covered in this chapter. Vascular and pigmented lesions of the skin are discussed in Chapter 50.

Warts

These are small epidermal tumours produced in response to papilloma virus infections of the skin. They are contagious to a limited degree. Those on the soles of the feet can cause discomfort on weight-bearing. Treatment of troublesome lesions involves destruction of the lesion by topical application of liquid nitrogen, salicylic acid or podophyllin paint, or curettage.

Molluscum contagiosum

This is caused by a pox virus, which produces clusters of pink papules with a central plug which can be squeezed out. They usually resolve after 2 months or may be treated like warts.

Epidermal and pilar cysts

These are common cysts of epidermal and pilar (=hair follicle= tricholemmal) origin, respectively. Although most

often seen in adults, they are not uncommon in children. Treatment is by complete surgical excision.

Dermoid cysts

These are most commonly found in the head and neck. Dermoid cysts contain epithelium and adnexal structures, such as sweat glands or hair follicles of varying degrees of differentiation. Nasal dermoids may have a small pit or sinus with associated hair growth. External angular dermoids appear in the lateral eyebrow region [Fig. 16.7]. They are sometimes located under the pericranium and appear hard and fixed. Treatment is by complete surgical excision; however, for nasal dermoids possible deep, intracranial extension should be excluded.

Pilomatrixoma

This relatively common skin appendage tumour occurs on the face, neck and upper extremities of young children. It is a hard, non-tender and irregular intradermal or subcutaneous lesion, which may appear white or yellow in colour through the skin [Fig. 51.1]. They enlarge slowly. It is characterised histologically by areas of calcification and 'ghost cells'. Excision is recommended. Multiple lesions should arouse suspicion of Gardner's syndrome.

Jones' Clinical Paediatric Surgery, 6th edition. By Hutson, O'Brien, Woodward and Beasley. Published 2008 by Blackwell Publishing, ISBN: 978-1-4051-6267-8.

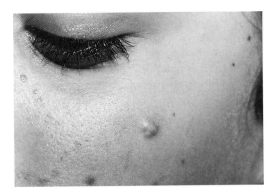

Figure 51.1 Pilomatrixoma.

Naevus sebaceous

Naevus sebaceous is present at birth and appears as a yellowish, slightly raised lesion, usually on the scalp or face. There is a 15–20% incidence of basal cell carcinoma developing during adulthood if it is left untreated. These lesions are best excised electively during early childhood.

Hypertrophic scars and keloids

Some children tend to produce thick red scars that take 1–2 years to involute to become acceptably pale and flat. This is more common on the earlobes, sternum and deltoid regions, particularly in Africans and Asians. A keloid continues to grow beyond the margins of the original wound [Fig. 51.2]. The appearance is often very unsatisfactory, and the scars are itchy and sometimes cause contractures. Management can be difficult and involves counselling parents (about the time course and expected outcome), intralesional corticosteroid injections, topical application of vitamin E cream, pressure (often applied through specially designed lycra garments) and the use of silicon gel sheeting.

Ganglia

Ganglia contain gelatinous synovial fluid and frequently arise from joints, particularly the wrist, principally from the scapholunate ligament. They also arise from tendon sheaths. They may be uncomfortable and can be treated

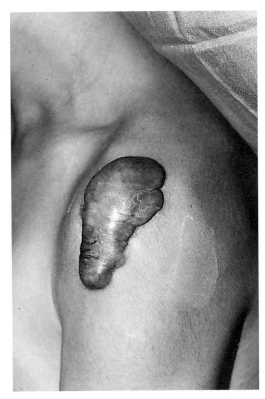

Figure 51.2 Keloid scar in an adolescent Asian male following a BCG vaccination.

with aspiration and corticosteroid injections followed by splintage, or by excision.

Neurofibromatosis

This autosomal dominant condition affects 1 in 3000 children, and may present as café-au-lait pigmented spots or soft tissue tumours. These consist of fibroblasts, Schwann cells and nerve fibres. Large plexiform lesions of the nerve trunks may be quite disfiguring. Neurofibrosarcoma occurs in approximately 5% of patients later in adulthood.

Fibromatosis

This is an idiopathic, self-limiting fibroblastic proliferation that infiltrates locally, and tends to recur, but never metastasises. Fibromatosis often affects the digits or palm, and may be aggressive (e.g. extra-abdominal desmoid).

Soft-tissue sarcomas

These make up 6–8% of all malignancies in childhood, with rhabdomyosarcoma and undifferentiated sarcoma being the most common. After diagnostic biopsy and complete staging, combined treatment with chemotherapy, wide excision, and sometimes radiotherapy is planned. Sophisticated reconstruction, often with microsurgically transferred tissues, may be required.

> **Key Points**
> - Unless a firm diagnosis of a benign tumour can be made, excision of a soft tissue lump to exclude malignancy is prudent.
> - Naevus sebaceous is best treated by excision to prevent basal cell carcinoma in adulthood.
> - Keloid scars may need local treatment.
> - A ganglion may be treated by aspiration and corticosteroid injection.

Further reading

Cohen K, Peacock EE (1990) Keloids and hypertrophic scars. In: McCarthy JG (ed) *Plastic Surgery Volume 1*, W.B. Saunders, Philadelphia, pp. 732–747.

Miranda EP, Mathes SJ (2006) Congenital defects of the skin, connective tissues, muscles, tendons and hands. In: Grosfeld JL, O'Neill JA Jr., Fonkalsrud EW, Coran AG (eds) *Pediatric Surgery*, 6th Edn. Mosby Elsevier, Philadelphia, pp. 2061–2078.

Zarem HA, Lowe NJ (1997) Benign growths and generalized skin disorders. In: Aston SJ, Beasley RW, Thorn CHM (eds) *Grabb and Smith's Plastic Surgery*, 5th Edn. Lippincott-Raven, Philadelphia, pp. 141–160.

Answers to Case Questions

52 Answers to Case Questions

Introduction

1 Antenatal diagnosis – surgical aspects

1.1 Regular ultrasounds to monitor progress; ongoing discussion with, and counselling by, paediatric surgeon.

1.2 Yes; antenatal ultrasound allows antibiotic prophylaxis and early postnatal investigation to be initiated before kidney becomes further damaged by infection and/or obstruction.

2.1 Chromosomal analysis and search for other major anomalies.

2.2 No: only rarely is time or mode of delivery important.

2 The care and transport of the newborn

1.1 Wrap the exposed viscera and abdomen in plastic wrap (be careful not to twist bowel); insert IV line for 4% dextrose and 1/5 (0.18%) normal saline; nil orally; nasogastric tube with aspiration; put baby in incubator; check for other anomalies; talk to parents about surgery and prognosis (good); obtain consent for transport and surgery; take photograph for parents.

2.1 Bronchopulmonary damage; pneumothorax.

2.2 Avoid high airway pressures during resuscitation and allow baby to breathe spontaneously. The key metabolic problems are respiratory.

3 The child in hospital

1.1 No. General anaesthetic is required to prevent fear and keep the patient still during surgery. Local anaesthetic is used for postoperative analgesia.

1.2 Removal of sutures (with blade or scissors) is frightening to children, because they assume it will be painful (which it is).

1.3 Allow regular washing and activity.

Jones' Clinical Paediatric Surgery, 6th edition. By Hutson, O'Brien, Woodward and Beasley. Published 2008 by Blackwell Publishing, ISBN: 978-1-4051-6267-8.

2.1 Fear of pain, staying overnight away from home and parents, unknown technology, unfamiliar people.

Neonatal emergencies

4 Respiratory distress in the newborn

1.1 Cystic lung disease (sequestration; cystic adenomatoid malformation; congenital tumour [e.g. teratoma]).

1.2 Excision.

2.1 Pneumothorax ± tension.

2.2 Intercostal drainage: formal catheter (fourth IC space, mid-axillary line) or needle (second IC space, mid-clavicular line) if urgent.

5 Diaphragmatic hernia

1.1 Diaphragmatic hernia.

1.2 X-ray of chest and abdomen (± insertion of NG tube to determine position of stomach).

1.3 Pulmonary hypoplasia and pulmonary hypertension are main intrinsic factors. Iatrogenic factors include excessive ventilation with pneumothorax, rough handling or premature surgical intervention prior to stabilisation.

2.1 No.

2.2 Insert nasogastric tube and apply gentle suction to keep bowel decompressed.

2.3 Tension pneumothorax.

6 Oesophageal atresia and tracheo-oesophageal fistula

1.1 Pass a stiff 10-French catheter gently via the mouth: arrested at 9–11 cm from gums confirms diagnosis of oesophageal atresia.

1.2 Yes: look for VATER/CHARGE and others.

1.3 Standard neonatal preoperative 'first aid', plus ten minutely suction of the oesophagus.

2.1 VATER: clinical examination and imaging.

2.2 Renal and cardiac ultrasonography, as well as a preoperative workup.

7 Bowel obstruction

1.1 Hirschsprung disease; small bowel atresia; volvulus neonatorum; meconium ileus.

1.2 Call the Neonatal Emergency Transport Service (NETS).

1.3 See under 'General Treatment'.

2.1 Rectal biopsy for histochemical tests and an examination for ganglion cells.

2.2 Neonatal primary pull-through (laparotomy/transanal ± laparoscopy) or colostomy above transition zone at diagnosis and pull-through operation at 3–6 months of age.

2.3 Initial prognosis is good and surgery is life saving, but there are some problems with long-term morbidity, especially faecal soiling, constipation and proximal gut function.

3.1 Duodenal atresia; volvulus neonatorum; high jejunal atresia.

3.2 Plain x-ray and barium meal.

3.3 Volvulus neonatorum is one of the most urgent conditions seen by paediatric surgeons.

8 Abdominal wall defects

1.1 Exomphalos.

1.2 Failure of correct formation of the umbilical ring with embryonic folding.

1.3 See Table 8.1

1.4 Aim to excise sac and umbilical cord and close defect primarily. Prognosis reasonable if no other anomalies present.

2.1 Yes, if 'first aid' is good.

2.2 Heat and water loss cause rapid hypothermia and dehydration.

2.3 Yes, but not very common, except for secondary atresia of the bowel compressed at level of defect in abdominal wall.

3.1 Bladder exstrophy.

3.2 Yes, but prognosis for urinary continence is guarded.

3.3 Each corpus cavernosum forms separately. Sexual function should be fair, but not normal (penis bent and short).

9 Spina bifida

1.1 Level and appearance at birth, motor and sensory levels, any secondary deformities, other abnormalities (e.g. hydrocephalus).

1.2 There is a high risk of Arnold-Chiari malformation and associated hydrocephalus.

1.3 Intellect should be reasonable, as long as hydrocephalus is controlled; walking is unlikely although hip flexion and adduction may be preserved.

2.1 Incontinence ± partial outlet obstruction, infection, stone, renal failure.

2.2 Clean intermittent catheter for urine (± reconstruction procedures); diet and washouts/laxatives for faeces.

10 Disorders of sexual development

1.1 Any child with (a) apparently enlarged clitoris; (b) apparent hypospadias with bifid scrotum and/or undescended testes; (c) truly ambiguous genitalia.

1.2 As much as possible, so they understand and can participate in decision-making.

1.3 Genital anomaly is a medical and social emergency, requiring urgent referral to a tertiary centre.

1.4 (a) Possible adult fertility; (b) relative degree of development of male versus female organs.

2.1 No.

2.2 Bifid 'scrotum' and/or bilateral or unilateral 'cryptorchidism'.

11 Anorectal anomalies

1.1 Same as for Case 1, Chapter 2.

1.2 E ither definitive surgery if low anomaly, or colostomy if high anomaly, then pull-through at about 3 months.

1.3 Outcome for faecal continence poor for more severe anomalies: bowel washouts ± diet and laxative treatment required. Less severe anomalies with better outlook, but soiling or constipation still common.

2.1 MRI.

2.2 Diet and laxatives or regular washouts (via anus or appendicostomy).

Head and neck

12 The scalp, skull and brain

1.1 Head circumference crosses the percentiles (hydrocephalus), or abnormal shape of skull.

2.1 Headaches are frequent or 'different'; there is significant child or parental anxiety; there are other signs of raised ICP or focal signs.

2.2 Some are benign (e.g. pilocystic astrocytoma, craniopharyngioma, pineocytoma) and may be cured with surgery. Germinoma and medulloblastoma are malignant, but prognosis is quite good with treatment. The rest do badly (e.g. brain stem glioma, pineoblastoma, disseminated medulloblastoma or ependymoma).

3.1 Not always. Neurosurgical referral is required.

4.1 Surgery is possible, but prognosis varies. Occipital lesions are worse than sincipital (because of blindness/ataxia/hydrocephalus). Genetic counselling is needed.

5.1 Plagiocephaly with 'sticky' lambdoid suture. Often improves but strip craniectomy is needed sometimes. Definite synostosis does need surgery.

13 The eye

1.1 Amblyopia may develop if squint ± poor vision is untreated.

1.2 Eye examination, including cover test and check of vision.

2.1 Yes: there is nystagmus which may be secondary to poor vision.

2.2 Vision and eye examination, referral to ophthalmologist.

3.1 Cause is nasolacrimal duct obstruction, which resolves in 95% by 1 year. Probing (under GA) reserved for persisting symptoms only.

3.2 Antibiotic drops only needed if secondary infection with conjunctivitis occurs.

4.1 History and examination should reveal cause, for example, foreign body.

14 The ear, nose and throat

1.1 A pale, opaque membrane occurs with fluid behind the membrane and/or inflammatory thickening.

1.2 Amoxycillin 40 mg/kg/day in × 3 doses for 5 days.

1.3 The infant has otitis media with effusion (± acute suppuration). The fluid in the middle ear reduces hearing.

2.1. Tonsillectomy plus adenoidectomy is recommended if attacks of tonsillitis are very frequent.

3.1 Physical examination to determine site of stridor plus degree of airway obstruction, followed by flexible laryngoscopy.

3.2 Nose blocked, stenosis, choanal atresia; glossoptosis; laryngomalacia; vocal cord lesions; subglottic stenosis; tracheomalacia.

15 Cleft lip, palate and craniofacial anomalies

1.1 Pierre Robin sequence with mandibular hypoplasia and secondary cleft palate.

1.2 Nurse prone ± airway for first few days. Long-term spontaneous resolution with growth.

2.1 4% if no parents affected.

2.2 16% if parents affected.

3.1 Apert syndrome.

3.2 Craniofacial surgery for synostosis, repair of fingers, genetic counselling.

3.3 Mental deficiency is present in a significant number of patients.

16 Abnormalities of the neck and face

1.1 Cervical lymphadenitis, abscess, sialectasis.

1.2 Once proven/suspected to contain pus: incision and drainage.

2.1 External angular dermoid; excision.

3.1 Thyroglossal cyst ± infection, ectopic thyroid, dermoid cyst, submental lymph node (goitre).

3.2 Sistrunk operation (removal of cyst, track including middle 1/3 of hyoid bone).

Abdomen

17 The umbilicus

1.1 No; spontaneous closure in >90% by 2 years of age.

1.2 If not closed by 2–3 years, because of increasing risk of incarceration.

1.3 Normal gap in abdominal wall of fetus for placental vessels (umbilical arteries × 2, umbilical vein × 1).

2.1 Residual necrotic tissue from cord stump colonised by skin organisms. Granulation tissue ('granuloma') is produced in response to subacute inflammation. Silver nitrate cauterisation or excision.

3.1 Extraperitoneal fat.

3.2 No.

3.3 Yes, if symptoms are troublesome.

18 Vomiting in the first months of life

1.1 Observe visible peristalsis and palpate pyloric tumour.

1.2 Refer to paediatric surgeon.

1.3 Serum electrolytes and acid–base looking for metabolic alkalosis.

2.1 Malrotation with volvulus.

2.2 Barium meal.

2.3 Ladd's operation (laparotomy and detorsion of bowel)–extremely urgent.

3.1 Gastro-oesophageal reflux.

3.2 Reduce handling after feeds, thickening feeds.

19 Intussusception

1.1 Intussusception.

1.2 Rectal examination, plain abdominal x-ray and abdominal ultrasound or gas enema.

1.3 7% risk.

2.1 Bowel obstruction secondary to intussusception (or other causes).

2.2 Resuscitation with IV fluids, nasogastric tube decompression, cross-match blood.

2.3 Operative reduction ± resection.

20 Abdominal pain: Appendicitis

1.1 Mesenteric adenitis, but should exclude urinary infection.

1.2 Urine micro and culture, rectal examination.

2.1 Appendicitis (retrocaecal/retroileal).

2.2 No, as you have already made a diagnosis.

21 Recurrent abdominal pain

1.1 Parents often worry that pains are caused by cancer, because of similar symptoms in an elderly relative.

1.2 Frequent short-lived pains, referred to periumbilical region, perhaps associated with stress in the child's life. Physical examination rarely shows anything other than constipation.

1.3 Surgeons' role is to exclude serious disease after careful history and physical examination, and then reassure.

22 Constipation

1.1 Needs diet (fluid and fibre increase) and laxative treatment. Rule out organic causes. (Tables 22.1, 22.2)

2.1 Needs exclusion of organic causes, especially Hirschsprung disease and slow transit constipation with intestinal neuronal dysplasia. Initial management includes enemas ± faecal disimpaction (under GA).

23 Bleeding from the alimentary canal

1.1 See Table 23.3.

1.2 Anal fissure, secondary to constipation.

1.3 Correct the constipation with diet and laxatives.

2.1 Meckel's diverticulum, duplication, peptic ulcer, varices.

24 Inflammatory bowel disease

1.1 Ulcerative colitis; barium enema, colonoscopy with biopsy, full blood examination and bacteriological cultures.

2.1 'Top-and-tail' endoscopy with biopsies, barium meal and follow-through, full blood examination, liver function tests, stool cultures.

2.2 Extent of disease; extra-intestinal signs and symptoms; histology.

25 The child with an abdominal mass

1.1 Hydronephrosis.

1.2 Renal ultrasound, DTPA scan ± cystoscopy with retrograde pyelogram to distinguish pelvi-ureteric junction obstruction from vesico-ureteric junction obstruction.

2.1 Wilms' tumour or neuroblastoma, once ultrasound confirms lesion is solid.

2.2 Biopsy/excision, chemotherapy ± radiotherapy.

3.1 Catecholamine measurements (VMA, HMA) in urine, CT scan, bone scan, bone marrow, FBE; neuroblastoma.

3.2 Prognosis is poor, but some still curable with chemotherapy and surgery.

26 Spleen, pancreas and biliary tract

1.1 Trauma (handle-bar, child abuse, MCA), bile duct stone, idiopathic.

1.2 Serum lipase level, epigastric peritonism and ileus, ultrasound/CT scan shows swollen gland.

1.3 A cystic cavity secondary to leakage of enzymes from the pancreatic duct.

2.1 Liver function tests, ultrasound, HIDA scan.

2.2 Stone is removed by laparotomy, laparoscopy or ERCP. Biliary atresia requires Kasai portoenterostomy.

27 Anus, perineum and female genitalia

1.1 Perianal abscess with fistula *in ano*; incision of abscess and tract.

2.1 Labial adhesions.

2.2 Separation with thermometer, paper clip or gentle pressure (± anaesthetic jelly). Regular application of vaseline and general measures to prevent nappy-rash.

28 Undescended testes and varicocele

1.1 Risk of subsequent ascent at 5–10 years of age.

1.2 If ascent occurs, orchidopexy is recommended once the testis no longer can reside spontaneously in the scrotum.

2.1 Disorders of sexual development; bilateral intra-abdominal testes; bilateral perinatal torsion/agenesis.

2.2 Hormone/chromosome tests; laparoscopy ± orchidopexy/orchidectomy.

3.1 6–12 months.

3.2 Not known for certain, but expected to be normal or near normal in most boys with early treatment.

29 Inguinal region and acute scrotum

1.1 Indirect inguinal hernia.

1.2 Inguinal herniotomy – many surgeons would do bilateral operation.

2.1 Torsion of testis or its appendages; epididymitis; idiopathic scrotal oedema.

2.2 No – this affects testis after puberty.

2.3 Exploration of scrotum, R/o appendage, or detorsion and fixation of (both) testes.

30 The penis

1.1 No, not necessary; normal washing (externally) is sufficient.

1.2 After 5 years in the majority of boys; partial adherence still normal up until adolescence.

2.1 Urethral meatus and glans visible in normal child on retraction or traction.

2.2 Topical corticosteroid cream or circumcision.

3.1 Neonatal circumcision not necessary for hygiene and procedure is dangerous.

3.2 Acceptable standard is general anaesthetic (after 6 months), full surgical technique, adequate postoperative analgesia.

3.3 Bleeding, infection, penile deformity, glanular/meatal ulceration, acute retention (pain).

4.1 6–12 months.

4.2 Fix chordee, put urethra on tip of glans, satisfactory cosmetic appearance, minimal complications.

4.3 Extensive mobilisation to fix chordee, foreskin advance to ventral surface, neourethra constructed, ± postoperative stenting/urinary diversion, one or two stages.

Urinary tract

31 Urinary tract infection

1.1 Urine micro and culture to confirm UTI, then renal ultrasound. Further tests only if ultrasound scan abnormal.

1.2 Low risk of anomaly, but still possible.

1.3 Perineal contamination secondary to poor perineal hygiene ± constipation with soiling.

2.1 Suprapubic aspirate for urine specimen.

2.2 Renal and bladder ultrasound scan, MCU ± DTPA or DMSA scan.

32 Vesico-ureteric reflux

1.1 Renal ultrasound, MCU ± DMSA scan.

1.2 Unpleasant and invasive, but gold standard for VUR, urethral and bladder anomalies.

1.3 Indirect MCU.

2.1 Both.

2.2 Should not (although scars become visible very slowly and may appear to be occurring later).

2.3 Failed medical treatment, anatomical anomalies, persisting VUR in prepubertal girls.

33 Urinary tract dilatation

1.1 Spontaneous resolution is common, especially in the less severe cases. Severe dilatation suggests progressive obstruction requiring treatment.

1.2 Pelvi-ureteric junction obstruction, vesico-ureteric junction obstruction, vesico-ureteric reflux, urethral obstruction.

1.3 Antibiotic prophylaxis, early ultrasound and MCU (<1–2 weeks) and MAG3/DTPA scan (2–6 weeks).

2.1 Vesico-ureteric obstruction, vesico-ureteric reflux, urethral obstruction.

2.2 MCU and renal ultrasound, especially in infants and preschool children. MCU less useful in older children.

34 The child with wetting

1.1 Each predisposes to the other.

1.2 Renal and bladder ultrasound, x-ray ± MCU, ± cystoscopy to document bladder anatomy, cystometry for bladder function.

1.3 Consider surgery for VU reflux if still present, bladder training, antibiotics ± anticholinergics.

2.1 Ectopic ureter in perineum.

2.2 Patch test (wet patch on sheet within 10 min) renal ultrasound, DTPA scan ± MRI.

2.3 Heminephroureterectomy.

3.1 Occult spina bifida: hairy/pigmented patch, lipoma, sinus, palpable defect in vertebral spines. Absent sacral segments.

3.2 Spinal ultrasound can identify the spinal cord and roots in babies, but later an MRI is required.

3.3 Clean intermittent catheterisation is mainstay of treatment.

35 The child with haematuria

1.1 Meatal ulcer.

1.2 Soak off scabs, apply vaseline, leave off nappy, treat nappy rash.

2.1 Ruptured kidney, Wilms' tumour, hydronephrosis.

2.2 Renal ultrasound: if minor renal trauma, then treat conservatively unless significant urine leak. Tumour, hydronephrosis: treat condition.

Trauma

36 Trauma in childhood

1.1 Airway, breathing, circulation; resuscitation; secondary (head-to-toe) survey; continued resuscitation; definitive care.

1.2 Detailed examination of all body systems to identify all injuries.

1.3 Airway obstruction (from tongue or blood) may depress conscious state.

2.1 Surgical examination and debridement under anaesthetic.

2.2 Tetanus management, excision of devitalised tissue, foreign bodies and blood clot.

37 Head injuries

1.1 See Table 37.1.

1.2 See Table 37.4.

2.1 See Table 37.2.

3.1 Acute left extradural haemorrhage.

3.2 Extremely urgent.

3.3 Determine the GCS; urgent resuscitation and X-match, CT, then craniotomy and removal of collection.

4.1 See Table 37.5.

5.1 Transient/prolonged amnesia after HI. No pathology with minor concussion; severe concussion with diffuse axonal injury (swelling on CT with haemorrhage in corpus callosum/dorsal brainstem) – may cause a persisting vegetative state.

38 Abdominal and thoracic injuries

1.1 Ruptured spleen.

1.2 ABC, correction of hypovolaemia, CT or U/S to confirm rupture, conservative treatment (unless uncontrollable haemorrhage, which is very rare).

2.1 The girl has a femur and intra-abdominal bleeding (liver or splenic rupture). The leg needs an air-splint and traction/fixation. After airway control and oxygen, the girl needs resuscitation with fluids and urgent transfusion. CT scan will demonstrate the injury; however, conservative treatment is likely unless there is bowel perforation.

39 Foreign bodies

1.1 No.

1.2 No.

2.1 Under GA with mosquito forcep inserted via a small incision guided with image intensifier.

40 The ingestion of corrosives

1.1 Immediate copious irrigation of face and mouth with water, and drinking copious water/milk.

1.2 Observation to see if drooling/dysphagia is present, and if so, oesophagoscopy to diagnose full-thickness oesophageal burn, which needs treatment. The aim is to prevent oesophageal stricture.

41 Burns

1.1 Remove clothing and immerse affected parts in cold water for 10–20 min, Commence IV (Hartmann's solution). Give IV morphine 0.05–0.1 mg/kg over 5 min. Wrap child in clean sheet and blanket. Take swabs of nose, throat, faeces and burn. Insert urinary catheter. Give maintenance fluids orally. Start IV rate at ($\frac{1}{2} \times$ 2–3 mL/kg/1% burn area over first 8 h, giving ½ estimated volume as 5% serum albumin and ½ Hartmann's solution. Call Burns Unit for advice and to arrange transfer.

2.1 Possible child abuse by deliberate immersion.

3.1 Possible inhalation injury with airway burn.

Orthopaedics

42 Neonatal orthopaedics

1.1 Callus of healing fracture of humerus secondary to birth injury.

1.2 Spontaneous healing with full recovery.

2.1 Dislocated hip with soft tissue oedema around capsule. Aspiration of joint revealed pus, consistent with diagnosis of septic dislocation of hip. Even with drainage, IV antibiotics and abduction bracing, there is a risk of proximal femoral growth arrest and short limb.

3.1 Birth injury to brachial plexus.

3.2 Spontaneous recovery with elbow movements at 6 weeks and shoulder movements normal by 3 months. Failure of recovery by 3 months suggests microsurgical repair is needed.

4.1 'Postural' club foot.

4.2 Normal function after a few weeks of stretching exercises.

5.1 Talipes calcaneovalgus may be associated with developmental dysplasia of hip.

6.1 Serial plaster casts commencing immediately. Surgical release of contracted tendons may be required at 6 months, if there is residual deformity.

43 Orthopaedics in the infant and toddler

1.1 The child has bow legs, which resolves over 6–12 months. Monitoring the deformity in the standing position with serial photographs, is useful.

2.1 Internal tibial torsion is common with mild bowing. Six-monthly reviews should demonstrate resolution by 3 years of age.

3.1 Developmental dysplasia of the hip.

3.2 Ortolani's test with confirmation by hip ultrasonography should have been done at birth, as she had all the risk factors for DDH.

4.1 Cerebral palsy with hemiparesis.

5.1 Osteomyelitis of proximal femur.

5.2 A hot area in right upper femur.

6.1 Child abuse.

6.2 Fracture of femoral shaft and a strong likelihood of other healing fractures, such as rib, skull and collarbone.

7.1 Osteogenesis imperfecta (Type 1); a skull x-ray would show multiple Wormian bones.

44 Orthopaedics in the child

1.1 Internal femoral torsion.

2.1 The gap is not excessive and spontaneous resolution is expected without surgery.

3.1 Simple orthotics may prolong shoe life, but makes little difference to the condition itself.

4.1 This is likely to be a supracondylar fracture with brachial artery compromise. There is a high risk of Volkman's ischaemia unless treatment is rapid and appropriate.

45 Orthopaedics in the teenager

1.1 Scoliosis.

1.2 Likely to show an intrinsic curvature ± rotational deformity.

1.3 Less than 20°: observe; 20°–40°: brace; greater than 40°: spinal fusion.

2.1 Slipped upper femoral epiphysis.

2.2 AP and lateral x-ray; ultrasonography may help diagnose secondary haemarthrosis.

2.3 Pinning of epiphysis *in situ* to prevent further chronic slippage.

3.1 Overuse syndrome affecting immature retropatellar cartilage.

3.2 No further tests needed if x-ray is normal, Arthroscopy is indicated occasionally.

3.3 Conservative; analgesics, restriction of provocative activities, gentle exercises.

4.1 Osteosarcoma or Ewing's tumour.

4.2 Imaging (plain x-ray, bone scan, CT/MRI) and biopsy.

4.3 Chemotherapy followed by tumour excision ± limb salvage.

46 The hand

1.1 Trigger thumb.

1.2 No.

1.3 Yes.

2.1 Erb's palsy; traction on branchial plexus during delivery; surgery if not resolved after 3 months.

Chest

47 The breast

1.1 Premature thelarche; remains static or resolves over 6–12 months.

1.2 Only if mastitis occurs, surgery for drainage of abscess (rare at this age).

2.1 Neonatal hypertrophy; clean skin with antiseptic, do not squeeze breast (milk production ceases spontaneously).

2.2 Either male or female (female hormones from mother).

48 Chest wall deformities

1.1 Chest wall deformities only cause *subtle* changes in cardiorespiratory function, except in severe deformity.

1.2 A chest x-ray, especially if there is a low protrusion.

1.3 Reassure there is no major functional limitation, and cosmetic surgery can be done if required (often delayed until adolescence).

49 Lungs, pleura and mediastinum

1.1 Staph. pneumonia, and may be developing Staph. empyema.

1.2 Flucloxacillin and gentamicin IV until cultures confirm sensitivity, regular x-ray review, ± surgical drainage of empyema.

2.1 Spontaneous pneumothorax; confirm with x-ray, needle or intercostal catheter if under tension; if no tension, observe in ward; diagnose and treat cause.

Skin and soft tissues

50 Vascular and pigmented naevi

1.1 No risk of melanoma.

1.2 Cosmetic treatment if needed.

2.1 Amblyopia of eye; deformity of face throughout preschool years; some residual scar.

2.2 Surgical excision or laser treatment. Occasionally need intralesional steroid injection or interferon treatment.

51 Soft tissue lumps

1.1 This is a naevus sebaceous, which needs excision in early childhood.

1.2 If untreated, 15–20% risk of basal cell carcinoma in adulthood.

2.1 Keloid; counselling, intralesional steroid injections, pressure via lycra or silicon gel sheeting.

Index